2012
YEAR BOOK OF
SURGERY®

The 2012 Year Book Series

Year Book of Anesthesiology and Pain Management™: Drs Chestnut, Abram, Black, Gravlee, Lien, Mathru, and Roizen

Year Book of Cardiology®: Drs Gersh, Cheitlin, Elliott, Gold, Graham, and Thourani

Year Book of Critical Care Medicine®: Drs Dries, Zanotti-Cavazzoni, Latenser, Martinez, Rincon, and Zwank

Year Book of Dermatology and Dermatologic Surgery™: Dr Del Rosso

Year Book of Diagnostic Radiology®: Drs Elster, Abbara, Oestreich, Offiah, Rosado de Christenson, Stephens, and Strickland

Year Book of Emergency Medicine®: Drs Hamilton, Bruno, Handly, Minczak, Mullin, Quintana, and Ramoska

Year Book of Endocrinology®: Drs Schott, Apovian, Clarke, Eugster, Meikle, Oetgen, Ovalle, Schteingart, and Toth

Year Book of Hand and Upper Limb Surgery®: Drs Yao, Adams, Isaacs, Lee, and Rizzo

Year Book of Medicine®: Drs Barker, Garrick, Gersh, Khardori, LeRoith, Panush, Talley, and Thigpen

Year Book of Neonatal and Perinatal Medicine®: Drs Fanaroff, Benitz, Donn, Neu, Papile, Polin, and Van Marter

Year Book of Neurology and Neurosurgery®: Drs Klimo, Minagar, Gandhi, House, Kevill, Liu, Mazia, Panagariya, Ragel, Riesenburger, Robottom, Schwendimann, Shafazand, Uhm, and Yang

Year Book of Obstetrics, Gynecology, and Women's Health®: Drs Dungan and Shulman

Year Book of Oncology®: Drs Arceci, Bauer, Chiorean, Gordon, Lawton, Murphy, Thigpen, and Tsao

Year Book of Ophthalmology®: Drs Rapuano, Cohen, Flanders, Hammersmith, Milman, Myers, Nagra, Nelson, Penne, Pyfer, Sergott, Shields, Talekar, and Vander

Year Book of Orthopedics®: Drs Morrey, Huddleston, Rose, Swiontkowski, and Trigg

Year Book of Otolaryngology-Head and Neck Surgery®: Drs Sindwani, Balough, Franco, Gapany, and Mitchell

Year Book of Pathology and Laboratory Medicine®: Drs Raab and Bissell

Year Book of Pediatrics®: Dr Stockman

Year Book of Plastic and Aesthetic Surgery™: Drs Miller, Gosman, Gurtner, Gutowski, Ruberg, Salisbury, and Smith

Year Book of Psychiatry and Applied Mental Health®: Drs Talbott, Ballenger, Buckley, Frances, Krupnick, and Mack

Year Book of Pulmonary Disease®: Drs Barker, Jones, Maurer, Spradley, Tanoue, and Willsie

Year Book of Sports Medicine®: Drs Shephard, Cantu, Feldman, Galea, Jankowski, Janssen, Lebrun, and Nieman

Year Book of Surgery®: Drs Copeland, Behrns, Daly, Eberlein, Fahey, Huber, Klodell, Mozingo, and Pruett

Year Book of Urology®: Drs Andriole and Coplen

Year Book of Vascular Surgery®: Drs Moneta, Gillespie, Starnes, and Watkins

2012

The Year Book of SURGERY®

Editor-in-Chief

Edward M. Copeland III, MD

Distinguished Professor of Surgery, Department of Surgery, University of Florida, Gainesville, Florida

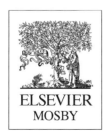

ELSEVIER
MOSBY

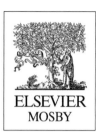

Vice President, Continuity: Kimberly Murphy
Editor: Jessica McCool
Production Supervisor, Electronic Year Books: Donna M. Skelton
Electronic Article Manager: Emily Ogle
Illustrations and Permissions Coordinator: Dawn Vohsen

Composition by TNQ Books and Journals Pvt Ltd, India

Editorial Office:
Elsevier
1600 John F. Kennedy Blvd.
Suite 1800
Philadelphia, PA 19103-2899

International Standard Serial Number: 0090-3671
International Standard Book Number: 978-0-323-08895-4

Printed and bound by CPI Group (UK) Ltd, Croydon, CR0 4YY

Transferred to Digital Print 2012

Editorial Board

Table of Contents

Journals Represented

JPEN Journal of Parenteral and Enteral Nutrition
Lancet
Laryngoscope
Liver Transplantation
New England Journal of Medicine
Plastic and Reconstructive Surgery
Regional Anesthesia and Pain Medicine
Stroke
Surgery
Thyroid
Transplantation
World Journal of Surgery
Wound Repair and Regeneration

STANDARD ABBREVIATIONS

The following terms are abbreviated in this edition: acquired immunodeficiency syndrome (AIDS), cardiopulmonary resuscitation (CPR), central nervous system (CNS), cerebrospinal fluid (CSF), computed tomography (CT), deoxyribonucleic acid (DNA), electrocardiography (ECG), health maintenance organization (HMO), human immunodeficiency virus (HIV), intensive care unit (ICU), intramuscular (IM), intravenous (IV), magnetic resonance (MR) imaging (MRI), ribonucleic acid (RNA), and ultrasound (US).

NOTE

Introduction

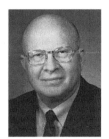

ALBERT RHOTON, MD

I was pleased to find in my possible selections for the YEAR BOOK OF SURGERY an editorial declaring Albert Rhoton, MD, as Neurosurgeon of the Year World Wide.[1] The article is short and gives him all the credit for the better understanding of the anatomy of the skull and its contents. I bring a different perspective in underlying the value of Dr Rhoton to medicine.

Dr Rhoton came to the University of Florida as Chairman of the Department of Neurosurgery in the late 1970s when the institution was not mentioned among the great medical schools in the United States. Dr Rhoton built his department into, if not the best, one of the best places for clinical care, training, and research in neurosciences in this country. His resolve for excellence was joined by several other notable surgeons, pediatricians, and anesthesiologists to bring a small school in the small university town of Gainesville, Florida, to the notice and admiration of our peers nationwide.

I came to the University of Florida in 1982, because these men had the vision to develop unparalleled training programs and were able to do so with the support of our university. Dr Rhoton has served as a role model for me from 1982 until today. We have both retired from the University of Florida but continue to be involved in medical school activities and are sought out for our clinical opinions. Dr Rhoton retired several years before me. I was impressed with the aplomb with which he left his job and therefore used him as a mentor for my own retirement from the university. He is almost too modest and has always put the success of the medical school foremost in his thoughts. Yes, we had the usual "in-fighting" as do any faculty members, but these debates were always resolved to everyone's satisfaction, even though compromises had to be made to move forward. On a local level, Dr Rhoton was just recognized for his accomplishments by the receipt of the President's Medallion, the greatest distinction that can be bestowed on a faculty member from within the University of Florida system.

Dr Rhoton has been honored by every national and international neurosurgical organization in existence. Many of us have also had the honor of some of these distinctions in our specialties. For me at least, Dr Rhoton led the way, and it is my honor to be able to thank him through this inclusion in the YEAR BOOK OF SURGERY.

Edward M. Copeland III, MD

Reference

1. Black PM. Al Rhoton as Neurosurgeon of the Year. *World Neurosurgery.* 2011;75: 162.

1 General Considerations

2010 SSO Presidential Address: Subspecialty Certificate in Advanced Surgical Oncology
Michelassi F (Cornell Univ, NY)
Ann Surg Oncol 17:3094-3103, 2010

Background.—In June 2009 the American Board of Surgery (ABS) unanimously approved the proposal for a subspecialty certificate in advanced surgical oncology. The process by which this was achieved was outlined, along with future steps.

Historical Perspective.—The principal objective of the ABS is to assess the education, training, and knowledge of surgeons and to issue certificates to those candidates who meet the board's requirements and complete prescribed examinations satisfactorily. Certification is voluntary and is pursued to support the public by guaranteeing certified surgeons are highly qualified and to support the diplomates by conferring on them recognition of their advanced skills, training, and knowledge. In the early 1980s the Society of Surgical Oncology (SSO) sought to approve training programs in surgical oncology and planned for a written certifying examination. This would lead toward a certificate of "added qualifications" in surgical oncology. The certification process was further refined by defining the certificate as not being a license that would exclude general surgeons from treating primary tumors but would be available to all persons who completed an Accreditation Council for Graduate Medical Education (ACGME)-n-approved training program in surgical oncology. In addition, the certificate would require 2 years of training covering core knowledge and enhancing clinical expertise in surgical oncology. Trainees would be required to be well-founded in all areas and to initiate investigation in one or more of them. Guidelines for the training programs in surgical oncology were set up, including participation in a minimum number of advanced surgical oncological operative cases before graduation and institutional leadership in oncology as a required skill. In 1989 surgical oncology was recognized by the ABS as a primary component of general surgery and pertinent questions and clinical scenarios were included in the examination process even though the ABS did not authorize certificates.

Surgical oncology consolidated and refined its professional and scientific status for about 15 years. This strengthened and enhanced the subspecialty certification movement. Specifically, it identified a body of scientific medical knowledge characteristic of surgical oncology and distinct from the knowledge characteristic of general surgery; it recognized the existence of a group of physicians whose practices focused on surgical oncology; and it was bolstered by the existence of a national society whose major interest was the practice of surgical oncology. In 1998 the ABS established the Surgical Oncology Advisory Council (SOAC) to report on issues relevant to surgical oncology, including training, maintenance of certification, and potential certification processes, and to provide a channel for formal communication with the surgical oncology community.

A questionnaire distributed in 2007 to the directors of the surgical oncology training programs revealed overwhelming support for pursuing a certificate of advanced practice in surgical oncology. An ABS Advisory Task Force was charged with investigating the appropriateness and timing of such a request. In late 2007 the task force expressed the belief that oversight by the ACGME would ensure objectivity and external credibility regarding the quality and uniformity of training programs. The ABS certification program would then create a formal, highly structured examination to objectively measure competence. Having a certification process was seen as a way to improve the quality of applicants attracted to surgical oncology training programs. The SOAC was sent a request for a certificate in surgical oncology. It would be available only to graduates of ACGME-accredited surgical oncology programs; no one would be "grandfathered" in.

Future Steps.—ACGME will accredit fellowships in surgical oncology. Program requirements are being developed. The Committee on Certification Sub-certification and Recertification (COCERT) is preparing a report for the ABS. In the future, all candidates who complete the surgical oncology training program approved by the ACGME will be eligible for evaluation for the subspecialty certificate in advanced surgical oncology. Both a written (qualifying) and an oral (certifying) examination will be conducted. Both examinations must be successfully passed to achieve subspecialty certification. Certificates will be time-limited and diplomates must comply with an American Board of Medical Specialties (ABMS)-n-approved maintenance of certification (MOC) program to retain the certification.

▶ This article catalogs the path taken to obtain the Subspecialty Certificate in Advanced Surgical Oncology. My name is mentioned along the way several times in the development process. Early on in my career as an academic surgeon, the buzz word was "fragmentation." In the 1980s many of us were against breaking general surgeries into fragments. Well, that "battle" has long since been lost, exampled by the advent of fellowships in minimally invasive surgery, surgical critical care, trauma, gastrointestinal surgery, breast, and endocrine surgery.

Now I am very much in favor of the surgical oncology certificate to prevent the fragmentation of surgical oncology. The military term would be to retreat and regroup or accept your losses and consolidate what remains. Unfortunately, the fragmentation of surgical oncology is proceeding down the same path as did general surgery. Categorical cancer institutions have surgical specialists dedicated to pancreas, hepatobiliary, soft tissue sarcoma, breast, and endocrine surgeries. The surgical oncology fellows rotate through these specialty services, each of which will probably soon want to have a more advanced fellow who has completed the qualifications for the advanced surgical oncology certificate that just was established. Where does all this subspecialization stop? Who can afford the time to proceed through these certifications to become an expert in a single organ requiring only a few operations? To me, it doesn't make sense. I am, however, a proponent of regionalization of difficult surgical procedures with established protocols for postoperative care. There are ample data that indicate that the hospital is almost as important as the surgeon in generating acceptable outcomes for difficult surgical procedures.

We have reached the stage in surgical education where we should take a lesson learned from our neurosurgical colleagues in the past, when a general surgical residency was required to matriculate through a neurosurgical residency. We train excellent neurosurgeons today with only an internship in general surgery. Does it really take 6 to 8 years to learn the principles of breast surgery? Why does vascular surgery require completion of a general surgery residency? In some institutions, if the wound created by the vascular surgeon dehisces, a general surgeon is called for the repair! We once said that a general surgery residency was needed to learn pre- and postoperative care, but now we have established fellowships in critical care, therefore eliminating the aforementioned reason.

I propose that we accept fragmentation and shorten the training needed to become competent in many of the fragments. For breast, that would be no more than an internship in general surgery and 3 additional years, in which patient management would be integrated with medical and radiation oncology, genetics, epidemiology, and physical therapy. Once these fragments are removed, there will still be a place for the well-trained general surgeon and surgical oncologist who is willing to complete the training necessary to become competent in the fragments and all of the practice of surgery that falls between them.

E. M. Copeland III, MD

A Policy-based Intervention for the Reduction of Communication Breakdowns in Inpatient Surgical Care: Results From a Harvard Surgical Safety Collaborative

Arriaga AF, Elbardissi AW, Regenbogen SE, et al (Harvard School of Public Health, Boston, MA; et al)
Ann Surg 253:849-854, 2011

Objective.—To develop and evaluate an intervention to reduce breakdowns in communication during inpatient surgical care.

Background.—Communication breakdowns are the second most common cause of avoidable surgical adverse events after technical errors.

Methods.—In a pre- and postintervention study, a random selection of patients on the surgical services of 4 teaching hospitals were observed according to 3 measures: (1) resident-attending communication of critical patient events (eg, transfer into the intensive care unit, unplanned intubation, cardiac arrest); (2) resident-attending notification regarding routine weekend patient status; and (3) frequency of weekend patient visits by an attending. All departments then developed and adopted a set of policy and education initiatives designed to increase prompt and consistent resident-attending communication (especially in critical events) and to improve regular attending visits with surgical patients. Specific reinforcement of the policies included a pocket information card for residents, as well as periodic reminders. Repeat audits of the surgical services were then conducted.

Results.—We reviewed information for 211 critical events and 1360 patients for the nature of resident and attending communication practices. After the intervention, the proportion of critical events not conveyed to an attending decreased from 33% (26/80) to 2% (1/47), and gaps in the frequency of attending notification of patient status on weekends were virtually eliminated ($P < 0.0001$); the proportion of weekend patients not visited by an attending for greater than 24 hours decreased by half (from 61% to 33%; $P = 0.0002$). Contact resulted in attending-led changes in patient management in one-third of cases.

Conclusions.—An intervention to improve surgical communication practices at 4 teaching hospitals led to significant reductions in potentially harmful communication breakdowns during inpatient care; significant alterations in patient management were noted in one-third of cases in which there was an adherence to recommended communication practices.

▶ This study puts some numbers to the problem with communication, and the numbers are scary if you are a patient in any hospital not using a system similar to the one described here. I am sure that patients in the Harvard-affiliated hospitals feel much safer now.

The work environment has changed over the past 10 years. Residents have to check out to each other more frequently or check out to a hospitalist, nurse practitioner, night float resident, etc. Ownership of the patient is diffused among many individuals, whereas in the past, the ownership was tightly maintained by physicians on the same surgical service. The gap in ownership was to be taken up by more responsibility from the attending surgeon. However, the attending surgeon cannot participate in decisions unless the attending surgeon is notified of the problem or is at the bedside.

After the intervention, attending physician weekend visits doubled. This finding means that the attending physicians before the intervention were still depending on notification of a patient problem from the on-call resident. I find this result interesting. The problems with resident communication with each other and with the attending physicians were corrected, yet the attending physicians still felt compelled to visit their patients more frequently on the weekend than before. The patients in the Harvard-affiliated hospitals got a double bonus: better resident coverage and more visits by their doctors.

I would like to congratulate the authors of this article for recognizing the patient care problems, setting up a mechanism for correction, and then having the courage to share their data with the rest of us.

E. M. Copeland III, MD

Acute Care Surgery Survey: Opinions of Surgeons About a New Training Paradigm

Tisherman SA, Ivy ME, Frangos SG, et al (Univ of Pittsburgh, PA; Bridgeport Hosp, CT; New York Univ; et al)
Arch Surg 146:101-106, 2011

Hypothesis.—The acute care surgery (ACS) 2-year training model, incorporating surgical critical care (SCC), trauma surgery, and emergency general surgery, was developed to improve resident interest in the field. We believed that analysis of survey responses about the new training paradigm before its implementation would yield valuable information on current practice patterns and on opinions about the ACS model.

Design.—Two surveys.

Participants.—Members of the Surgery Section of the Society of Critical Care Medicine and SCC program directors.

Interventions.—One survey was sent to SCC program directors to define the practice patterns of trauma and SCC surgeons at their institutions, and another survey was sent to all Surgery Section of the Society of Critical Care Medicine members to solicit opinions about the ACS model.

Main Outcome Measures.—Practice patterns of trauma and SCC surgeons and opinions about the ACS model.

Results.—Fifty-seven of 87 SCC program directors responded. Almost all programs are associated with level I trauma centers with as many as 15 trauma surgeons. Most of these trauma surgeons cover SCC and emergency general surgery. Sixty-six percent of surgical intensive care units are semiclosed; 89.0% have surgeons as directors. Seventy percent of the staff in surgical intensive care units are surgeons. One hundred fifty-five of approximately 1100 Surgery Section of the Society of Critical Care Medicine members who responded to the other survey did not believe that the ACS model would compromise surgical intensive care unit and trauma care or trainee education yet would allow surgeons to maintain their surgical skills. Respondents were less likely to believe that the ACS fellowship would be important financially, increase resident interest, or improve patient care.

Conclusions.—In academic medical centers, surgical intensivists already practice the ACS model but depend on many nonsurgeons. Surgical intensivists believe that ACS will not compromise care or education and will help maintain the field, although the effect on resident interest is unclear.

▶ The University of Florida has had a level I trauma center for 6 years. Prior to this, all general surgeons incorporated trauma care into their regular call schedule of 1 night in 9. Procedures that would interrupt the surgical schedule the next day were placed on the schedule of the individual on call when the patient was seen initially and no operating room was set vacant awaiting a trauma victim. Thus, any interruption in the daily schedule was only for the surgeon on call. Continuity of care was no issue because the acute care patient became the patient of the on-call surgeon. Resident training was not interrupted because trauma critical care patients were incorporated into the daily activities of a service that had a stable complement of resident and attending surgeons (3-4 residents and 3 attendings, thus 1 attending surgeon on call once every ninth night if there were 3 general surgical services). I am unaware in the 20 years of this type of rotation that any trauma patient received suboptimal treatment. We were a level II trauma center and were not the sole referral hospital for trauma or critical care. In fact, a level I trauma center exists 80 miles away equipped with a helicopter as was/is our hospital. Our surgical residents had responsibility for their patients in the intensive care unit (ICU), but the ICU was run by anesthesiologists with critical care experience. This system worked to the advantage of everyone.

With the advent of a level I trauma center, 5 trauma surgeons were hired and no general surgeons with other interests were required to take emergency call. Our service is a trauma, critical care, emergency surgery unit as described in this article. It works fine as long as there are enough trauma surgeons and they can supplant the existing critical care anesthesiologist. Herein lies the rub. Both anesthesia and surgical faculty members have been hired with the fee for service of nonoperative trauma patients in the ICU built into the business plan to pay doctors. The beauty for the surgical oncologist, for example, is no emergency room call!

The advantage for trauma surgeons is that they are on call every fifth night; one of them can be responsible for inpatients each week, freeing up the other 4, and the residents rotating through the service have no other inpatient responsibilities and then can function as a team for a set period. They are not responsible for other attending surgeons and vice versa. Clearly trauma service is the best organized service in our training program. In the past, we had a predominance of chief residents applying for surgical oncology fellowships and no trauma fellowships, and now the fellowship applications are completely reversed. Residents gravitate to organized services with distinct mentorship. The need to cross-cover other services and have residents be responsible for a myriad of attending surgeons creates both anxiety and disorganization.

So all things work well until the ratio of the number of trauma surgeons and trauma victims becomes skewed. A level I trauma center attracts trauma patients because it alleviates surrounding hospitals from the responsibility of providing adequate trauma care. If the number of trauma surgeons does increase to meet the needs of additional patients, trauma surgeons will seek other employment, further skewing the ratio. I don't need to elaborate on the problems this situation creates. For example, surgical oncologists have been hired with the understanding that they will not need to take emergency call.

For academic training centers in metropolitan cities, few of these problems will arise, and the trauma patient volume might be needed to fill hospital beds. For academic programs in more rural areas, planning for a level I trauma center needs to be done very carefully because once a level I trauma center is established, there is no turning back.

E. M. Copeland III, MD

Choosing "The Best"

Linehan DC, Jaques D (Washington Univ School of Medicine, St Louis, MO)
Arch Surg 146:604-605, 2011

Background.—When a patient looks for the best hospital or best physician to manage his or her particular problem, perhaps cancer, they often turn to rating systems if they have no access to recommendations of trusted friends or health care professionals. The hospital and provider recommendations offered by these rating systems were evaluated.

Method.—The risk-adjusted 30-day mortality of patients having one of three surgical procedures for cancer was compared for institutions designated "best hospitals" and all other hospitals to determine if outcomes were truly better at the designated hospitals. A media-based hospital rating system was compared with an Internet-based system to determine the quality of care in the 50 best hospitals in each ranking in relation to the outcomes from all other hospitals.

Results.—The two rating systems shared little concordance in terms of which hospitals were best, with few hospital appearing on both lists. A significantly lower risk-adjusted mortality was found in the *US News and World Report* best hospital list for all three procedures but only because "best hospital" translated to highest volume of cases. It is reasonable to expect centers that specialize in certain procedures to have better outcomes and lower mortality rates than nonspecialized institutions. Weaknesses of the study include the use of the 30-day mortality to measure the quality of care because this is a highly imperfect metric, especially in cancer care. In addition, both rating systems use Medicare data, which are relevant only to persons over age 65 years. This database lacks robust clinical detail, undermining the validity of risk stratification. Persons choosing a "best hospital" may also have to travel further to receive care, sometimes past high-volume hospitals that offer comparable mortality. The gravest concern is for patients who have no choice; they will be suboptimally cared for in a hospital that has poor outcomes because of its low volume of experience with complex procedures.

Conclusions.—Both outcome measures and ranking systems are part of the health care system and will become more prevalent with health care reform. By 2014 the number of publicly reported quality metrics will increase from the current 25 to 355 performance measures. The term *meaningful use* is applied to assessing the depth of deployment of health care information technology. It may more appropriately be applied to the complete understanding of how these quality measures will be used and what they will mean. It is hoped that health care will be allowed the time and resources to manage the causes of adverse outcomes and be less focused on collecting data and making explanations. It is important to develop and validate scientifically rigorous ways to measure quality and adjust for risk based on relevant patient-specific variables rather than rely on commercially available media-based and Internet-based rankings.

▶ I have waited for this evaluation of the "best hospitals" for some time and am reminded of this wait when driving down the road and see a billboard advertising some hospital that I have never heard of as being rated as "the best" by some poll (or who knows, maybe by no poll!). For patients who go to the "best hospital," there is still no guarantee that they will get the most qualified doctor.

I have commented for some time now that the disparity between the best and worst doctors in this country is widening. Data from the American Board of Surgery oral examination has shown that the gap between the pass rate for foreign-trained medical graduates and North American—trained graduates is ever widening. My observation over the last few years is that the judgmental and technical gap between the best and least good chief residents in our own surgical programs is widening as well.

I am not a fan of the bureaucracy created by the quality of care initiatives that are currently thrust upon us, but I must say, the public does need some kind of accurate "report card" that defines gradations between the best and the worst hospitals and the physicians who practice within them.

E. M. Copeland III, MD

Continuity of care in a rural critical access hospital: Surgeons as primary care providers
Rossi A, Rossi D, Rossi M, et al (Hopedale Med Complex, IL)
Am J Surg 201:359-362, 2011

Background.—The question of volume and outcomes has perfused the surgical literature. Hopedale Hospital is a critical access hospital located in central Illinois. The authors elected to review surgical outcomes to establish quality benchmarks for similar facilities. They also propose a practice model in which general surgeons provide primary care.

Methods.—The authors consecutively reviewed retrospectively 100 each of 5 commonly performed procedures. These included carotid endarterectomy, laparoscopic cholecystectomy, laparoscopic Nissen fundoplication, hysterectomy, and inguinal hernia repair. Demographic data, c-morbidities, and outcomes up to 30 days postoperatively were summarized.

Results.—The overall complication rate was 4%. This exceeded any benchmarks found in a surgical literature review through Medline.

Conclusions.—Critical access hospitals are capable of producing excellent surgical outcomes. Having a surgeon totally involved in perioperative management may contribute to the improved outcomes. This practice model could be used to recruit medical students into surgical training, perhaps alleviating shortages of rural surgeons and primary care physicians simultaneously.

▶ For those of you who have been readers for a while, you know that I have made many comments about hospital ease of access, size, and volume, as these parameters relate to surgical outcomes. For the past 1.5 years, I have been on the Board of Directors of Highlands-Cashiers Hospital, a critical access hospital in the city of Highlands, North Carolina, and located in the mountains of this state. I have recently become a member of the Quality Assurance Committee, which oversees the multiple quality measures of both the hospital and a nursing center. The nursing staff, administration, and physicians function as a team and are proud of the excellent quality numbers that are collected monthly. There is total transparency among these groups. Complications, although few, are presented in a form, such as morbidity and mortality conferences, that would make many university surgical programs both envious and proud. Our surgical complication rates are less than the 4% reported here.

Our patient satisfaction rating is often in the 99th percentile. Considering that our hospital volume swells during the summer months because of the easy access of our community to Floridians and Georgians, our satisfaction rating is even more impressive since so many of our summer residents and patients come from affluent neighborhoods in Atlanta, Miami, Orlando, Sarasota, Gainesville, and points west like New Orleans and Dallas. These patients have access to the best and most well-organized medical services available in their communities where hospitals are in stiff competition for patients, and hospital amenities often make the difference.

How can this track record be so good? The answers are the same as in the current article by Rossi and coworkers. Continuity of care is easily maintained among patients and physicians. Our emergency room is state of the art in which stabilization and evacuation to a neighboring large medical center can be done swiftly and safely if the medical circumstance requires it. The surgical staff is well qualified to handle emergencies that require on-site resolution. Our medical and surgical staff members are chosen carefully to exhibit the same philosophies of excellent patient care and communication that have evolved over the last few years with the leadership of a dedicated CEO and team of nursing directors.

I am one of those warm weather residents of Highlands, North Carolina, who seeks the comfort of cool, pleasant days in the mountains. For an older patient population, access to health care is one of the most important factors in choosing a home. Actually, all of this information sounds so good, I am thinking about going back to work!

E. M. Copeland III, MD

Effects of duty hours and time of day on surgery resident proficiency

Brandenberger J, Kahol K, Feinstein AJ, et al (Phoenix Integrated Surgical Residency, AZ; Banner Good Samaritan Med Ctr, Phoenix, AZ; et al)
Am J Surg 200:814-819, 2010

Background.—Night floats have evolved in the era of limited resident work hours. This study was designed to define the effect of restricted nighttime duty hours on the psychomotor and cognitive skills of surgery residents.

Methods.—To quantify the effect of fatigue on the skills of residents on day-shift and night-float rotations, residents were asked to complete visuo-haptic simulations before and after 12-hour duty periods and to rate their fatigue level with questionnaires.

Results.—Both groups showed significant decrements in proficiency measures after their shifts compared with baseline. The night-float group showed more significant declines ($P < .05$) in all areas assessed than the day-shift group. The night-float group was significantly less proficient in cognitive tasks after their shifts compared with the day-shift group.

Conclusions.—The deterioration of surgical proficiency is to a degree dependent on the time of day during which call occurs, not solely on the length of call.

▶ One impact of the 80-hour work week has been the evolution of the night-float system of resident 24-hour coverage of inpatients. I have selected many articles that have catalogued this evolution. In every study cited, the interruption of continuity of care has been a hypothetical problem of night float. Some studies have confirmed the hypothesis and others have not. Even in most studies that confirmed a deficiency in communication among the day and the night shifts, the more rested residents during the night have theoretically compensated for any oversight in communication.

Now comes this study that says the cognitive ability of the night-shift residents is inferior to that of their counterparts working during the day. The unknown is what the cognitive ability of the day-shift residents would be if they were to work all 24 hours and then be tested at the end of the night shift. Similarly, aren't the night-shift residents the same ones who are on day-shift rotations?

Nevertheless, the study has merit. I am not sure that residents' cognitive abilities are totally dependent on the sun or the moon (I am aware of the diurnal variation of steroid metabolism). Their cognitive ability may be more dependent on the knowledge of the patients' problems; their level of industriousness during the night; their activity level during the day, which dictates their level of awareness, interest, and concern during the night; and whether night-shift residents are of equivalent stamina, intellect, and resourcefulness as their day-shift counterparts.

As an example, I am aware of residents who elect to change specialties early in their residency and finish the year as the night-shift resident. Actually, working only at night might be a good thing because the diurnal variation of metabolism would adapt to night work. Testing the cognitive ability of emergency physicians who shift from day to night regularly would be interesting, as would the same evaluation of workers who hold two 8-hour-a-day jobs.

In the years to come, when all the appropriate evaluations of the night-float system, as it is currently practiced, are tabulated, I think that it will be deemed deleterious to patient care. I feel the same way about the 8-hour-shift hospitalist, but this is a topic for another day.

E. M. Copeland III, MD

Mental Practice Enhances Surgical Technical Skills: A Randomized Controlled Study

Arora S, Aggarwal R, Sirimanna P, et al (Imperial College London, UK; et al)
Ann Surg 253:265-270, 2011

Objective.—To assess the effects of mental practice on surgical performance.

Background.—Increasing concerns for patient safety have highlighted a need for alternative training strategies outside the operating room. Mental practice (MP), "the cognitive rehearsal of a task before performance," has been successful in sport and music to enhance skill. This study investigates whether MP enhances performance in laparoscopic surgery.

Methods.—After baseline skills testing, 20 novice surgeons underwent training on an evidence-based virtual reality curriculum. After randomization using the closed envelope technique, all participants performed 5 Virtual Reality (VR) laparoscopic cholecystectomies (LC). Mental practice participants performed 30 minutes of MP before each LC; control participants viewed an online lecture. Technical performance was assessed using video Objective Structured Assessment of Technical Skills—based global ratings scale (scored from 7 to 35). Mental imagery was assessed using a previously validated Mental Imagery Questionnaire.

Results.—Eighteen participants completed the study. There were no intergroup differences in baseline technical ability. Learning curves were demonstrated for both MP and control groups. Mental practice was superior to control (global ratings) for the first LC (median 20 vs 15, $P = 0.005$), second LC (20.5 vs 13.5, $P = 0.001$), third LC (24 vs 15.5, $P < 0.001$), fourth LC (25.5 vs 15.5, $P < 0.001$) and the fifth LC (27.5 vs 19.5, $P = 0.00$). The imagery for the MP group was also significantly superior to the control group across all sessions ($P < 0.05$). Improved imagery significantly correlated with better quality of performance (ρ 0.51–0.62, $Ps < 0.05$).

Conclusions.—This is the first randomized controlled study to show that MP enhances the quality of performance based on VR laparoscopic cholecystectomy. This may be a time- and cost-effective strategy to augment traditional training in the OR thus potentially improving patient care.

▶ One of the appeals of surgical oncology was the expectation that I would be able to use my anatomic skills by operating in almost all parts of the body. This expectation was realized except for certain specialized areas such as the brain. While faculty members at the University of Texas MD Anderson Cancer Hospital in the 1970s and early 1980s, we 4 general surgeons rotated as 2-man teams by doing gastrointestinal surgery for 6 months and then soft tissue surgery for 6 months. Unlike today when cancer surgeons tend to specialize in 1 organ, such as the breast or colon, or in one disease, such as melanoma or sarcoma, our group preferred the variety of anatomic areas in which we operated. For example, soft tissue sarcomas occur all over the body. At the time, we did the orthopedic oncology as well. Operations like hemipelvectomies did not come along that often, which required a review of the anatomy and mental preparation for the operation—almost always the evening before. The same could be said for operating in the popliteal space, on the sole of the foot, or in the obturator fossa.

The point I am making is that mental preparation of the operation to be done was routine in the past, at least for the surgeons with whom I spent my formative years. Thus, the outcome of the current study was predictable. Nevertheless, I am excited that mental preparation before a procedure has been proven of value in a randomized controlled trial, even if the operation chosen is repetitive and relatively simple from the anatomic and technical standpoint. The old adage that there are no "minor" or "routine" operations, especially if they are to be done on you, should still be held in utmost respect.

E. M. Copeland III, MD

Special Report: Suicidal Ideation Among American Surgeons
Shanafelt TD, Balch CM, Dyrbye L, et al (Mayo Clinic, Rochester, MN; American College of Surgeons, Chicago, IL; et al)
Arch Surg 146:54-62, 2011

Background.—Suicide is a disproportionate cause of death for US physicians. The prevalence of suicidal ideation (SI) among surgeons and their use of mental health resources are unknown.

Study Design.—Members of the American College of Surgeons were sent an anonymous cross-sectional survey in June 2008. The survey included questions regarding SI and use of mental health resources, a validated depression screening tool, and standardized assessments of burnout and quality of life.

Results.—Of 7905 participating surgeons (response rate, 31.7%), 501 (6.3%) reported SI during the previous 12 months. Among individuals 45 years and older, SI was 1.5 to 3.0 times more common among surgeons than the general population ($P<.02$). Only 130 surgeons (26.0%) with recent SI had sought psychiatric or psychologic help, while 301 (60.1%) were reluctant to seek help due to concern that it could affect their medical license. Recent SI had a large, statistically significant adverse relationship with all 3 domains of burnout (emotional exhaustion, depersonalization, and low personal accomplishment) and symptoms of depression. Burnout (odds ratio, 1.910; $P<.001$) and depression (odds ratio, 7.012; $P<.001$) were independently associated with SI after controlling for personal and professional characteristics. Other personal and professional characteristics also related to the prevalence of SI.

Conclusions.—Although 1 of 16 surgeons reported SI in the previous year, few sought psychiatric or psychologic help. Recent SI among surgeons was strongly related to symptoms of depression and a surgeon's degree of burnout. Studies are needed to determine how to reduce SI among surgeons and how to eliminate barriers to their use of mental health resources.

▶ Older surgeons, those aged 45 years or older, had a higher rate of suicidal ideation than did their peers in corresponding age groups from the general population. I am not a psychologist but will offer an opinion as to why. Surgeons delay short-term goals to attain long-term goals. While in training, their counterparts in age, intelligence, and ability to compete for "good" jobs are enjoying life, making a good living, and, by comparison, "living the good life." The long-term goals that have been delayed by the physicians in training are to be able to fulfill their altruistic goals of providing health care for the public while eventually also being able to "live the good life." It is only after age 45 that some physicians realize this combination of goals will not be attained, and this realization can be depressing.

Physicians younger than 45 years had the same incidence of suicidal ideation as did their general-public counterparts. These physicians had progressed through the new 80-hour training paradigm, and many were currently or are anticipating being employees of the health care system. My prediction is that their suicidal ideation rates will continue to reflect that of their age groups and will not increase as has occurred in the current 45 and older age groups. The former groups have only somewhat delayed short-term goals and may also have fewer "good life" anticipations than the latter group.

The big question is this: will the public be better off from the health care standpoint with these younger physicians than with the older ones? The younger docs may have a better life, but will their patients?

E. M. Copeland III, MD

The Role of Surgical Champions in the American College of Surgeons National Surgical Quality Improvement Program — A National Survey

Raval MV, Bentrem DJ, Eskandari MK, et al (American College of Surgeons, Chicago, IL; Northwestern Univ Feinberg School of Medicine, Chicago, IL; et al)
J Surg Res 166:e15-e25, 2011

Background.—The American College of Surgeons National Surgical Quality Improvement Program (ACS NSQIP) empowers surgeons and medical centers to reliably collect, analyze, and act on clinically collected outcomes data. How individual ACS NSQIP leaders designated as Surgeon Champions (SC) utilize the ACS NSQIP at the hospital level and the obstacles they encounter are not well studied.

Materials and Methods.—All SC representing the 236 hospitals participating in the ACS NSIQP were invited to complete a survey designed to assess the role of the SC, data use, continuous quality improvement (CQI) efforts, CQI culture, and financial implications.

Results.—We received responses from 109 (46.2%) SC. The majority (72.5%) of SC were not compensated for their CQI efforts. Factors associated with demonstrable CQI efforts included longer duration of participation in the program, frequent meetings with clinical reviewers, frequent presentation of data to administration, compensation for Surgical Champion efforts and providing individual surgeons with feedback (all $P < 0.05$). Almost all SC stated ACS NSQIP data improved the quality of care that patients received at the hospital level (92.4%) and that the ACS NSQIP provided data that could not be obtained by other sources (95.2%). All SCs considered future funding for participation in the ACS NSQIP secure.

Conclusions.—Active use of ACS NSQIP data provide SC with demonstrable CQI by regularly reviewing data, having frequent interaction with clinical reviewers, and frequently sharing data with hospital administration and colleagues. SC thus play a key role in successful quality improvement at the hospital level.

▶ The National Surgical Quality Improvement Program has now been around for more than 10 years. It had its roots in the Veterans Administration (VA) quality improvement initiative. From the outset, at the VA, private, and public hospitals, quality was demonstrated to improve on the local level. The hindrance for universal acceptance of the program was the initial cost of implementing the program, primarily the cost of hiring a dedicated nurse to abstract the necessary data from patients' charts. Most hospital administrators did not consider the results on a local level to justify the costs.

Dr Clifford Ko, the Director of Research and Optimal Patient Care Division of the American College of Surgeons, and his colleagues have worked diligently over the last several years to convert the data into meaningful information at the individual surgeon and procedure level. The survey reported here attests to their success. A 42% response to a survey is better than most questionnaire responses and, even if the 58% of nonresponders felt that NSQIP was of no value, the results in improvement in the 42% responders would indicate that the lack of positive results in the 58% of nonresponders was the fault of the nonresponders, not the program. I would hope that all surgeons would welcome a 42% increase in quality in their institutions.

Obamacare may be modified after the next presidential election, depending on the outcome. However, the quality improvement portions should remain. Who can be against quality improvement? Tying reimbursement from federal insurance programs to demonstrated quality improvement will ensure that such quality measures are instituted, measured, and reported. The electronic medical record will be a reality before 2014, especially if hospitals want to be reimbursed by the government for instituting the electronic medical record. Quality measures will become more easily retrieved.

Dr Ko and his colleagues have perfected a program that works, and the drill down to even more definable quality issues is on the horizon. To not institute NSQIP in hospitals with moderate to large volumes of surgical patients is to have your head in the sand.

E. M. Copeland III, MD

Unsupervised Procedures by Surgical Trainees: A Windfall for Private Insurance at the Expense of Graduate Medical Education
Feinstein AJ, Deckelbaum DL, Madan AK, et al (Univ of Arizona College of Medicine, Phoenix; McGill Univ, Montreal, Quebec, Canada; Univ of Miami, FL)
J Trauma 70:136-140, 2011

Background.—Surgical faculty cannot always be present while trainees perform minor procedures. Fees are not obtained for these unsupervised services because Medicare rules do not allow residents and fellows to bill. Medicare already supplements hospitals via medical education funds and thus reimbursement for trainee services would constitute double billing. Private insurance companies, however, do not supplement trainees' salaries and thus benefit when they are not charged for these procedures. The objective is to determine whether significant revenue is lost to private insurers for unsupervised procedures performed by surgical trainees.

Methods.—We retrospectively evaluated a prospective database of procedures performed by residents and fellows from March 1998 through 2007. All procedures were entered by the trainees into a computerized electronic note system. Unsupervised procedures were not billed to insurance carriers.

Results.—During the study period, 14,497 minor procedures were performed without attending supervision, of which 13,343 had valid current procedural terminology codes. Total charges for these procedures would have been $10,096,931. For patients with private insurance companies (PICs), $6,876,000 could have been billed. Using our historic collection ratios, $2,269,083 in revenue was lost, or $232,726 annually.

Conclusions.—Trainees perform a significant number of unsupervised procedures on patients with private insurance without charge. This pro bono service represents a significant amount of lost income for teaching institutions. Private insurance companies benefit financially from Medicare billing regulations without contributing to education. Billing for these services might help offset the costs of graduate medical education (Table 1).

▶ I once wondered how much revenue our department of surgery lost from such procedures as central line placements, arterial lines, central line replacements, as listed in Table 1. The lost revenue was comparable to the figures quoted in this article. My solution was to hire a person to be sure that the procedures (most of which were done on the inpatient floor) were supervised, and an appropriate bill was submitted regardless of the source of insurance. The revenue easily paid the salary of the person hired, and faculty supervision for

TABLE 1.—Unsupervised Procedures Performed

Procedure	Current Procedural Terminology	Charge	N	Total $
Central venous catheter (guidewire change)	36580	$1,080	3292	$3,555,360
Arterial line	36620	$290	2689	$779,810
Central venous catheter (new site)	36556	$1,090	2248	$2,450,320
Chest tube/catheter insertion	32551	$865	1014	$877,110
Pulmonary artery catheter	93503	$760	863	$655,880
Tracheal intubation	31500	$440	850	$374,000
Suture of laceration	12032	$440	740	$325,600
Hemodialysis access	36800	$600	541	$324,600
Bronchoscopy	31622	$820	241	$197,620
Diagnostic ileoscopy/colonoscopy	45330	$280	228	$63,840
Percutaneous transplant liver biopsy	47000	$480	125	$60,000
Peritoneal lavage	49080	$410	81	$33,210
Ventriculostomy placement	61107	$1,525	70	$106,750
Thoracentesis	32421	$335	56	$18,760
Peripherally inserted venous catheter mid/l n/stick	36569	$1,220	53	$64,660
Lumbar puncture	62270	$350	50	$17,500
Paracentesis	49080	$410	42	$17,220
Cardiopulmonary resuscitation	92950	$580	31	$17,980
Percutaneous tracheostomy	31600	$1,100	28	$30,800
Abdominal wound exploration	20102	$740	26	$19,240
Hickman/port removal	36589	$640	18	$11,520
Lumbar drain placement	62272	$450	14	$6,300
Cervical tongs placement	20660	$1,000	13	$13,000
Thoracotomy	32110	$6,364	9	$57,276
Esophagogastroduodenoscopy percutaneous gastrostomy	43246	$1,265	6	$7,590
Epidural catheter	62319	$670	6	$4,020
Complex abdominal wound care	97606	$45	3	$135
Cricothyroidotomy	31605	$1,025	2	$2,050
Pacemaker, insertion	33206	$1,825	2	$3,650
Pericardiocentesis	33010	$565	2	$1,130
Total			13,343	$10,096,931

these elective procedures was not onerous when well organized by the person in charge.

The argument can be made that faculty supervision of these "minor" procedures takes the faculty member away from more financially productive activities. I did not find this to be the case. In fact, in today's world, many trauma services are organized with a different trauma surgeon in charge of the inpatient floor on a weekly basis, while the other trauma surgeons take call and operate. Having this "patient rounding" trauma surgeon and his or her team well organized on the inpatient floor should make appropriate faculty member coverage of these elective procedures quite easy.

Since trauma surgery has been organized as described above, the specialty has become relatively more popular because it appeals now to "lifestyle" friendly surgeons. Making rounds for a week without on-call responsibilities is not especially taxing to the psyche nor is taking calls for 24 hours and not having any further responsibility for the patient upon whom the operation is performed. There are institutions that find that fiscal support for the trauma surgeons working the described schedules is difficult unless the trauma surgeon also participates in critical care, which of course then makes trauma surgery less "lifestyle" friendly. It seems to me that collecting the fees from the unsupervised procedures described in this article would help eliminate the need for rotations of the trauma surgeons on a critical care service, if that were an issue.

E. M. Copeland III, MD

Women in Surgery Residency Programs: Evolving Trends from a National Perspective
Davis EC, Risucci DA, Blair PG, et al (American College of Surgeons, Chicago, IL)
J Am Coll Surg 212:320-326, 2011

Background.—Similar numbers of men and women are currently graduating from United States (US) medical schools; therefore, surgery residency programs need to attract graduates of both genders. This study compared gender distributions of allopathic US medical graduates (USMG) from academic years 1999-2000 through 2004-2005. In addition, the gender distributions of USMG and international medical graduates (IMG; analyzed separately) entering accredited general surgery (GS) programs and USMG entering other surgical specialty programs were compared across academic years 2000-2001 through 2005-2006.

Study Design.—Data were extracted from the American College of Surgeons Resident Master File and the Association of American Medical Colleges FACTS Website and Data Warehouse. Chi-square statistics compared gender distributions across years for all USMG graduating and applying to GS programs each year between 1999-2000 and 2004-2005 and for USMG and IMG entering training between 2000-2001 and 2005-2006.

Results.—During the study period, the proportion of women increased significantly ($p < 0.001$) among USMG (43% to 47%), USMG applying to GS programs (27% to 33%), and USMG entering GS residencies (32% to 40%); the percentages of women among IMG entering GS residencies ranged from 11% to 18%, with no apparent linear increase. Proportions of women among USMG entering training increased in most surgical specialties examined.

Conclusions.—The gender gap among USMG entering GS training appears to be closing, concurrent with that of USMG overall during the study period. Surgery programs must continue to recruit and retain women to attract the best and brightest trainees (Table 1).

▶ I have been given an interesting perspective on many aspects of health care "reform," tort "reform," work-hour restrictions, and women in medicine—especially in surgery.

This excellent article from the American College of Surgeons and the American Association of Medical Colleges codifies the successes with the attraction of women into the discipline of general surgery. No doubt, limitation of work

TABLE 1.—Percent of Women among USMG Entering Surgery Programs by Specialty: Academic Years 2000-2001 Through 2005-2006

Specialty	2000–2001		2001–2002		2002–2003		2003–2004		2004–2005		2005–2006	
	n	%	n	%	n	%	n	%	n	%	n	%
General surgery	282	32	282	31	259	31	300	32	355	34	384	40
Neurosurgery	22	14	8	6	22	18	22	13	20	12	18	11
Obstetrics/gynecology	766	78	748	76	776	80	692	79	709	81	726	82
Ophthalmology	151	36	137	33	138	34	134	34	148	36	153	39
Orthopaedic surgery	55	9	60	10	66	11	68	11	78	12	84	13
Otolaryngology	53	19	64	23	59	26	60	25	73	30	75	30
Plastic surgery	40	21	49	26	41	22	34	18	40	21	48	24
Urology	32	13	40	18	47	22	50	23	46	21	53	25

hours, an increase in female faculty members who can serve as mentors, and the sheer increase in the percentage of female medical students matriculating through US medical schools all have contributed to the increase of female applicants to general surgery programs. (I consider the increase in applicants even more important than the increase in female residents.)

Surgery is now more attractive to women. The programs put in place to attract women into surgery are working. A somewhat silent reason for the increase is the ability to limit the scope of practice that has evolved in the practice of general surgery. Breast, laparoscopic, bariatric, and stint vascular surgery are examples. Trauma surgery has also become organized to allow a schedule-friendly lifestyle. There are some increases in the number of women selecting otolaryngology and obstetrics and gynecology, but not a dramatic actual increase in numbers (Table 1). In the past, women interested in a specialty with a technical component chose these specialties. General surgery has invaded these subspecialties' "turf." I am not at all surprised. Women have always been interested in general surgery. Lifestyle limitations prevented them from becoming general surgeons. No longer! We can begin to congratulate ourselves on attracting an extremely qualified gender into what was a male-dominated specialty in the recent past.

The lack of increase in international medical graduate applicants can also be attributed to increased numbers of qualified female US medical graduate applicants into the surgical specialties.

E. M. Copeland III, MD

An Acute Care Surgery Rotation Contributes Significant General Surgical Operative Volume to Residency Training Compared With Other Rotations
Stanley MD, Davenport DL, Procter LD, et al (Univ of Kentucky College of Medicine, Lexington)
J Trauma 70:590-594, 2011

Background.—Surgical resident rotations on trauma services are criticized for little operative experience and heavy workloads. This has resulted in diminished interest in trauma surgery among surgical residents.

Acute care surgery (ACS) combines trauma and emergency/elective general surgery, enhancing operative volume and balancing operative and nonoperative effort. We hypothesize that a mature ACS service provides significant operative experience.

Methods.—A retrospective review was performed of ACGME case logs of 14 graduates from a major, academic, Level I trauma center program during a 3-year period. Residency Review Committee index case volumes during the fourth and fifth years of postgraduate training (PGY-4 and PGY-5) ACS rotations were compared with other service rotations: in total and per resident week on service.

Results.—Ten thousand six hundred fifty-four cases were analyzed for 14 graduates. Mean cases per resident was 432 ± 57 in PGY-4, 330 ± 40 in PGY-5, and 761 ± 67 for both years combined. Mean case volume on ACS for both years was 273 ± 44, which represented 35.8% (273 of 761) of the total experience and exceeded all other services. Residents averaged 8.9 cases per week on the ACS service, which exceeded all other services except private general surgery, gastrointestinal/minimally invasive surgery, and pediatric surgery rotations. Disproportionately more head/neck, small and large intestine, gastric, spleen, laparotomy, and hernia cases occurred on ACS than on other services.

Conclusions.—Residents gain a large operative experience on ACS. An ACS model is viable in training, provides valuable operative experience, and should not be considered a drain on resident effort. Valuable ACS rotation experiences as a resident may encourage graduates to pursue ACS as a career.

▶ I don't have to be convinced that a trauma/critical care rotation for residents or students is important. In the not-too-distant future, the trauma surgeon is going to be the only one who is comfortable and qualified to do many of the difficult intra-abdominal operations done today and exampled by complicated intraperitoneal abscesses, complicated enterocutaneous fistulae, and bowel obstructions caused by dense adhesions.

I chose oncologic surgery for several reasons, and one was because I got to operate all over the human body. In other words, I was not limited to 1 cavity, 1 extremity, or 1 organ as is now the ever-growing tendency for residents finishing their general surgery training. In fact, today, many of these singular organ operations are done without even palpating the offending diseases because the operations are done off of a television screen.

Laparoscopy is a great technical advance, and studies have shown that the metabolic response to trauma from these procedures is much less than from open laparotomy, thus leading to shortened recovery times and a quicker return to normal society. Nevertheless, surgeon comfort in a "difficult" abdomen may soon become a lost art.

Were I a resident today, I would choose trauma/acute care as my specialist. I enjoy treating the metabolic response to trauma whether it is normal or abnormal. Likewise, trauma surgery would allow me to operate on injuries to almost all parts of the body. I would develop a technical and judgmental comfort zone with difficult operations that don't follow the text book descriptions. The importance of this study is the confirmation of my choice of specialty if I had a second life!

E. M. Copeland III, MD

Adhesive-Enhanced Sternal Closure to Improve Postoperative Functional Recovery: A Pilot, Randomized Controlled Trial

Fedak PWM, Kieser TM, Maitland AM, et al (Univ of Calgary, Alberta, Canada; et al)
Ann Thorac Surg 92:1444-1450, 2011

Background.—We previously established a proof-of-concept in a human cadaveric model where conventional wire cerclage was augmented with a novel biocompatible bone adhesive that increased mechanical strength and early bone stability. We report the results of a single-center, pilot, randomized clinical trial of the effects of adhesive-enhanced closure of the sternum on functional postoperative recovery.

Methods.—In 55 patients undergoing primary sternotomy, 26 patients underwent conventional wire closure and were compared with 29 patients who underwent adhesive-enhanced closure, which consisted of Kryptonite biocompatible adhesive (Doctors Research Group Inc, Southbury, CT) applied to each sternal edge in addition to conventional 7-wire cerclage. Patients were monitored postoperatively at 72 hours, weekly for 12 weeks, and then after 12 months for incisional pain, analgesic use, and maximal inspiratory capacity measured by spirometry. Standardized assessment tools measured postoperative physical disability and health-related quality of life.

Results.—No adverse events or sternal complications from the adhesive were observed early or after 12 months. Incisional pain and narcotic analgesic use were reduced in adhesive-enhanced closure patients. Inspiratory capacity was significantly improved, postoperative health-related quality of life scores normalized more rapidly, and physical disability scores were reduced. Computed tomography imaging was suggestive of sternal healing.

Conclusions.—Adhesive-enhanced closure is a safe and simple addition to conventional wire closure, with demonstrated benefits on functional recovery, respiratory capacity, incisional pain, and analgesic requirements. A large, multicenter, randomized controlled trial to examine the potential of the adhesive to prevent major sternal complications in higher risk patients is warranted.

▶ Sternal wound dehiscence, infection, and instability lead to additional morbidity in postoperative patients after cardiac procedures. Various attempts have been made to improve sternal healing, but the standard of care remains wire sternal closure. These authors performed a prospective randomized trial to evaluate adhesive-enhanced sternal wire closure compared with sternal wire closure alone. Importantly, postoperative inspiratory capacity was improved and pain was decreased in the treated group. No adverse effects such as sternal infections were observed. This is an important study despite the small numbers of patients entered. It demonstrated no harm and showed some potential beneficial effects, which is the purpose of conducting a Phase II—type trial. As the authors concluded, a multicenter, large, prospective, randomized trial is indicated, which can measure multiple additional parameters to evaluate the true efficacy of this adhesive applied to the sternal wound edges after cardiac procedures.

J. M. Daly, MD

2 Trauma

Formulated collagen gel accelerates healing rate immediately after application in patients with diabetic neuropathic foot ulcers

Blume P, Driver VR, Tallis AJ, et al (Affiliated Foot Surgeons, New Haven, CT; Boston Univ Med Ctr and School of Medicine, MA; Associated Foot and Ankle Specialists, Phoenix, AZ; et al)

Wound Repair Regen 19:302-308, 2011

We assessed the safety and efficacy of Formulated Collagen Gel (FCG) alone and with Ad5PDGF-B (GAM501) compared with Standard of Care (SOC) in patients with $1.5-10.0\,cm^2$ chronic diabetic neuropathic foot ulcers that healed <30% during Run-in. Wound size was assessed by planimetry of acetate tracings and photographs in 124 patients. Comparison of data sets revealed that acetate tracings frequently overestimated areas at some sites. For per-protocol analysis, 113 patients qualified using acetate tracings but only 82 qualified using photographs. Prior animal studies suggested that collagen alone would have little effect on healing and would serve as a negative control. Surprisingly trends for increased incidence of complete closure were observed for both GAM501 (41%) and FCG (45%) vs. Standard of Care (31%). By photographic data, Standard of Care had no significant effect on change in wound radius (mm/week) from during Run-in to Week 1 (-0.06 ± 0.32 to 0.78 ± 1.53, $p=$ ns) but both FCG (-0.08 ± 0.61 to 1.97 ± 1.77, $p<0.002$) and GAM501 (-0.02 ± 0.58 to 1.46 ± 1.37, $p<0.002$) significantly increased healing rates that gradually declined over subsequent weeks. Both GAM501 and FCG appeared to be safe and well tolerated, and alternate dosing schedules hold promise to improve overall complete wound closure in adequately powered trials.

▶ This is an interesting trial in many respects. First, the problem of patients developing diabetic foot ulcers is enormous. Second, their treatment methods are unclear, and the outcomes are unsatisfactory. Third, the morbidity and mortality related to long-term care are substantial. Thus, a multitude of studies, many including growth factors applied locally to the wound area, have been conducted in an effort to improve the healing process.

The conduct and results of this study bear close reading. The authors described a statistical need for 20 patients, but only 129 were randomized. Importantly, the trial was interrupted, and different treatment protocols and endpoints were substituted as stated after the trial results were reviewed in a blinded fashion, yet with site investigators reporting early rapid healing rates, which then slowed.

In addition, methods of measurement appeared unreliable, as both photographs and outline drawings of the ulcer sizes were done. Clearly, the gel impregnated with the growth factor vector was no better than the gel alone, but both appeared better when the new (first week healing) was added as an endpoint.

This is an interesting article about an important topic, but reader beware: read the article carefully.

J. M. Daly, MD

Marked reduction in wound complication rates following decompressive hemicraniectomy with an improved operative closure technique

Sughrue ME, Bloch OG, Manley GT, et al (Univ of California at San Francisco)
J Clin Neurosci 18:1201-1205, 2011

Although decompressive hemicraniectomy with dural expansion and bone flap removal is a potentially life-saving procedure, concerns remain regarding the morbidity associated with this approach. We and others have noted the high rate of wound complications resulting from this technique, often associated with cerebrospinal fluid (CSF) absorption problems. Here, we present our experience with an improved technique for wound closure after unilateral decompressive hemicraniectomy with a wide cruciate durotomy. Data for all patients who underwent a decompressive hemicraniectomy at our institution from October 2005 to October 2009 were gathered prospectively. Starting in mid 2008, we adopted an alternate approach to operative wound closure, which involved skin closure with a running Monocryl absorbable stitch, and prolonged subgaleal drainage. We compared the rates of wound complication using this approach with those obtained with earlier conventional closure techniques. Over a 1 year period, we dramatically reduced the rate of wound complications in patients undergoing hemicraniectomy at our hospital using this new (Monocryl technique, 0% $(n = 29)$ compared to other techniques, 35% $(n = 98)$, chi-squared $[\chi^2]$ $p < 0.001$). Patients closed using our new technique experienced markedly reduced rates of wound infection $(p < 0.01)$, and CSF leak $(p < 0.05)$, compared to other, more standard, techniques. Thus, attention to closure of hemicraniectomy wounds can markedly reduce the rate of wound complications, thus improving the risk-to-benefit ratio of this procedure.

▶ This interesting article documents a group of neurosurgeons who noted the unacceptably high wound infection rate in patients undergoing major craniectomy and made changes in the manner of closure in an attempt to reduce infectious complications and cerebrospinal fluid leaks. They used a meticulous closure technique, making certain that there were no leaks around drain sites. They also closed the wounds with a continuous monocryl suture, making sure wound approximations were appropriate. In the last 29 patients using this technique, there were no wound infections noted. The important part of this article is the recognition of a clinical problem, the determination to fix it, the uniformity of all surgeons in the group in the manner of addressing the problem, and the prospective database that was used to assess the outcomes. As the authors pointed out, further cases are likely to result in some wound infections. Critics would argue that to prove their points about wound closure techniques, they should perform a randomized trail of each of the components of the closure technique. I agree with those points yet applaud the authors for tackling a problem together and solving a major cause of morbidity and mortality.

J. M. Daly, MD

Faster Wound Healing With Topical Negative Pressure Therapy in Difficult-to-Heal Wounds: A Prospective Randomized Controlled Trial

de Laat EHEW, van den Boogaard MHWA, Spauwen PHM, et al (Radboud Univ Nijmegen Med Centre, The Netherlands; et al)
Ann Plast Surg 67:626-631, 2011

Objective.—A randomized clinical trial was conducted to determine the effectiveness and safety of topical negative pressure therapy in patients with difficult-to-heal wounds.

Methods.—A total of 24 patients were randomly assigned to either treatment with topical negative pressure therapy or treatment with conventional dressing therapy with sodium hypochlorite. The study end point was 50% reduction in wound volume. The maximum follow-up time was 6 weeks.

Results.—The median treatment time to 50% reduction of wound volume in the topical negative pressure group was 2.0 weeks (interquartile range = 1) versus 3.5 weeks (interquartile range = 1.5) in the sodium hypochlorite group ($P < 0.001$). The unadjusted hazard rate ratio for the time until 50% wound volume reduction was 0.123 ($P < 0.001$). After adjustment for relevant baseline characteristics in a Cox proportional hazards model treatment group, membership was found as the only and statistically significant indicator for the time to 50% wound volume reduction (hazard rate ratio of 0.117 [$P < 0.001$]). Subgroup analysis of spinal cord injured patients with severe pressure ulcers showed similar statistically significant results as in the total wound group.

Conclusion.—Topical negative pressure resulted in almost 2 times faster wound healing than treatment with sodium hypochlorite, and is safe to use in patients with difficult-to-heal wounds.

▶ Topical negative pressure (TNP) is a superb method to manage chronically slow to heal wounds. Its use after open abdominal and soft tissue wounds has increased many-fold. This interesting prospective, randomized trial compared TNP with standard of care using sodium hypochlorite for wound treatment, an effort to decrease wound bacterial counts and debride the wound itself. As stated, TNP resulted in a median 2-week period for 50% reduction in the size of the wound compared with a median 3.5-week timeframe for the sodium hypochlorite solution, a significant reduction in duration of therapy.

The major problem with TNP is the nursing expertise required to properly apply the bandage and seal around the wound. In addition, the equipment can be bulky and noisy, certainly limiting mobility of the patient. Nevertheless, a median 1.5-week reduction in healing time is quite important and would make a great difference in the patient's quality of life.

J. M. Daly, MD

Acceleration of diabetic-wound healing with PEGylated rhaFGF in healing-impaired streptozocin diabetic rats

Huang Z, Lu M, Zhu G, et al (Wenzhou Med College, China)
Wound Repair Regen 19:633-644, 2011

Molecular modification with polyethylene glycol (PEGylation) is an effective approach to improve protein biostability, in vivo lifetime and therapeutic potency. In the present study, the recombinant human acid fibroblast growth factor (rhaFGF) was site-selectively PEGylated with 20 kDa mPEG-butyraldehyde. Mono-PEGylated rhaFGF was purified to near homogeneity by Sephadex G 25-gel filtration followed by a Heparin Sepharose TM CL-6B affinity chromatography. PEGylated rhaFGF has less effect than the native rhaFGF on the stimulation of 3T3 cell proliferation in vitro; however, its relative thermal stability at normal physiological temperature and structural stability were significantly enhanced, and its half-life time in vivo was significantly extended. Then, the physiological function of PEGylated rhaFGF on diabetic-wound healing was evaluated in type 1 diabetic Sprague Dawley rats. The results showed that, compared with the group of animal treated with native rhaFGF, the group treated with PEGylated rhaFGF exhibited better therapeutic efficacy with shorter healing time, quicker tissue collagen generation, earlier and higher transforming growth factor (TGF)-β expression, and dermal cell proliferation. In addition, in vivo analysis showed that both native and PEGylated rhaFGF were more effective in the wound healing in the diabetic group compared with the nondiabetic one. Taken together, these results suggest that PEGylation of rhaFGF could be a more effective approach to the pharmacological and therapeutic application of native rhaFGF.

▶ This interesting experimental study used polyethylene glycol (PEGylation) to stabilize recombinant human acid fibroblast growth factor in an attempt to increase its therapeutic potency and bioavailability. The experimental compound had less effect on 3Ts cell populations in vitro, but its half-life time in vivo was markedly prolonged. The authors then used an in vivo model of diabetic rats that had been shown previously to exhibit impaired wound healing. They found that the experimental compound when administered to these animals resulted in shorter healing time and increased collagen generation as well as improved dermal cell proliferation.

Recombinant human fibroblast growth factor (rHFGF) has been administered systemically and topically in an effort to enhance wound healing. Topically, it seems to improve wound healing that is impaired but does not accelerate healing in normal animals. This new experimental compound seems to further improve the efficacy and bioavailability of rHFGF and should continue to be tested, perhaps moving rapidly to human phase I clinical trials.

J. M. Daly, MD

Aminated β-1,3-D-glucan has a dose-dependent effect on wound healing in diabetic *db/db* mice
Berdal M, Appelbom HI, Eikrem JH, et al (Univ of Tromsø, Norway)
Wound Repair Regen 19:579-587, 2011

Inflammatory responses are common in diabetes and are operative in angiopathy, neuropathy, and wound healing. There are indications of incomplete macrophage activation in diabetes and reduced expression of growth factors. We have previously found that up to 15 topical applications of the macrophage-stimulant, aminated β-1,3-D-glucan (AG), improved wound healing in *db/db* mice. The present open-label study was undertaken to examine dose-dependent effects of AG over 40 days in *db/db* mice. AG was given as a single dose (group 1), one dose every 10th day (group 2), five initial doses on consecutive days (group 3), and ≥15 doses (group 4). Controls were *db/db* mice receiving platelet-derived growth factor + insulin-like growth factor-1 (group 5), topical placebo (NaCl 9 mg/mL) and insulin (group 6), placebo (group 7), and a nondiabetic group receiving placebo (group 8). Seven to 14 animals were allocated to each group. Percentage wound closure 17 days after surgery in groups 1 and 2 were (mean ± standard error of the mean) 25.5 ± 5.3 and 32.2 ± 6.3, respectively. Corresponding closure in groups 3, 4, and 5 was 55.7 ± 5.0, 57.3 ± 5.0, and 55.6 ± 4.8, respectively ($p < 0.05$ vs. groups 1 and 2). Groups 6, 7, and 8 closed 32.0 ± 4.5, 38.2 ± 5.3, and $98.5 \pm 0.4\%$, respectively. Significant association between the number of AG-dosages and wound closure indicates dose-related effects in *db/db* mice.

▶ It is well known that wound healing is decreased significantly in diabetic subjects compared with controls. It is thought that the inflammatory response in the wound itself is diminished in diabetic subjects compared with normal individuals. Interestingly, this appears to be due to diminished macrophage activation and reduced expression of growth factors. It is thought that administration of agents that stimulate wound macrophages will therefore improve wound healing in diabetic mice.

This randomized, prospective animal study showed that administration of insulin alone to diabetic mice did not improve wound healing compared with the placebo-treated diabetic animal. All diabetic animals exhibited decreased wound healing of an open dorsal skin wound compared with nondiabetic controls. Administration of β-1, 3-D-glucan improved wound healing in all treated animals. As the doses of glucan were increased, wound healing continued to improve. It was critically important, however, that the agent was administered during the early phases of wound healing for it to exhibit a maximum affect.

The ability to better heal wounds and diabetic subjects is the Holy Grail of many investigators. However, it is unclear at this time as to whether stimulants, growth factors themselves, cellular therapy to stimulate macrophages, and other cells in the region of the wound will be individually or collectively important in improving wound healing in diabetic subjects.

J. M. Daly, MD

Bone Marrow–Derived Mesenchymal Stem Cells Enhanced Diabetic Wound Healing Through Recruitment of Tissue Regeneration in a Rat Model of Streptozotocin-Induced Diabetes
Kuo Y-R, Wang C-T, Cheng J-T, et al (Chang Gung Univ College of Medicine, Kaohsiung, Taiwan, China; Natl Sun Yat-sen Univ, Kaohsiung, Taiwan, China)
Plast Reconstr Surg 128:872-880, 2011

Background.—This study investigated whether bone marrow–derived mesenchymal stem cell therapy has effectiveness in the enhancement of diabetic wound healing through tissue regeneration.

Methods.—The authors used a dorsal skin defect (6×5 cm) in a streptozotocin-induced diabetes rodent model. Forty male Wistar rats were divided into four groups: group I, nondiabetic rats (controls); group II, diabetic controls receiving no mesenchymal stem cells; group III, rats receiving 1×10^7 stem cells per dose (subcutaneously administered in eight areas surrounding wound margin) on day 7; and group IV, rats receiving stem cells on days 7 and 10. Wound healing was assessed clinically. Histologic examination was performed with hematoxylin and eosin staining. CD45, Ki-67, prolyl 4-hydroxylase, epidermal growth factor, and vascular endothelial growth factor were evaluated with immunohistochemical analysis.

Results.—Overall clinical results showed that wound size was significantly reduced in mesenchymal stem cell–treated rats as compared with controls. Complete wound-healing time was statistically shorter in rats treated once as compared with controls (6.6 ± 1.13 weeks versus 9.8 ± 0.75 weeks; $p < 0.001$). It was significantly shorter in rats treated with mesenchymal stem cells twice as compared with rats treated once (5.2 ± 0.75 weeks versus 6.6 ± 1.13 weeks; $p = 0.026$). Histologic analysis revealed significant reduction in topical proinflammatory reaction and suppression of CD45 expression in the mesenchymal stem cell group as compared with the control group. On immunohistochemistry analysis, significant increases in epidermal growth factor, vascular endothelial growth factor, prolyl 4-hydroxylase, and Ki-67 expression were noted in the treated group as compared with the control group.

Conclusions.—Mesenchymal stem cells significantly enhanced diabetic wound healing. Treatment with them is associated with increases of biomarkers in tissue regeneration.

▶ The authors carried out an experimental study to evaluate mesenchymal stem cell therapy as a means of providing growth factors and other substrates locally to enhance wound healing. They chose a standard dorsal wound healing model in rats and evaluated wound size over time as well as histologic analyses. Mesenchymal stem cell—treated animals were injected either once on day 7 or twice on days 7 and 10 after wounding. They noted significantly faster wound contraction time with 1 injection and even shorter healing time when 2 injections were given. Topical proinflammatory reaction was less, which was an interesting finding. Indeed, they also noted increased vascular endothelial growth factor and epidermal growth factor by histochemical analyses in the wound edges of mesenchymal-treated animals.

It will be important to compare stem cell therapy with the best available biochemical therapy applied topically to wounds in normal and compromised subjects to determine the most efficacious approaches to use going forward.

J. M. Daly, MD

Arginase inhibition promotes wound healing in mice
Kavalukas SL, Uzgare AR, Bivalacqua TJ, et al (Sinai Hosp of Baltimore, MD; The Johns Hopkins Med Institutions, Baltimore, MD)
Surgery 151:287-295, 2012

Objective.—Arginase plays important regulatory roles in polyamine, ornithine, and nitric oxide syntheses. However, its role in the healing process has not been delineated. In this study, we used a highly potent and specific inhibitor of arginase, namely 2(S)-amino-6-boronohexanoic acid NH4 (ABH) to evaluate the role of arginase function in wound healing.

Materials and Methods.—ABH or saline was applied topically to full thickness, dorsal, excisional wounds in C57BL/6 mice every 8 hours for 14 days post surgery and the rate of wound closure was estimated planimetrically. Wound tissue was harvested from mice sacrificed on postoperative days 3 and 7 and examined histologically. The extent of epithelial, connective, and granulation tissue present within the wound area was estimated histomorphometrically. The effect of ABH on wound arginase activity, production of nitric oxide metabolites (NO_x), and presence of smooth muscle actin positive cells (myofibroblasts) was evaluated.

Results.—While arginase activity was inhibited in vivo, the rate of wound closure significantly increased 7 days post-surgery, ($21 \pm 4\%$: $P < .01$; Student t test) in ABH treated animals. This was accompanied by an early increase in wound granulation tissue and accumulation of NO_x followed by enhanced re-epithelialization and localization of myofibroblasts beneath the wound epithelium.

Conclusion.—Arginase inhibition improves excisional wound healing and may be used to develop therapeutics for early wound closure.

▶ The importance of the biochemical milieu in tissue after wounding needs to be better understood to rationally change topical therapies directed at accelerating wound healing. In this experiment, the authors evaluated the role of arginase in the healing wound inhibited arginase activity. They hypothesized that greater amounts of arginine would then be available for cellular proliferation. A potent arginase inhibitor was administered every 8 hours to the wound area after a full-thickness excision in mice. At 7, 10, and 14 days, there was significant improvement in wound healing in the arginase inhibitor—treated animals. There was also improvement in the development of granulation tissue and myofibroblast proliferation in treated animals. However, although at 14 days a statistical difference in healing was noted between groups, both groups of animals on average healed quite well with few numerical differences.

Thus, this experiment showed that arginase inhibition administered topically every 8 hours in the area of the wound may have benefit in accelerating the healing process. It will be important to test this hypothesis in animals that demonstrate impaired wound healing, such as those treated with radiation or those with diabetes mellitus. Studies such as this demonstrate the need to better understand the biochemical milieu within the healing wound so that steps may be taken to alter it and accelerate wound healing, particularly in those with impaired function.

J. M. Daly, MD

Acceleration of cutaneous healing by electrical stimulation: Degenerate electrical waveform down-regulates inflammation, up-regulates angiogenesis and advances remodeling in temporal punch biopsies in a human volunteer study

Sebastian A, Syed F, Perry D, et al (The Univ of Manchester, UK; et al)
Wound Repair Regen 19:693-708, 2011

We previously demonstrated the beneficial effect of a novel electrical stimulation (ES) waveform, degenerate wave (DW) on skin fibroblasts, and now hypothesize that DW can enhance cutaneous wound healing *in vivo*. Therefore, a punch biopsy was taken from the upper arm of 20 volunteers on day 0 and repeated on day 14 (NSD14). A contralateral upper arm biopsy was taken on day 0 and treated with DW for 14 days prior to a repeat biopsy on day 14 (ESD14). A near-completed inflammatory stage of wound healing in ESD14, compared to NSD14 was demonstrated by up-regulation of interleukin-10 and vasoactive intestinal peptide using quantitative real time polymerase chain reaction and down-regulation of CD3 by immunohistochemistry (IHC) ($p < 0.05$). In addition to up-regulation ($p < 0.05$) of mRNA transcripts for re-epithelialization and angiogenesis, IHC showed significant overexpression ($p < 0.05$) of CD31 (15.5%), vascular endothelial growth factor (66%), and Melan A (8.6 cells/0.95 mm^2) in ESD14 compared to NSD14 (9.5%, 38% and 4.3 cells/0.95 mm^2, respectively). Furthermore, granulation tissue formation (by hematoxylin and eosin staining), and myofibroblastic proliferation demonstrated by alpha-smooth muscle actin (62.7%) plus CD3+ T lymphocytes (8.1%) showed significant up-regulation ($p < 0.05$) in NSD14. In the remodeling stage, mRNA transcripts for fibronectin, collagen IV (by IHC, 14.1%) and mature collagen synthesis (by Herovici staining, 71.44%) were significantly up-regulated

($p < 0.05$) in ESD14. Apoptotic (TUNEL assay) and proliferative cells (Ki67) were significantly up-regulated ($p < 0.05$) in NSD14 (5.34 and 11.9 cells/ 0.95 mm^2) while the proliferation index of ESD14 was similar to normal skin. In summary, cutaneous wounds receiving DW electrical stimulation display accelerated healing seen by reduced inflammation, enhanced angiogenesis and advanced remodeling phase.

▶ Electrical stimulation of wounds to enhance wound healing is not a new concept. Previous reports evaluated bone healing subjected to electrical stimulation and found beneficial effects especially in nonhealing types of fractures. These authors used a novel electrical stimulation waveform, degenerate wave (DW), on skin punch biopsy sites on the arms of 20 volunteers. Each patient served as his or her own control. The study demonstrated up-regulation of mRNA transcripts for re-epithelialization and angiogenesis. In addition, granulation tissue formation and myofibroblastic proliferation were enhanced by electrical stimulation using DW.

It would be interesting to use this method experimentally to determine if these molecular markers and histologic changes correlated with breaking/bursting strengths in different animal models. While other methods to enhance wound healing have been shown to do so in malnourished, steroid-treated, diabetic or older individuals, this method showed positive results in well-nourished healthy young volunteers. Further work is needed to investigate these interesting results.

J. M. Daly, MD

Chronic wound fluid—thinking outside the box
Widgerow AD (Univ of the Witwatersrand, Johannesburg, South Africa)
Wound Repair Regen 19:287-291, 2011

Chronic wounds are associated with an altered wound milieu that results from an imbalance in extracellular matrix (ECM) homeostasis. This alteration is characterized by an increased destruction and degradation of components of the ECM with a concomitant lack of synthesis of these elements. Traditionally wound fluid has been considered a reflection of the internal wound milieu. It has been used to monitor and reflect on the chronic status of a wound or to measure the efficacy of wound treatment. However, on closer inspection of chronic wound fluid, certain components of the fluid, particularly matrix metalloproteinases (MMPs) and their subcomponents (MMP-9) have been found to exist at higher levels in wound fluid than in the corresponding wound. There is mounting evidence that much of the destructive effects observed in chronic wounds may be compounded by components of the wound exudate which are corrosive in nature resulting in a continuum of ECM breakdown. Isolation of these components has identified MMPs, in particular MMP-9 as dominant in this destructive process. Additionally an association has been made between high bacterial levels and elevated MMP9 in chronic wounds. Agents that have efficacy against MMP-9 and significant antibacterial potency thus provide a dual defense against chronic wounds. It is likely that these agents cause a change in the chronic wound fluid components that more closely resemble the balance of proteases and growth factors seen acute wounds, thus triggering a positive wound healing process. Nanocrystalline silver appears to fulfill these criteria. A strategy is suggested whereby wound fluid is directly targeted to diminish the corrosive wound fluid elements in an attempt to break the ongoing destructive inflammatory cycle. This presents a relatively new treatment paradigm attempting to influence wound healing by working from without to initiate changes within.

▶ This interesting article hypothesizes that chronic wound fluid is actually deleterious to the wound itself. The authors suggest that there are substances within chronic wound fluid that inhibit the wound from continuing to heal. They note, for example, that chronic wound fluid contains metalloproteinase, particularly metalloproteinase 9. They believe that high concentrations of this metalloproteinase in fact inhibit continued healing in the wound. They also note that nanocrystalline silver is one substance that may inhibit metalloproteinase 9 and therefore be useful as a topical application in chronic wounds that do not heal.

The management of patients with chronic wounds is a dilemma. The use of moderate lower pressure vacuum applied to the area of the wound has been shown to be of benefit. In addition, this mechanical means to accelerate wound healing also removes chronic wound fluid from the area of the wound. Thus, it may be possible to target metalloproteinase 9 as well as to remove chronic wound fluid using a low-pressure vacuum in an attempt to maximize the healing of these difficult wounds and improve patient outcomes.

J. M. Daly, MD

A Multisite Assessment of the American College of Surgeons Committee on Trauma Field Triage Decision Scheme for Identifying Seriously Injured Children and Adults

Newgard CD, the WESTRN investigators (Oregon Health & Science Univ, Portland; et al)
J Am Coll Surg 213:709-721, 2011

Background.—The American College of Surgeons Committee on Trauma (ACSCOT) has developed and updated field trauma triage protocols for decades, yet the ability to identify major trauma patients remains unclear. We estimate the diagnostic value of the Field Triage Decision Scheme for identifying major trauma patients (Injury Severity Score [ISS] ≥16) in a large and diverse multisite cohort.

Study Design.—This was a retrospective cohort study of injured children and adults transported by 94 emergency medical services (EMS) agencies to 122 hospitals in 7 regions of the Western US from 2006 through 2008. Patients who met any of the field trauma triage criteria (per EMS personnel) were considered triage positive. Hospital outcomes measures were probabilistically linked to EMS records through trauma registries, state discharge data, and emergency department data. The primary outcome defining a "major trauma patient" was ISS ≥16.

Results.—There were 122,345 injured patients evaluated and transported by EMS over the 3-year period, 34.5% of whom met at least 1 triage criterion and 5.8% had ISS ≥16. The overall sensitivity and specificity of the criteria for identifying major trauma patients were 85.8% (95% CI 85.0% to 86.6%) and 68.7% (95% CI 68.4% to 68.9%), respectively. Triage sensitivity and specificity, respectively, differed by age: 84.1% and 66.4% (0 to 17 years); 89.5% and 64.3% (18 to 54 years); and 79.9% and 75.4% (≥55 years). Evaluating the diagnostic value of triage by hospital destination (transport to Level I/II trauma centers) did not substantially improve these findings.

Conclusions.—The sensitivity of the Field Triage Decision Scheme for identifying major trauma patients is lower and specificity higher than previously described, particularly among elders.

▶ The American College of Surgeons, the Injury Control Center of the Centers for Disease Control and Prevention, the American College of Emergency Physicians, and nearly a dozen other professional organizations have worked together to develop a trauma triage and transport tool (Fig 1 in the original article) that could be used by all prehospital care providers and trauma systems in this country. This study examines decisions about field triage in routine civilian trauma care and should not be confused with the triage of mass casualties or the military definition of triage. In the settings discussed in this article, field triage refers only to the decisions made by prehospital personnel about the severity of injury and the likelihood of benefit in selectively bypassing closer hospitals in favor of trauma centers. The authors have evaluated more than 122 000 trauma patients for the accuracy of the triage tool, demonstrating that one-third met at least 1 of the criteria for a major trauma patient. However, only 5.8% of the total population proved to have an injury severity score (ISS) of 16 or greater. This is usually considered the best single indicator when a major trauma patient would benefit from care at a level 1 trauma center. The tool identified 6091 and missed 1009 of these patients. This resulted in a sensitivity of 80% to 89% and a specificity of 64% to 75%, depending on the age of the patient. The triage tool does not miss many severely injured patients, but it appears to overidentify the severely injured 26% to 35% of the time. The outcome of interest should be the ability of this tool to identify a major trauma patient who would benefit from trauma center care. This has been shown to be clearly true for patients with an ISS of 16 or greater, with greater survival benefit to the more severely injured, but it has not been well defined in the elderly, children, patients with an ISS of 9 to 15, or those with complex injury patterns.

D. W. Mozingo, MD

American College of Surgeons' Committee on Trauma Performance Improvement and Patient Safety Program: Maximal Impact in a Mature Trauma Center

Sarkar B, Brunsvold ME, Cherry-Bukoweic JR, et al (Univ Hosp, Ann Arbor)
J Trauma 71:1447-1454, 2011

Background.—To examine the impact of an ongoing comprehensive performance improvement and patient safety (PIPS) program implemented in 2005 on mortality outcomes for trauma patients at an established American College of Surgeons (ACS)-verified Level I Trauma Center.

Methods.—The primary outcome measure was in-hospital mortality. Age, Injury Severity Score (ISS), and intensive care unit admissions were used as stratifying variables to examine outcomes over a 5-year period (2004—2008). Institution mortality rates were compared with the National Trauma Data Bank mortality rates stratified by ISS score. Enhancements to our comprehensive PIPS program included revision of trauma activation criteria, development of standardized protocols for initial resuscitation, massive transfusion, avoidance of over-resuscitation, tourniquet use, pelvic fracture management, emphasis on timely angiographic and surgical inter-vention, prompt spine clearance, reduction in time to computed tomography imaging, reduced dwell time in emergency department, evidence-based traumatic brain injury management, and multidisciplinary efforts to reduce healthcare-associated infections.

Results.—In 2004 (baseline data), the in-hospital mortality rate for the most severely injured trauma patients (ISS >24) at our trauma center was 30%, consistent with the reported mortality rate from the National Trauma Data Bank for patients with this severity of injury. Over 5 years, our

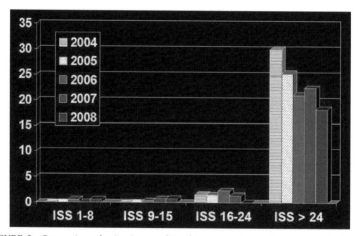

FIGURE 2.—Progressive reduction in mortality of trauma patients with ISS >24. (Reprinted from Sarkar B, Brunsvold ME, Cherry-Bukoweic JR, et al. American college of surgeons' committee on trauma performance improvement and patient safety program: maximal impact in a mature trauma center. *J Trauma.* 2011;71:1447-1454, with permission from Lippincott Williams & Wilkins.)

mortality rate decreased significantly for severely injured patients with an ISS >24, from 30.1% (2004) to 18.3% (2008), representing a 12% absolute reduction in mortality ($p = 0.011$). During the same 5-year time period, the proportion of elderly patients (age >65 years) cared for at our trauma center increased from 23.5% in 2004 to 30.6% in 2008 ($p = 0.0002$). Class I trauma activations increased significantly from 5.5% in 2004 to 15.5% in 2008 based on our reclassification. A greater percentage of patients were admitted to the intensive care unit (25.8% in 2004 to 37.3% in 2007 and 30.4% in 2008). No difference was identified in the rate of blunt (95%) or penetrating (5%) mechanism of injury in our patients over this time period. Trauma Quality Improvement Program confirmed improved trauma outcomes with observed-to-expected ratio and 95% confidence intervals of 0.64 (0.42–0.86) for all patients, 0.54 (0.15–0.91) for blunt single-system patients, and 0.78 (0.51–1.06) for blunt multisystem patients.

Conclusion.—Implementation of a multifaceted trauma PIPS program aimed at improving trauma care significantly reduced in-hospital mortality in a mature ACS Level I trauma center. Optimal care of the injured patient requires uncompromising commitment to PIPS (Fig 2).

▶ The authors of this selection reported a 12% absolute reduction in mortality for severely injured trauma patients after the implementation of a comprehensive process improvement and patient safety program at their level I trauma center (Fig 2). Optimal care of patients is feasible by targeting processes that contribute to preventable death, excess morbidity, and poor outcomes. This process requires ongoing reassessment and allocation of resources, as trauma care is by nature broad and varied to manage the diverse range of injuries encountered among varied patient populations. The authors have documented that implementation of a multifaceted trauma process improvement and patient safety program aimed at improving trauma care significantly reduced in-hospital mortality in a mature American College of Surgeons level I trauma center. This publication provides a solid framework for other trauma centers to improve patient outcomes through enhanced process improvement. The protocols critiqued in this process, such as massive transfusion, central venous access, fluid resuscitation, and radiologic screening, as well as others, are critical elements to ensure quality outcomes.

D. W. Mozingo, MD

An Acute Care Surgery Model Improves Timeliness of Care and Reduces Hospital Stay for Patients with Acute Cholecystitis

Lau B, DiFronzo LA (Kaiser Permanente Los Angeles Med Ctr, CA)
Am Surg 77:1318-1321, 2011

In October 2009, an acute care surgery (ACS) model was implemented to facilitate urgent surgical consults. This study examines the impact of ACS on the timeliness of care and length of hospitalization for patients with acute cholecystitis. A retrospective cohort study was performed of patients presenting to the emergency department (ED) with acute cholecystitis who underwent early cholecystectomy. Patients with choledocholithiasis, pancreatitis, biliary colic, or cholelithiasis without cholecystitis were excluded. There were two study cohorts: ACS (October 2009 to July 2010) and pre-ACS (October 2008 to September 2009). Primary outcome measures were length of stay (LOS) and time from the ED to the operating room (OR). One hundred fifty-two cases were identified: 71 in the ACS group and 81 in the pre-ACS group. Patient demographics were similar. The ACS group had a significantly shorter average time from the ED to the OR (24.6 vs 35.0 hours, P = 0.0276). Overall LOS was reduced by a mean of 14.7 hours in the ACS group (mean 3.23 vs 2.63 days, P = 0.11). There was no significant difference in OR time (2.45 vs 2.38 hours, P = 0.562). There was a significant decrease in after-hours cases in the ACS group (5.6 vs 21%, P = 0.004) and a decrease in complication rates (18.5 vs 7.0%, P = 0.032). In conclusion, the ACS model decreased time from the ED to the OR, decreased after-hours cases, decreased length of hospitalization, and decreased complications for patients with acute cholecystitis.

▶ The acute care surgery (ACS) model was initiated to combine trauma and urgent nontrauma general surgery because of a trend to reduce costs and maximize surgical resources. ACS has gained popularity in recent years; however, relatively few studies have evaluated the effects on patient care for emergency general surgery cases. In this article, the authors chose to evaluate the impact of the ACS model on outcomes of patients with acute cholecystitis, a common surgical problem.

In recent years, a number of studies have demonstrated not only the safety and efficacy but also the benefits of an early cholecystectomy on decreased length of stay and complication rates. By implementing the ACS model, there is potential to not only treat patients with acute cholecystitis with an early cholecystectomy but also to reduce health care costs and improve patient outcomes. Implementation of an ACS model significantly decreased time to overall recovery, decreased complications, and showed a trend toward a decrease in overall length of stay. The changes observed in resident involvement, namely those of increased junior resident participation, may have additional implications in this model regarding resident education and is worthy of further investigation.

D. W. Mozingo, MD

Comparison of Nonoperative Management With Renorrhaphy and Nephrectomy in Penetrating Renal Injuries
Bjurlin MA, Jeng EI, Goble SM, et al (Cook County Hosp, Chicago, IL; Univ of Illinois at Chicago, IL; American College of Surgeons, Chicago, IL; et al)
J Trauma 71:554-558, 2011

Background.—We reviewed our experience with penetrating renal injuries to compare nonoperative management of penetrating renal injuries with renorrhaphy and nephrectomy in light of concerns for unnecessary explorations and increased nephrectomy rates.

Methods.—In this retrospective study, we reviewed the records of 98 penetrating renal injuries from 2003 to 2008. Renal injuries were classified according to the American Association for the Surgery of Trauma and analyzed based on nephrectomy, renorrhaphy, and nonoperative management. Patient characteristics and outcomes measured were compared between management types. Continuous variables were summarized by means and compared using t test. Categorical variables were compared using χ^2 test.

Results.—Nonoperative management was performed in 40% of renal injuries, followed by renorrhaphy (38%) and nephrectomy (22%). Of renal gunshot wounds (n = 79), 26%, 42%, and 32% required nephrectomy, renorrhaphy, and were managed nonoperatively, respectively. No renal stab wound (n = 16) resulted in a nephrectomy and 81% were managed conservatively. Renal injuries managed nonoperatively had a lower incidence of transfusion (34 vs. 95%, $p < 0.001$), shorter mean intensive care unit (ICU) (3.0 vs. 9.0 days, $p = 0.028$) and mean hospital length of stay (7.9 vs. 18.1 days, $p = 0.006$), and lower mortality rate (0 vs. 20%, $p = 0.005$) compared with nephrectomy but similar to renorrhaphy (transfusion: 34 vs. 36%, $p = 0.864$; mean ICU: 3.0 vs. 2.8 days, $p = 0.931$; mean hospital length of stay: 7.9 vs. 11.2 days, $p = 0.197$; mortality: 0 vs. 6%, $p = 0.141$). The complication rate of nonoperative management was favorable compared with operative management.

Conclusions.—Selective nonoperative management of penetrating renal injuries resulted in a lower mortality rate, lower incidence of blood transfusion, and shorter mean ICU and hospital stay compared with patients managed by nephrectomy but similar to renorrhaphy. Complication rates were low and similar to operative management (Fig 1).

▶ Nonoperative management of select penetrating renal injuries continues to be an expanding field of investigation. In this study, the authors describe their

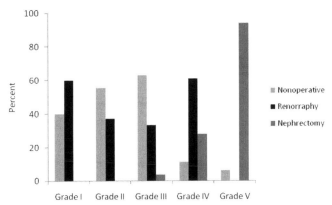

FIGURE 1.—Incidence of nonoperative management, renorrhaphy, and nephrectomy of penetrating renal injury grades I to V. (Reprinted from Bjurlin MA, Jeng EI, Goble SM, et al. Comparison of nonoperative management with renorrhaphy and nephrectomy in penetrating renal injuries. *J Trauma.* 2011;71:554-558.)

experience with the nonoperative management of penetrating renal injuries compared with renal injuries managed with nephrectomy and renorrhaphy. In their hands, nonoperative management was used successfully in 40% of all penetrating renal trauma patients, 81% of stabs wounds, and 32% of gunshot wounds (GSW). Fig 1 is included in this selection highlighting the differences in the selective management of these 2 injuries.

The authors defined nonoperative management as no active surgical intervention of a penetrating renal injury to control hemorrhage. This definition allowed patients who sustained an intraperitoneal injury to undergo an exploratory laparotomy when indicated, while the renal injury remained nonoperative. However, this may have also inflated the rate of renorrhaphy over nonoperative management because 60% of grade I renal GSWs were classified as renorrhaphy. Renal exploration and repair was performed in these 6 cases of grade I injuries because of already being in the abdomen for associated injuries. Although prior studies have demonstrated that operations on other intra-abdominal organs impart a higher risk of nephrectomy regardless of renal injury grade, no grade I or II and only 1 grade III injury resulted in nephrectomy.

D. W. Mozingo, MD

Early Vasopressor Use in Critical Injury Is Associated With Mortality Independent From Volume Status
Plurad DS, Talving P, Lam L, et al (LAC + USC Dept of Surgery)
J Trauma 71:565-572, 2011

Background.—Complications of excessive crystalloid after critical injury have increased interest in vasopressor support. However, it is hypothesized that vasopressor use in patients who are under-resuscitated is associated with death. We performed this study to determine whether volume status is associated with increased mortality in the critically injured exposed to early vasopressors.

Methods.—The intensive care unit database at a Level I center was queried for all adult admissions surviving for >24 hours from January 1, 2001, to December 31, 2008. Patients with spinal cord injury and severe traumatic brain injury were excluded. The vasopressor group [Vaso (+)] was exposed to dopamine, epinephrine, phenylephrine, norepinephrine, or arginine vasopressin within 24 hours of admission. Demographic and injury data were studied including intensive care unit admission central venous pressure. Hypovolemia [Hypov (+)] was considered an admission central venous pressure ≤ 8 mm Hg. The Vaso (+) group was analyzed to determine whether Hypov (+) was independently associated with death.

Results.—Of 1,349 eligible patients, 26% (351) were Vaso (+). Mortality was 43.6% (153) in the Vaso (+) versus 4.2% (42) in the Vaso (−) group (17.60 [12.10−25.60], <0.01). Vasopressor exposure was associated with death independent of injury severity. In Vaso (+) patients, Hypov (+) was not associated with mortality, whereas Emergency Department admission Glasgow Coma Scale ≤ 8 and multiple vasopressor use were.

TABLE 4.—Variables Independently Associated With Death in Population Overall

Variable	OR, 95% CI	p
Vasopressor use	11.51 (7.76−17.09)	<0.01
GCS ≤8	4.10 (2.74−6.12)	<0.01
ISS ≥35	2.71 (1.74−4.22)	<0.01
Age ≥55 yr	2.30 (1.51−3.51)	<0.01

Other variables entered: Gender, mechanism (blunt), chest AIS >3, ED and ICU admission hypotension (SBP <90 mm Hg), BMI >30 kg/m², Hypov (+), ICU admit CPK >5 k.

Conclusions.—Vasopressor exposure early after critical injury is independently associated with death and mortality is increased regardless of fluid status. Although it is not advisable to withhold support with impending cardiovascular collapse, use of any vasopressor during ongoing resuscitation should be approached with extreme caution regardless of volume status (Table 4).

▶ Excessive crystalloid administration to the critically injured trauma patient causes pulmonary dysfunction, abdominal and extremity compartment syndromes, coagulopathy, and increased mortality. Although the concept of temporary use of vasoconstrictor agents following trauma is old, there has been renewed interest in volume-sparing resuscitation strategies in hemorrhagic shock. This clinical evidence shows an independent association between vasopressor exposure and mortality and is included as Table 4. It is difficult to determine whether vasopressor use is truly detrimental to outcomes after hemorrhagic shock or if it is simply a marker for increased physiologic injury. Acute cardiovascular support in hemorrhagic shock remains controversial. Critics view the practice as a simplistic, overly used, and potentially harmful solution having no good evidence-based guidelines for its initiation or endpoints. However, it is suggested that a subpopulation of patients who have adequate filling pressures may glean a relative benefit from vasopressors. The authors performed this study to examine the pattern of use of these agents in a cohort of critically injured and determine the effect of volume status on mortality in patients who were exposed to vasopressors early in their course of illness. This study found a similar risk of mortality in critically injured patients who required early vasopressors regardless of indicators of resuscitation. Further prospective studies are needed to determine whether the theoretical benefits of vasopressor support in hemorrhagic shock can be substantiated and evidence-based strategies can be developed.

D. W. Mozingo, MD

Eliminating Preventable Death on the Battlefield

Kotwal RS, Montgomery HR, Kotwal BM, et al (US Army Special Operations Command, Fort Bragg, NC; et al)
Arch Surg 146:1350-1358, 2011

Objective.—To evaluate battlefield survival in a novel command-directed casualty response system that comprehensively integrates Tactical Combat Casualty Care guidelines and a prehospital trauma registry.

Design.—Analysis of battle injury data collected during combat deployments.

Setting.—Afghanistan and Iraq from October 1, 2001, through March 31, 2010.

Patients.—Casualties from the 75th Ranger Regiment, US Army Special Operations Command.

Main Outcome Measures.—Casualties were scrutinized for preventable adverse outcomes and opportunities to improve care. Comparisons were made with Department of Defense casualty data for the military as a whole.

Results.—A total of 419 battle injury casualties were incurred during 7 years of continuous combat in Iraq and 8.5 years in Afghanistan. Despite higher casualty severity indicated by return-to-duty rates, the regiment's rates of 10.7% killed in action and 1.7% who died of wounds were lower than the Department of Defense rates of 16.4% and 5.8%, respectively, for the larger US military population ($P = .04$ and $P = .02$, respectively). Of 32 fatalities incurred by the regiment, none died of wounds from infection, none were potentially survivable through additional prehospital medical intervention, and 1 was potentially survivable in the hospital setting. Substantial prehospital care was provided by nonmedical personnel.

Conclusions.—A command-directed casualty response system that trains all personnel in Tactical Combat Casualty Care and receives continuous feedback from prehospital trauma registry data facilitated Tactical Combat Casualty Care performance improvements centered on clinical outcomes that resulted in unprecedented reduction of killed-in-action deaths, casualties who died of wounds, and preventable combat death. This data-driven approach is the model for improving prehospital trauma care and casualty outcomes on the battlefield and has considerable implications for civilian trauma systems.

▶ The authors of this study are to be commended for documenting the ability of focused process improvement to increase combat casualty care to the highest level of achievement. The deficiencies of civilian Advanced Trauma Life Support training were noted and addressed quickly. In 1996, the Tactical Combat Casualty Care guidelines were published. They took into account issues unique to battle, such as the prevention of additional casualties, mission completion, and the tactical challenges of evacuations under fire, and focused medically on the 3 major causes of preventable death: hemorrhage from extremity wounds, tension pneumothorax, and airway compromise. The Special Operations units implemented them quickly. The next intervention was the inclusion of medical training as one of the Big Four priorities for every member of the 75th Ranger Regiment. Among the Rangers, all were trained as first responders, 10% as emergency medical technicians, and 3% as combat medics. Thus, every member of the regiment was responsible for casualty care of his or her fellow soldiers, and battle commanders also had medical knowledge and training that could be taken into consideration when making tactical decisions. This is different from the majority of the Armed Forces in which only the medics are relied on for initial casualty care. The Rangers developed a robust prehospital registry to be able to track events and improve processes. The outstanding survival rates attained by using this system are truly remarkable.

D. W. Mozingo, MD

Impact of Interhospital Transfer on Outcomes for Trauma Patients: A Systematic Review

Hill AD, Fowler RA, Nathens AB (Univ of Toronto, Ontario, Canada)
J Trauma 71:1885-1901, 2011

Background.—Evidence suggests that there may be an association between transfer status (direct admission or interhospital transfer) and outcomes in trauma patients. The purpose of this study was to systematically review the current evidence of the association between transfer status and outcomes for patients.

Methods.—Systematic search of Medline and EMBASE databases to identify eligible control trials or observational studies that examined the impact of transfer status on trauma patient outcomes. Data were extracted on study design, quality, participants, outcomes, and risk estimates reported. Pooled odds ratio based on data from retrieved studies was calculated using a random effect model.

Results.—Thirty-six observational studies were identified. There were no significant differences in length of stay (LOS) between transfer and direct admissions although costs were marginally higher for transferred patients, (relative increase, 1.09; 95% confidence interval, 1.08−1.09). We found no significant association between transfer status (transfer vs. direct) and in-hospital mortality (pooled odds ratio, 1.06; 95% confidence interval, 0.90−1.25); however, heterogeneity of the studies was high ($I^2 = 82\%$).

Conclusion.—Available evidence suggests there is no difference in mortality between transfer and direct admissions. However, the significant heterogeneity across studies precludes deriving any definitive conclusions regarding the impact of interhospital transfer on mortality after major trauma. Moreover, most studies excluded patients dying at outlying hospitals, which may underestimate the association of transfer status with mortality. Prospective studies that address the limitations of the current evidence, including use of population-based trauma registries, are warranted to establish whether the process of interhospital transfer to higher level care when compared with direct admission to a trauma center negatively impacts clinical outcomes for trauma patients.

▶ The centralization of specialized trauma resources within a few dedicated hospitals has consequences regarding the initial triage and transport of trauma patients. Importantly, some critically injured patients are initially triaged to and receive care at outlying hospitals before transfer to a higher-level hospital for definitive care. The initial transfer of these patients to more proximal hospitals increases the time to definitive care. This is particularly true for patients in rural settings who are not close to centers resourced to manage their care needs. The impact of the delay in receiving definitive care may have significant implications for patient outcomes. This is consistent with evidence from other critically ill patient populations that suggests transfer patients have higher mortality and longer lengths of stay than direct admissions. There is little debate regarding the necessity of interfacility transfer, particularly when faced with challenges of geography. The authors of this selection review the Medline and EMBASE databases and identified 36 studies on this topic in the literature. They were unable to show a definitive difference between length of stay or in-hospital survival in direct admit versus transfer patients, although transfer patients had slightly higher hospital costs. This type of analysis is confounded by being unable to analyze the population of trauma patients managed at non-trauma center hospitals. Such an analysis would include not only those transferred to a higher-level facility but also those who were admitted locally or died during their initial attempts at resuscitation. This needs to be a geographically based population study.

D. W. Mozingo, MD

Impact of preinjury warfarin and antiplatelet agents on outcomes of trauma patients

Bonville DJ, Ata A, Jahraus CB, et al (Albany Med College, NY)

Surgery 150:861-868, 2011

Background.—Warfarin and antiplatelet agents (WAA) are prevalent among trauma patients, but the impact of these agents on patient outcomes has not been clearly defined. In this study, we examined the impact of pre-injury WAA on outcomes in trauma patients.

Methods.—A 40-month (September 2004 to December 2007) retrospective review of data in the trauma registry at a New York State level 1 trauma center was performed. Patients on WAA were compared to those not on these medications. The primary outcome of interest was mortality, and the secondary outcomes of interest were as length of stay (LOS) and disposition on discharge. A separate analysis was done for patients with intracranial hemorrhage (ICH). The chi-square test, the Student t test, and the modified Poisson regression analysis were used to estimate the incident risk ratios for the outcomes.

TABLE 2.—Comparison of the Effect of Preinjury Warfarin and Antiplatelet Agents (WAA) Combinations on the Risk of Mortality*

	% Died	Unadjusted Risk Ratio	Adjusted Risk Ratio
None	6.2		
Any WAA	13.6	2.2 (1.7, 2.9)[†]	1.4 (0.8, 2.3)
Warfarin	24.1	3.9 (2.5, 6.1)[†]	3.2 (1.6, 6.6)[‡]
Aspirin only	12.3	2.0 (1.3, 3.0)[‡]	1.7 (0.8, 3.3)
Clopidogrel only	9.3	1.5 (0.6, 4.1)	
Aspirin + clopidogrel only	9.7	1.6 (0.7, 3.5)	
Warfarin + aspirin only	5.0	0.8 (0.1, 5.8)	

*The reference category is patients with no WAA.
[†]$P < .001$.
[‡]$P < .01$.

TABLE 3.—Comparison of Secondary Outcomes (Means and Proportions) by the Use of Preinjury Warfarin and Antiplatelet Agents (WAA) Medications

Outcome	Any WAA (%)	Warfarin Only (%)	None (%)	P Value*	P Value[†]
Mortality					
Patients with ICH	15.4	28.9	5.8	<.001	<.001
Patients without ICH	11.8	18.0	6.3	<.01	<.01
Intracranial hemorrhage	49.8	57.1	30.5	<.001	<.001
LOS >10, d	29.4	28.6	23.3	<.01	NS
ICU stay, d	8.1 (0.7)	9.8 (1.7)	6.9 (0.3)	NS	NS
Discharge to home	48.2	42.0	74.4	<.001	<.001

ICH, Intracranial hemorrhage; *LOS*, length of stay; *ICU*, intensive care unit.
*Any WAA vs none.
[†]Warfarin vs none.

Results.—A total of 3,436 trauma patients were identified, of whom 456 were taking anticoagulants (warfarin, $n = 91$ patients; aspirin, $n = 228$; clopidogrel, $n = 43$; and various combinations, $n = 94$). Patients on warfarin were 3.1 times more likely to die (relative risk [RR], 3.2; 95% confidence interval [CI], 1.6—6.6), after adjusting for potential confounders. Aspirin and clopidogrel were not associated with increased mortality, but WAA were associated with increased risk of ICH (49.8% vs 30.5%; RR, −1.6; 95% CI, 1.4—1.9). WAA did not affect LOS or disposition. Among patients with ICH, only warfarin increased mortality (28.9% vs 5.8%; RR, −3.1; 95% CI, 1.3—7.2).

Conclusion.—Preinjury warfarin treatment was found to be an independent risk factor for mortality. WAA agents increased risk of ICH. Among those patients with ICH, only warfarin was associated with increased mortality. Antiplatelet agents did not affect mortality or LOS (Tables 2 and 3).

▶ The percentage of Americans on warfarin and other antiplatelet agents continues to increase with the trend toward longer life expectancies and the increased numbers of baby boomers advancing in age. The authors of this selection have identified markedly worse outcomes in those patients taking warfarin, but not in antiplatelet agents as shown in Tables 2 and 3, included in this selection. Whether warfarin plays a mechanistic role in adverse outcomes or merely acts as a marker for significant comorbidities that lead to worse outcomes remains controversial. Possible mechanisms of the association between preinjury warfarin therapy and increased mortality include exsanguinations or more severe injury patterns due to coagulopathy, complications secondary to blood product transfusions, and complications related to more sever intracranial hemorrhage. Early use of fresh frozen plasma, prothrombin complex concentrates, or even recombinant factor VIIa may be warranted in selected patients within this population. The use of rapid thromboelastography and aggressive management protocols in controlled studies could help determine the optimal approach to these patients.

D. W. Mozingo, MD

Interhospital Transfers of Acute Care Surgery Patients: Should Care for Nontraumatic Surgical Emergencies be Regionalized?
Santry HP, Janjua S, Chang Y, et al (Univ of Massachusetts—UMass Memorial Med Ctr, Worcester; St Elizabeth's Med Ctr, Brighton, MA; Massachusetts General Hosp, Boston)
World J Surg 35:2660-2667, 2011

Background.—Patients with major nontraumatic surgical emergencies (NTSEs) are commonly transferred from small hospitals to tertiary care centers. We hypothesized that transferred patients (TRANS) have worse outcomes than patients with similar diagnoses admitted directly to a tertiary center (DIRECT).

Methods.—We reviewed all patients admitted to the acute care surgery service of our tertiary center (September 1, 2006—October 31, 2009) with one of eight diagnoses indicating a major NTSE. Patients transferred for reasons other than the severity of illness were excluded. Univariate and multivariable analyses compared TRANS and DIRECT patients.

Results.—Of 319 patients eligible for analysis, 103 (34%) were TRANS and averaged 3.8 days in the referring hospital before transfer. Compared to DIRECT patients, TRANS patients were more likely to be obese (18.5 vs. 8.0%, $P = 0.006$) and have cardiac (24 vs. 14%, $P = 0.022$) or pulmonary (25 vs. 12%, $P = 0.003$) co-morbidities. TRANS patients were also more likely to present to the tertiary center with hypotension (9 vs. 2%, $P = 0.021$), tachycardia (20 vs. 13%, $P = 0.036$), anemia (83 vs. 58%, $P < 0.001$), and hypoalbuminemia (50 vs. 14%, $P < 0.001$). TRANS patients had higher mortality (4.9 vs. 0.9%, $P = 0.038$) and longer hospital stay (8 with 5—13 days vs. 5 with 3—8 days, $P < 0.001$).

Conclusions.—TRANS patients comprised a significant portion of the population with major NTSEs admitted to the acute care surgery service of our tertiary center. They presented with greater physiologic derangement and had worse outcomes than DIRECT patients. As is currently

TABLE 1.—Complex Nontraumatic Surgical Emergency Patients Admitted to a Tertiary Care Hospital's Acute Care Surgery Service

Diagnosis	DIRECT Patients[a] (n = 216)	TRANSFER Patients[b] (n = 103)	ICD-9 Code
Pancreatitis and its complications	29 (13.4%)	22 (21.4%)	577.0–577.9
Cholangitis	3 (1.4%)	2 (1.9%)	576.1
Bowel obstruction including intussusception and volvulus)*	116 (53.7%)	34 (33.1%)	560.0–560.9, 552.0–552.9
Necrotizing fasciitis*	4 (1.9%)	18 (17.5%)	728.86, 785.4
Perforated viscus, peritonitis, and intraperitoneal abscess	15 (6.9%)	11 (10.7%)	569.83, 531.1, 532.6, 567.22, 540.1, 569.5
Ischemic colitis/enteritis*	2 (0.9%)	6 (5.8%)	557.0, 557.1, 557.9
Perforated diverticulitis*	46 (21.3%)	10 (9.7%)	562.11, 562.13, 562.12
Clostridium difficile colitis	1 (0.5%)	0	008.45

ICD-9 International Classification of Diseases, 9th revision.
[a]Patients admitted directly to the tertiary care hospital via the emergency department.
[b]Patients transferred to the tertiary care hospital from outlying community hospitals.
*χ^2 test: $P < 0.001$ between groups.

established for trauma care, regionalization of care for NTSEs should be considered (Table 1).

▶ This selection was chosen because many trauma centers currently incorporate emergency general surgery into their practice as part of an acute care surgery (ACS) program. The authors suggest eight diagnoses that, when coupled with significant comorbidities and physiologic derangement, may be appropriate as an initial dialogue regarding regionalization of care for patients with nontraumatic surgical emergencies. This list is included as Table 1. This study indicates that a significant portion of complex surgical emergency admissions to a tertiary care facility's ACS team consists of transfers from referring hospitals. These patients differ from patients with similar diagnoses admitted directly to the tertiary care facility and deserve focus and analysis. Transfer patients have worse outcomes than directly admitted patients, which is a cause for alarm. These outcomes may very well result from delays in transfer, inadequate initial care, or simply more serious disease. It is likely that a delay of nearly 4 days before transfer to definitive care has caused harm to these patients. These findings speak strongly for a critical evaluation of this issue.

D. W. Mozingo, MD

Lactate in Trauma: A Poor Predictor of Mortality in the Setting of Alcohol Ingestion
Herbert HK, Dechert TA, Wolfe L, et al (Virginia Commonwealth Univ, Richmond; Hosp of the Univ of Pennsylvania, Philadelphia)
Am Surg 77:1576-1579, 2011

Resuscitation end point markers such as lactate and base deficit (BD) are used in trauma to identify and treat a state of compensated shock. Lactate and BD levels are also elevated by alcohol. In blunt trauma patients with positive blood alcohol levels, lactate may be a poor indicator of injury. Retrospective data were collected on 1083 blunt trauma patients with positive blood alcohol levels admitted a Level I trauma center between 2003 and 2006. Patients were stratified by Injury Severity Score, age, gender, and Glasgow Coma Score. Logistic regression analyses were used to assess lactate and BD as independent risk factors for mortality. Seventy-four per cent of patients had an abnormal lactate level compared with 28 per cent with abnormal BD levels. In patients with mild injury, lactate levels were abnormal in more than 70 per cent of patients compared with less than 20 per cent of patients with abnormal BD levels. Linear regression showed lactate is not a significant predictor of mortality. Regardless of Injury Severity Score, lactate appeared to be more often abnormal than BD in the setting of alcohol ingestion. Additionally, because BD, and not lactate, was shown to be an independent predictor of mortality, lactate may not be a reliable marker of end point resuscitation in this patient population (Fig 3, Table 1).

▶ Markers used for the endpoint of resuscitation, such as lactate and base deficit, are used in trauma to identify and guide treatment of shock. During systemic hypoperfusion, the imbalance of tissue oxygen delivery causes anaerobic cellular metabolism followed by subsequent mitochondrial dysfunction and glycolysis. This process produces lactic acid quantified by elevated lactate and base deficit levels. Clinically, base deficit and lactate levels have been found

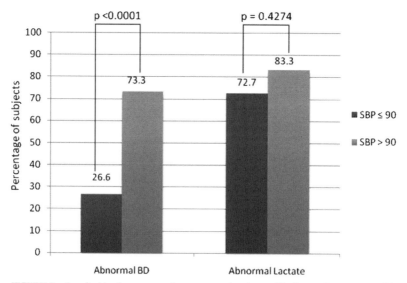

FIGURE 3.—Systolic blood pressure and percentage of patients with abnormal versus normal base deficit and lactate. (Reprinted from Herbert HK, Dechert TA, Wolfe L, et al. Lactate in trauma: a poor predictor of mortality in the setting of alcohol ingestion. *Am Surg*. 2011;77:1576-1579. © Southeastern Surgical Congress.)

TABLE 1.—Logistic Regression for Mortality

Effect	Odds Ratio	95% Confidence Limit		P
Base deficit	0.769	0.680	0.858	0.0002
Age	1.052	1.018	1.087	0.0013
Injury Severity Score	1.125	1.018	1.087	<0.0001
Lactate	0.978	0.758	1.261	0.7849

to correlate well with length of intensive care unit stay, transfusion requirements, injury severity, and mortality. Lactic acidosis also occurs following the consumption of alcohol as it is oxidized to form acetaldehyde. Through this metabolism, NAD is reduced to NADH, allowing the reduction of pyruvate to lactate, thereby inducing lactic acidosis.

In this selection, the authors have identified a number of patients who had relatively minor injuries, alcohol ingestion, and significantly elevated initial lactate levels. They sought to determine if using lactate was appropriate or if an alternative marker such as base deficit should guide initial resuscitation. No previously published studies have compared the accuracy of lactate with base deficit levels in the setting of alcohol ingestion. Fig 3 and Table 1 are included to demonstrate the lack of correlation between initial serum lactate and base deficit and the poor correlation of lactate with mortality.

D. W. Mozingo, MD

Management of Gunshot Pelvic Fractures With Bowel Injury: Is Fracture Debridement Necessary?

Rehman S, Slemenda C, Kestner C, et al (Temple Univ Hosp, Philadelphia, PA)
J Trauma 71:577-581, 2011

Background.—Low-velocity pelvic gunshot injuries occur commonly in urban trauma centers, occasionally involving concomitant intestinal viscus injury leading to potential fracture site contamination. Surgical debridement of the fractures may be necessary to prevent osteomyelitis, although not routinely performed in many centers. The purpose of this study was to determine whether fracture debridement should be done to prevent osteomyelitis in these injuries.

Methods.—A 5-year retrospective review of all patients older than 12 years with low-velocity gunshot pelvic fractures was performed at an urban Level I trauma center. Medical records and radiographs/computed tomographic scans were reviewed, and data regarding fracture location, concomitant intestinal viscus injury, orthopedic surgical intervention, antibiotic treatment, and bone and/or joint infection were recorded.

Results.—Of a total of 103 patients identified, 19 had expired within 48 hours and were excluded, resulting in a total of 84 study subjects for review. Fifty of 84 patients (59%) had a perforated viscus with 31 large bowel injuries and 30 small bowel injuries. Eighteen patients (21%) had intra-articular fractures, 15 of which involved the hip joint. Orthopedic surgical fracture debridement was done only in intra-articular fractures with retained bullet fragments (seven cases). Deep infection occurred in one patient with a missile injury to the hip joint with concomitant intestinal spillage. Immediate joint debridement was performed in this case, but successful missile fragment removal was not achieved until the second debridement after 48 hours. No infections occurred in any extra-articular fractures, regardless of the presence of intestinal spillage.

Conclusions.—Extra-articular gunshot pelvic fractures do not require formal orthopedic fracture debridement even in cases with concomitant intestinal viscus injury. However, debridement with bullet removal should be done in cases with intra-articular involvement, particularly if there are retained bullet fragments in the joint, to prevent deep infection.

▶ Some controversy still exists regarding the need of bone debridement when pelvic low-velocity gunshot wounds are potentially contaminated by concomitant bowel injury and spillage of intestinal contents. The results of this study suggest that orthopedic debridement of extra-articular pelvic fractures resulting from low-velocity gunshot injuries is not required, even in cases with extra luminal intestinal spillage. Exploratory laparotomy with intestinal repair and washout by the trauma surgeon and antibiotic treatment is a sufficient treatment; however, retained intra-articular hip joint bullet fragments do increase the risk of infection, as has been suggested in other studies. Arthrotomy of the affected joint and debridement should be performed in these cases.

D. W. Mozingo, MD

Relationship Between Leapfrog Safe Practices Survey and Outcomes in Trauma

Glance LG, Dick AW, Osler TM, et al (Univ of Rochester School of Medicine, NY; RAND Health, Pittsburgh, PA; Univ of Vermont Med College, Burlington; et al)
Arch Surg 146:1170-1177, 2011

Objective.—To examine the association between hospital self-reported compliance with the National Quality Forum patient safety practices and trauma outcomes in a nationally representative sample of level I and level II trauma centers.

Design.—Retrospective cohort study using the Nationwide Inpatient Sample.

Setting.—Level I and level II trauma centers.

Patients.—Trauma patients.

Main Outcome Measures.—Multivariate logistic regression models were estimated to examine the association between clinical outcomes (in-hospital mortality and hospital-associated infections) and the National Quality

Forum patient safety practices. We controlled for patient demographic characteristics, injury severity, mechanism of injury, comorbidities, and hospital characteristics.

Results.—The total score on the Leapfrog Safe Practices Survey was not associated with either mortality (adjusted odds ratio [aOR], 0.92; 95% confidence interval [CI], 0.79-1.06) or hospital-associated infections (1.03; 0.82-1.29). Full implementation of computerized physician order entry was not associated with reduced mortality (aOR, 1.03; 95% CI, 0.75-1.42) or with a lower risk of hospital-associated infections (0.94; 0.57-1.56). Full implementation of intensive care unit physician staffing was also not predictive of mortality (aOR, 1.13; 95% CI, 0.90-1.28) or of hospital-associated infections (1.04; 0.76-1.42).

Conclusion.—In this nationally representative sample of level I and level II trauma centers, we were unable to detect evidence that hospitals reporting better compliance with the National Quality Forum patient safety practices had lower mortality or a lower incidence of hospital-associated infections.

▶ The authors of this selection were unable to demonstrate that trauma outcomes were improved in hospitals with better self-reported performance on the Leapfrog Hospital Survey. These findings do not, however, confer that adherence to the National Quality Forum (NQF) patient safety practices does not result in improved outcomes. It is possible that self-reported measures of hospital-wide adherence with the NQF safety practices may not reliably capture actual clinical practice in differing clinical settings. The authors suggest adding those NQF patient safety practices considered most relevant to trauma outcomes to the American College of Surgeons Committee on Trauma Verification Program. They also suggested that some of the process measures based on patient safety practices could become part of the required data collection in the American College of Surgeons Trauma Quality Improvement Program that was recently created to benchmark trauma care. In this way, actual compliance with the NQF patient safety practices could be measured more accurately. Using these data, a core group of safety best practices might be identified.

D. W. Mozingo, MD

The Development of a Urinary Tract Infection Is Associated With Increased Mortality in Trauma Patients

Monaghan SF, Heffernan DS, Thakkar RK, et al (Rhode Island Hosp, Providence)
J Trauma 71:1569-1574, 2011

Background.—In October 2008, Medicare and Medicaid stopped paying for care associated with catheter-related urinary tract infections (UTIs). Although most clinicians agree UTIs are detrimental, there are little data to support this belief.

Methods.—This is a retrospective review of trauma registry data from a Level I trauma center between 2003 and 2008. Two proportional hazards regressions were used for analyses. The first predicted acquisition of UTI as a function of indwelling urinary catheter use, adjusting for age, diabetes, gender, and injury severity. The second predicted hospital mortality as a function of UTI, covarying for age, gender, chronic obstructive pulmonary disease, congestive heart failure, hypertension, diabetes, pneumonia, and injury severity.

Results.—After excluding patients who stayed in the hospital <3 days and those with a UTI on arrival, 5,736 patients were included in the study. Of these patients, 680 (11.9%) met criteria for a UTI, with 487 (71.6%) indwelling urinary catheter-related infections. Predictors of UTI included the interaction between age and gender ($p = 0.0018$), Injury Severity Score ($p = 0.0021$), and indwelling urinary catheter use ($p < 0.001$). The development of a UTI predicted the risk of in-hospital death as a patient's age increased ($p = 0.002$). Similar results were seen when only catheter-associated UTIs are included in the analysis.

Conclusions.—Indwelling urinary catheter use is connected to the development of UTIs, and these infections are associated with a greater mortality as the age of a trauma patients increases (Table 6).

▶ Urinary tract infections are the most common nosocomial infection, and most are believed to be related to indwelling urinary catheters. Much work has been done on the prevention and treatment of catheter-related urinary tract infections, but little is known about the impact of a catheter-related urinary tract infection on outcomes of hospitalized patients. Surgical patients, especially trauma patients, are particularly prone to catheter-related urinary tract infections. The authors of this article conducted a retrospective review of all trauma patients over a 5-year period and evaluated factors that predicted urinary tract infection and whether the development of a urinary tract infection had a significant impact on morbidity or mortality. Table 6 is included that demonstrates the effect of age and urinary

TABLE 6.—Factors to Predict In-Hospital Mortality (CA-UTI Patients)

Parameter	$p > \chi^2$	HR
Age (yr)	<0.001	
Female	0.6469	0.936
CA-UTI	0.0447	
Age and CA-UTI interaction	0.0062	
Chronic obstructive pulmonary disease	0.5673	1.160
Congestive heart failure	0.0085	1.725
Hypertension	0.0303	0.723
Diabetes mellitus	0.5249	0.878
Pneumonia	0.4986	0.866
ISS	<0.001	1.045

Results from proportional hazard regression model to predict hospital mortality. Items included in the analysis are CA-UTI, age, gender, chronic obstructive pulmonary disease, congestive heart failure, hypertension, diabetes mellitus, pneumonia, ISS, and the interaction between age and CA-UTI. Other interactions between variables were tested and only included if found to be significant.

tract infection on mortality in this study. Despite the new push to minimize the usage of urinary catheters, there will always be a need for them in certain hospitalized patients. Trauma patients who develop a urinary tract infection may have more dramatic immunologic derangements following trauma, and this immune dysfunction may lead to the observed increased association with mortality. The authors also demonstrate that the risk of development of a urinary tract infection independently correlates with the degree of injury severity. In this case, any decision to deny payment for the secondary diagnosis of catheter-related urinary tract infection in trauma patients should be reconsidered.

D. W. Mozingo, MD

Timing is Everything: Delayed Intubation is Associated with Increased Mortality in Initially Stable Trauma Patients
Miraflor E, Chuang K, Miranda MA, et al (UCSF-East Bay)
J Surg Res 170:286-290, 2011

Background.—The indications for immediate intubation in trauma are not controversial, but some patients who initially appear stable later deteriorate and require intubation. We postulated that initially stable, moderately injured trauma patients who experienced delayed intubation have higher mortality than those intubated earlier.

Methods.—Medical records of trauma patients intubated within 3 h of arrival in the emergency department at our university-based trauma center were reviewed. Moderately injured patients were defined as an ISS < 20. Early intubation was defined as patients intubated from 10–24 min of arrival. Delayed intubation was defined as patients intubated ≥25 min after arrival. Patients requiring immediate intubation, within 10 min of arrival, were excluded.

Results.—From February 2006 to December 2007, 279 trauma patients were intubated in the emergency department. In moderately injured patients, mortality was higher with delayed intubation than with early intubation, 11.8% *versus* 1.8% ($P = 0.045$). Patients with delayed intubations had greater frequency of rib fractures than their early intubation counterparts, 23.5% *versus* 3.6% ($P = 0.004$). Patients in the delayed intubation group had lower rates of cervical gunshot wounds than the early intubation group, 0% *versus* 10.7% ($P = 0.048$) and a trend toward fewer of skull fractures 2.9% *versus* 16.1%, ($P = 0.054$).

Conclusions.—These findings suggest that delayed intubation is associated with increased mortality in moderately injured patients who are initially stable but later require intubation and can be predicted by the presence of rib fractures (Figs 2 and 3).

▶ The indications for immediate endotracheal intubation of severely injured patients are well accepted. However, in a stable patient with moderate injury severity, the decision to intubate can be challenging. The authors of this article

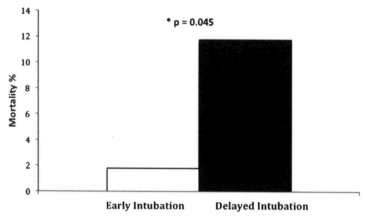

FIGURE 2.—Mortality in moderately injured patients by timing of intubation. Moderately injured patients (ISS < 20) intubated late had a higher mortality, 11.8%, than those intubated early, 1.8% ($P = 0.045$). The mortality risk reduction with earlier intubation was 85%. (Reprinted from The Journal of Surgical Research, Miraflor E, Chuang K, Miranda MA, et al. Timing is everything: delayed intubation is associated with increased mortality in initially stable trauma patients. *J Surg Res.* 2011;170:286-290. © 2011, with permission from Elsevier.)

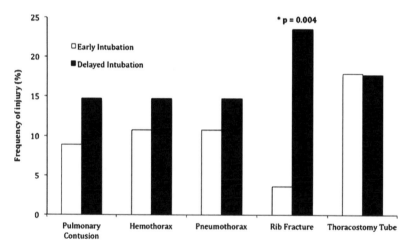

FIGURE 3.—Frequency of pulmonary contusion, hemothorax, pneumothorax, rib fracture, and thoracostomy tube by timing of intubation in moderately injured patients (ISS < 20). Patients in the delayed intubation group had a greater frequency of rib fractures, 23.5% *versus* 3.6%, ($P = 0.004$). (Reprinted from The Journal of Surgical Research, Miraflor E, Chuang K, Miranda MA, et al. Timing is everything: delayed intubation is associated with increased mortality in initially stable trauma patients. *J Surg Res.* 2011;170:286-290. © 2011, with permission from Elsevier.)

sought to determine whether the timing of intubation of initially stable, moderately injured trauma patients affected mortality. For moderately injured patients (ISS < 20), mortality was higher for patients whose intubation was delayed compared with those who were intubated earlier (11.8% vs 1.8%). The observed reduction in overall mortality was 10%, and the relative risk reduction was 85%. Figs 2 and 3 from this article demonstrate the severity of chest injury in this population, as well as the marked difference in mortality in the delayed intubation group. The presence of rib fractures may help clinicians predict delayed respiratory failure in the moderately injured patient. When faced with moderately injured patients who have sustained thoracic trauma resulting in multiple rib fractures, the clinician should consider earlier intubation, particularly in the elderly.

D. W. Mozingo, MD

Traumatic Injury of the Colon and Rectum: The Evidence vs Dogma
Steele SR, Maykel JA, Johnson EK (Madigan Army Med Ctr, Ft Lewis, WA; Univ of Massachusetts Med School, Worcester; Eisenhower Army Med Ctr, Ft. Gordon, GA)
Dis Colon Rectum 54:1184-1201, 2011

Background.—The treatment of traumatic injuries to the colon and rectum is often driven by dogma despite the presence of evidence suggesting alternative methods of care.

Objective.—This is an evidence-based review in the format of a review article to determine the ideal treatment of noniatrogenic traumatic injuries to the colon and rectum to improve the care provided to this group of patients. Recommendations and treatment algorithms were based on consensus conclusions of the data.

Data Sources.—A search of MEDLINE PubMed and the Cochrane Database of Collected Reviews was performed from 1965 through December 2010.

Study Selection.—Authors independently reviewed selected abstracts to determine their scientific merit and relevance based on key-word combinations regarding colorectal trauma. A directed search of the embedded references from the primary articles was also performed in select circumstances. We then performed a complete evaluation of 108 articles and 3 additional abstracts.

Main Outcome Measures.—The main outcomes were morbidity mortality and colostomy rates.

Results.—Evidence-based recommendations and algorithms are presented for the management of traumatic colorectal injuries.

Limitations.—Level I and II evidence was limited.

Conclusions.—Colorectal injuries remain a challenging clinical entity associated with significant morbidity. Familiarity with the different methods to approach and manage these injuries including "damage control" tactics when necessary will allow surgeons to minimize unnecessary complications and mortality (Fig 1).

▶ The authors of this selection are to be commended for their exhaustive review of the literature and forcing evidence-based assimilation of colorectal injuries

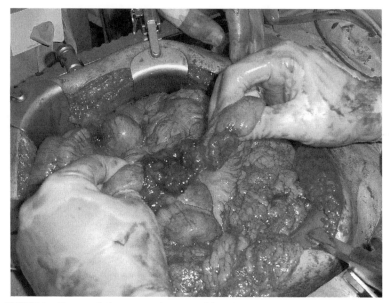

FIGURE 1.—Photograph depicting an obvious small-bowel injury with an injury to the medial wall of the cecum and ileocolic artery secondary to cavitation from a high-velocity projectile. (Reprinted from Steele SR, Maykel JA, Johnson EK. Traumatic injury of the colon and rectum: the evidence vs dogma. *Dis Colon Rectum*. 2011;54:1184-1201, with permission from The ASCRS.)

and their management. These injuries remain a challenging clinical entity associated with significant morbidity. Familiarity with the different methods for approaching and managing colorectal injuries, including damage control tactics when necessary, will allow the surgeon to minimize unnecessary complications and mortality. Evolution in care and extensive outcomes research over the last few decades have demonstrated that almost all civilian and military colon injuries can be repaired primarily with a low anastomotic leak rate that appears to be independent of the method of repair. Excellent discussions on the management of rectal injuries and the changing approach to these challenging injuries are included. Fig 1 is included as an example of the summary of an evidence-based guideline for a typical injury. Similar algorithms appear for rectal injury.

D. W. Mozingo, MD

Validating the Western Trauma Association Algorithm for Managing Patients With Anterior Abdominal Stab Wounds: A Western Trauma Association Multicenter Trial

Biffl WL, Kaups KL, Pham TN, et al (Denver Health Med Ctr/Univ of Colorado; Community Regional Med Ctr/Univ of California-San Francisco; Harborview Med Ctr/Univ of Washington, Seattle; et al)
J Trauma 71:1494-1502, 2011

The optimal management of stable patients with anterior abdominal stab wounds (AASWs) remains a matter of debate. A recent Western Trauma Association (WTA) multicenter trial found that exclusion of peritoneal penetration by local wound exploration (LWE) allowed immediate discharge (D/C) of 41% of patients with AASWs. Performance of computed tomography (CT) scanning or diagnostic peritoneal lavage (DPL) did not improve the D/C rate; however, these tests led to nontherapeutic (NONTHER) laparotomy (LAP) in 24% and 31% of cases, respectively. An algorithm was proposed that included LWE, followed by either D/C or admission for serial clinical assessments, without further imaging or invasive testing. The purpose of this study was to evaluate the safety and efficacy of the algorithm in providing timely interventions for significant injuries.

Methods.—A multicenter, institutional review board-approved study enrolled patients with AASWs. Management was guided by the WTA AASW algorithm. Data on the presentation, evaluation, and clinical course were recorded prospectively.

Results.—Two hundred twenty-two patients (94% men, age, 34.7 years ± 0.3 years) were enrolled. Sixty-two (28%) had immediate LAP, of which 87% were therapeutic (THER). Three (1%) died and the mean length of stay (LOS) was 6.9 days. One hundred sixty patients were stable and asymptomatic, and 81 of them (51%) were managed entirely per protocol. Twenty (25%) were D/C'ed from the emergency department after (−) LWE, and 11 (14%) were taken to the operating room (OR) for LAP when their clinical condition changed. Two (2%) of the protocol group underwent NONTHER LAP, and no patient experienced morbidity or mortality related to delay in treatment. Seventy-nine (49%) patients had deviations from protocol. There were 47 CT scans, 11 DPLs, and 9 laparoscopic explorations performed. In addition to the laparoscopic procedures, 38 (48%) patients were taken to the OR based on test results rather than a change in the patient's clinical condition; 17 (45%) of these patients had a NONTHER LAP. Eighteen (23%) patients were D/Ced from the emergency department. The LOS was no different among patients who had immediate or delayed LAP. Mean LOS after NONTHER LAP was 3.6 days ± 0.8 days.

Conclusions.—The WTA proposed algorithm is designed for cost-effectiveness. Serial clinical assessments can be performed without the added expense of CT, DPL, or laparoscopy. Patients requiring LAP generally manifest early in their course, and there does not appear to be

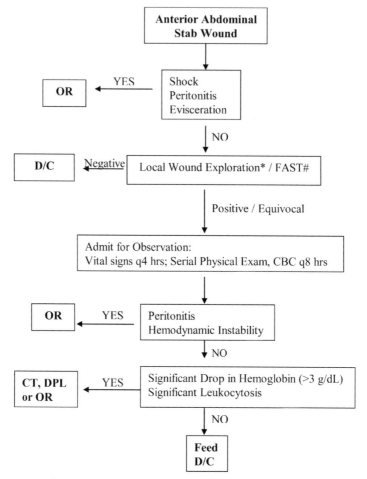

FIGURE 1.—Clinical pathway for management of patients with AASWs. *Consider CT scan if patient is morbidly obese (BMI > 30) or wound tract is long and tangential. #FAST demonstrating hemoperitoneum may be used as evidence of peritoneal penetration, obviating the need for LWE. CBC, complete blood count. (Reprinted from Biffl WL, Kaups KL, Pham TN, et al. Validating the western trauma association algorithm for managing patients with anterior abdominal stab wounds: a western trauma association multicenter trial. *J Trauma.* 2011;71:1494-1502.)

any morbidity related to a delay to OR. These data validate this approach and should be confirmed in a larger number of patients to more convincingly evaluate the algorithm's safety and cost-effectiveness compared with other approaches (Fig 1).

▶ Over a 30-month period, 4 participating institutions prospectively collected data on patients with anterior abdominal wall stab wounds. The treatment algorithm, included as Fig 1 in this review, defined the workup and treatment of patients presenting with anterior abdominal wall stab wounds. This algorithm, developed by the Western Trauma Association, represented a consensus of opinion regarding cost-effective and safe treatment of these patients. There are some limitations to this study, such as the self-reporting by surgeons of the therapeutic benefit of the operation as well as subsequent complications. Without controlled data collection, it is possible that the therapeutic benefit of certain operations was overstated and complications were underreported. It is also possible that some of the patients discharged from the emergency department were not included in the study. The numbers of patients are still relatively small to draw firm conclusions; however, one of the notable findings is that the data were extremely consistent with the previous Western Trauma Association study as well as the published literature on anterior abdominal wall stab wounds. The authors concluded from their study that the Western Trauma Association algorithm outlines a management strategy that minimizes unnecessary testing and nontherapeutic laparotomies without any demonstrable detrimental effect in terms of delayed diagnosis or operative intervention. Further evaluation of this algorithm is needed in larger populations of patients to confirm its use as a cost-effective approach to patients with anterior abdominal wall stab wounds.

D. W. Mozingo, MD

3 Burns

A Randomized Comparison Study of Aquacel Ag and Glucan II as Donor Site Dressings With Regard to Healing Time, Cosmesis, Infection Rate, and Patient's Perceived Pain: A Pilot Study
Bailey S, Carmean M, Cinat M, et al (Univ of California Irvine)
J Burn Care Res 32:627-632, 2011

This study was undertaken to compare pain, healing time, infection rate, and cosmetic outcome between Aquacel Ag (Convatec) and Glucan II (Brennan Medical) as donor site dressings. The authors performed a prospective, randomized, patient-controlled study. Eligible patients had two donor sites harvested. One site was dressed with Aquacel Ag and the other site with Glucan II. Patients were followed at set time points for 6 months to determine the rate of epithelialization, patient's perceived pain, infection rate, and the cosmetic outcome. A total of 20 patients were enrolled in the study. All patient data were collected through reepithelialization. The average time to wound healing for Aquacel Ag was 12.5 ± 2.07 days compared with Glucan II 12.7 ± 1.99 days. Perceived pain scores for each donor site were recorded. On postoperative day 5, patients reported significantly less pain with the Aquacel Ag site (Aquacel Ag 1.75 vs Glucan II 2.5, $P = .02$). Three donor sites showed clinical signs of infection (two Glucan II and one Aquacel Ag) prompting culture and dressing removal. There was no statistically significant difference in cosmetic outcomes of the donor sites at any time point. When comparing Aquacel Ag and Glucan II, our study has determined that there is no significant difference with regard to healing time, infection rates, and cosmetic outcomes. Both dressings are comparable with regard to ease of application and postoperative care.

▶ It is important in burned, critically ill patients to utilize autologous donor sites for maximum coverage and cosmesis. It is also important that donor sites heal quickly with as little pain and maximum function as possible. This study evaluated the use of 2 donor site dressings in a prospective, randomized trial. The study design used only 20 patients. Nevertheless, healing times were nearly identical. However, the study dressings were only in place for 8 days when they were removed, and a local antibiotic was applied for both groups. The Aquacel Ag group experienced less early donor-site pain, which is of real benefit to the patient. However, little other benefit was noted.

Studies such as these may seem mundane, yet they serve a real purpose in that they attempt to define the potential benefits of new therapies for patients with major burns. In fact, it is incumbent on us to conduct these trials so that we do not blindly accept that which is new as better than older methods of treatment.

J. M. Daly, MD

An Open, Parallel, Randomized, Comparative, Multicenter Study to Evaluate the Cost-Effectiveness, Performance, Tolerance, and Safety of a Silver-Containing Soft Silicone Foam Dressing (Intervention) vs Silver Sulfadiazine Cream
Silverstein P, Heimbach D, Meites H, et al (Paul Silverstein Burn Ctr, OK; Harborview Med Ctr, Seattle, WA; et al)
J Burn Care Res 32:617-626, 2011

An open, parallel, randomized, comparative, multicenter study was implemented to evaluate the cost-effectiveness, performance, tolerance, and safety of a silver-containing soft silicone foam dressing (Mepilex Ag) vs silver sulfadiazine cream (control) in the treatment of partial-thickness thermal burns. Individuals aged 5 years and older with partial-thickness thermal burns (2.5–20% BSA) were randomized into two groups and treated with the trial products for 21 days or until healed, whichever occurred first. Data were obtained and analyzed on cost (direct and indirect), healing rates, pain, comfort, ease of product use, and adverse events. A total of 101 subjects were recruited. There were no significant differences in burn area profiles within the groups. The cost of dressing-related analgesia was lower in the intervention group ($P = .03$) as was the cost of background analgesia ($P = .07$). The mean total cost of treatment was $309 vs $513 in the control ($P < .001$). The average cost-effectiveness per treatment regime was $381 lower in the intervention product, producing an incremental cost-effectiveness ratio of $1688 in favor of the soft silicone foam dressing. Mean healing rates were 71.7 vs 60.8% at final visit, and the number of dressing changes were 2.2 vs 12.4 in the treatment and control groups, respectively. Subjects reported significantly less pain at application ($P = .02$) and during wear ($P = .048$) of the Mepilex Ag dressing in the acute stages of wound healing. Clinicians reported the intervention dressing was significantly easier to use ($P = .03$) and flexible ($P = .04$). Both treatments were well tolerated; however, the total incidence of adverse events was higher in the control group. The silver-containing soft silicone foam dressing was as effective in the treatment of patients as the standard care (silver sulfadiazine). In addition, the group of patients treated with the soft silicone foam dressing demonstrated decreased pain and lower costs associated with treatment.

▶ Products that can be applied topically to burn wounds to accelerate wound healing or diminish the incidence of infection are important in the care of these often critically ill burn patients. This trial studied one such product, a silver-containing soft silicon foam compared with standard therapy with silver sulfadiazine cream in 101 burn patients. Randomization achieved its end in that average burn surface area was similar between groups. The experimental group demonstrated significantly less pain and less need for dressing changes (probably related to less pain in this group). Adverse effects were more commonly seen in the control group. Importantly, the authors sought to identify costs involved in using this new therapy and noted less cost in the experimental group than the control group, perhaps because of fewer dressing changes. They also noted greater ease of application of the foam product. Given this apparent benefit, it will be important to reproduce these results in a larger, multi-center trial in which patients with burns on greater than 20% of the body are included and measurements of wound healing and infection are carried out.

J. M. Daly, MD

Effect of 12-week isokinetic training on muscle strength in adult with healed thermal burn
Ebid AA, Omar MTA, Abd El Baky AM (Cairo Univ, Giza, Egypt)
Burns 38:61-68, 2012

Introduction.—Severe burns result in marked and prolonged skeletal muscle catabolism and weakness, which persist despite "standard" rehabilitation programmes of occupational and physical therapy. Therefore, the objectives of this study were of twofold: to quantify the long-term effects of burns on leg muscle strength and to assess whether adults with thermal burn would benefit from the isokinetic training programme.

Materials and Methods.—Burned adult patients, with 35—55% total body surface area (TBSA) burned, were assessed at 6 months after burn in respect to leg muscle strength at $150°$ s^{-1}, using isokinetic dynamometry. Non-burned adults were assessed similarly, and served as controls. The burned adults participated in the resistance training programme 3 times weekly. The isokinetic exercise programme was begun with 60% of the average peak torque. Intensity of isokinetic exercise was increased from one set to five sets during the first through fifth sessions and remained at six sets for the remaining 6th to 24th sessions. Finally, a dose of 10 sets was applied for the 25th to the 36th sessions. Each set consisted of five repetitions of concentric contraction in angular velocities of $150°$ s^{-1} for knee extensors, and flexors. All exercise sessions were preceded by a 5-min warm-up period on the treadmill.

Results.—Subjects with burns more than 35% of TBSA produced significantly less torque, work, and power in the quadriceps and hamstring than control subjects (20.5%, 15.2%, $p < 0.05$). Three months after isokinetic programme, muscle strength further increased by 17.9% ± 10.1% compared to the baseline measurement for burned patients but continued to be below the concurrent age-matched, non-burned adult.

Conclusion.—We found that adults with severe burns, relative to non-burned adults, had significantly lower peak torque as well as total work performance using the extensors and flexors muscles of the thigh.

Participation in isokinetic training resulted in a greater improvement in extensor and flexor muscle strength in adults with healed thermal burn compared to base line values.

▶ Major burn injury has a multitude of deleterious effects including loss of the skin barrier, which invites infection and sepsis, and loss of muscle strength due to catabolism, inactivity, and a deficit of nutrition relative to needs. This study sought to determine the potential beneficial effects of exercise on muscle strength in burned patients. As noted, peak torque and work performance were below that of unburned control subjects as expected, but importantly, iso-kinetic training significantly improved work performance in the flexor and extensor muscle groups. Results of this study can be extrapolated to many situations in hospitalized patients. Rehabilitation by exercise is vitally important in a patient's recovery, and professional training can lead to marked improvement in well-being and perhaps earlier discharge (although this was not studied in the report). Unfortunately, all too often, physical therapy professionals are not available for this training because of cost constraints in hospitals.

J. M. Daly, MD

Gastric Emptying and Intestinal Transit of Various Enteral Feedings Following Severe Burn Injury

Sallam HS, Kramer GC, Chen JDZ (Univ of Texas Med Branch, Galveston)
Dig Dis Sci 56:3172-3178, 2011

Background.—Burn-induced delayed gastric emptying and intestinal transit limits enteral feeding/resuscitation.

Aims.—To study (1) the effects of burn injury on gastric emptying and intestinal transit at different time points following enteral feeding/fluids, and (2) the effects of enteral resuscitative fluids on gastric emptying, intestinal transit, and plasma volume expansion.

Methods.—Rats were randomized into sham-burn and burn groups. They were either enterally untreated or treated by a gavage of one or multiple doses of oral rehydration solution (ORS) or, Vivonex®, all mixed with phenol red as a marker, at different time points from 1 to 6 h after burn. Gastric emptying, intestinal transit and hematocrit values were assessed. Gastric emptying of a semi-solid methylcellulose meal served as a standard control for gastric emptying studies.

Results.—We found that (1) burn did not alter the gastric emptying of ORS, but delayed its intestinal transit at all time points; (2) burn delayed the gastric emptying of both methylcellulose or Vivonex and the intestinal transit of Vivonex, 6 h after burn; and (3) multiple doses of ORS normalized the elevated post-burn hematocrit values. The percentage of plasma volume expansion at 6 h resulting from the multiple-dose ORS was superior to that of Vivonex by 50%. Addition of Erythromycin to Vivonex improved its gastric emptying, intestinal transit, and plasma volume expansion.

Conclusions.—Burn delays the gastric emptying of semi-solids, but not the ORS. Enteral electrolyte solution (ORS) and feeding (Vivonex) provided plasma volume expansion. Prokinetic drugs may be able to maximize the effectiveness of early post-burn feeding.

▶ After burn injury, the standard of care is that patients receive intravenous fluids containing electrolytes and dextrose. The Parkland formula documented decades ago describes the amount of fluids and electrolytes that burn patients should receive based on their size and the size of the burn injury. However, there are circumstances in which individuals are burned and live in areas in which intravenous access and appropriate electrolyte solutions may not be readily available. Therefore, it is important to try to determine the best method of oral rehydration of burn patients as well as whether nutritional solutions can be of benefit, because many individuals in underdeveloped countries are malnourished. In this study, after burn injury, rats were randomized to receive either oral rehydration solution or Vivonex, and gastric emptying as well as intestinal transit times were measured. Interestingly, there was no decrease in mean gastric emptying with the use of oral rehydration solution. Yet at the same time, there was a decrease in intestinal transit using the oral rehydration solution. Using Vivonex, gastric emptying was delayed, but intestinal transit was normal. The burn injury itself did decrease both gastric emptying and intestinal transit time. Thus, the model appeared appropriate.

These studies are important because they provide alternatives to the standard intravenous regimens that have been used to care for burn patients when these solutions or access are not available. It may be that some combination of oral rehydration solution and nutritional solutions may be of maximal benefit. Unfortunately, this concept of hybrid solutions was not tested in the this study.

J. M. Daly, MD

Novel biodegradable composite wound dressings with controlled release of antibiotics: Results in a guinea pig burn model
Elsner JJ, Egozi D, Ullmann Y, et al (Tel-Aviv Univ, Israel; RAMBAM Med Ctr, Haifa, Israel; et al)
Burns 37:896-904, 2011

Approximately 70% of all people with severe burns die from related infections despite advances in treatment regimens and the best efforts of nurses and doctors. Silver ion-eluting wound dressings are available for overcoming this problem. However, there are reports of deleterious effects of such dressings due to cellular toxicity that delays the healing process, and the dressing changes needed 1—2 times a day are uncomfortable for the patient and time consuming for the stuff. An alternative concept in wound dressing design that combines the advantages of occlusive dressings with biodegradability and intrinsic topical antibiotic treatment is described herewith. The new composite structure presented in this article is based on a polyglyconate mesh and a porous poly-(DL-lactic-CO-glycolic acid) matrix loaded with gentamicin developed to provide controlled release of antibiotics for three weeks. *In vivo* evaluation of the dressing material in contaminated deep second degree burn wounds in guinea pigs ($n = 20$) demonstrated its ability to accelerate epithelialization by 40% compared to an unloaded format of the material and a conventional dressing material. Wound contraction was reduced significantly, and a better quality scar tissue was formed. The current dressing material exhibits promising results, does not require frequent bandage changes, and offers a potentially valuable and economic approach to treating the life-threatening complication of burn-related infections.

▶ Sepsis is one of the major complications of major burns related to the loss of the skin barrier to invading micro-organisms. Coverage of the burned areas is important to restore this integrity and to reduce the rate of severe infection, which can convert second-degree to third-degree burns. The use of autologous skin is often limited by the size and location of the burned areas. Thus, the use of artificial skin or composite dressings that reduce the occurrence of infection is important.

This article describes a new composite dressing that can incorporate antibiotics and presumably growth factors that has mechanical substance, yet degrades biologically by hydrolysis when the wound is healing. This study in animals found that when slow release of gentamycin occurred in the wound gel matrix, the wound healed the quickest. Fast release of the antibiotic was also beneficial compared with results in controls. The antibiotic used does have nephrotoxic effects, but others could be substituted. It will be important to perform prospective, randomized animal trials comparing different antibiotic regimens and also compare with silver nitrate or sulfamylon standard dressings to address efficacy.

J. M. Daly, MD

Influence of Topically Applied Antimicrobial Agents on Muscular Microcirculation

Goertz O, Hirsch T, Ring A, et al (Ruhr-Univ Bochum, Germany; et al)
Ann Plast Surg 67:407-412, 2011

Bacterial infections cause major complications in wound healing. Local antiseptics are used for daily wound care; however, their potential toxic effects on the vasculature have not yet been thoroughly investigated. The aim of this study was to assess the effects of antiseptics on microcirculation. Investigations were performed on a standardized cremaster muscle model on rats (n = 60). The arteriolar diameter and functional capillary density (FCD) were investigated using transillumination microscopy before and 60 and 120 minutes after application of each of the following antimicrobial agents: alcohol, hydrogen peroxide, imipenem, octenidine dihydrochloride, polyhexanide, and ethacridine lactate. Although polyhexanide caused a significant arteriolar dilatation (106.25 ± 3.23 vs. $88.54 \pm 6.74 \, \mu m$ [baseline value]) and increase of FCD compared with baseline value (12.65 ± 0.82 vs. 9.10 ± 0.50 n/0.22 mm^2), alcohol led to a significant decrease of both parameters (90.63 ± 10.80 vs. 52.09 ± 7.69 and 5.35 ± 0.54 vs. 1.68 ± 0.48) and was the only agent that caused arteriolar thrombosis. The FCD also increased significantly after treatment with hydrogen peroxide (10.55 ± 0.33 vs. 12.30 ± 0.48) and octenidine (6.82 ± 0.63 vs. 12.32 ± 0.63). However, no positive effect on arteriolar diameter could be found. Ethacridine lactate and imipenem did not impact either parameter. In addition to reducing bacteria, an antiseptic should be nontoxic, especially to the microcirculation. Polyhexanide seems to have a positive influence on vessel diameter and capillary density, whereas alcohol reduces both parameters. If the antimicrobial efficacy is comparable, the antiseptic with less toxic effects should be chosen, especially in critically perfused wounds.

▶ Wound healing is often delayed in patients with diabetes mellitus, past radiation therapy, severe malnutrition, chronic smoking history, and other causes. Topical agents are often applied in these situations in an effort to control bacterial counts and help to accelerate wound healing. Yet little is known about the physiologic responses to these agents in wounds. In an attempt to learn these responses, the authors used a standard mouse cremaster muscle model to which they applied multiple agents and sought to determine the effects of these agents on microcirculation. Alcohol application was the most deleterious, while polyhexanide was the least deleterious to the microcirculation. This surrogate marker (microcirculation) needs to be supplemented by further studies of the immunologic, oxygen delivery, and cellular effects of these agents. In addition, the direct effects of these agents on bacterial counts and rates of wound healing need to be characterized.

J. M. Daly, MD

Deficiency of CX3CR1 delays burn wound healing and is associated with reduced myeloid cell recruitment and decreased sub-dermal angiogenesis
Clover AJP, Kumar AHS, Caplice NM (Univ College Cork, Ireland)
Burns 37:1386-1393, 2011

The development of a good blood supply is a key step in burn wound healing and appears to be regulated in part by myeloid cells. CX3CR1 positive cells have recently been identified as myeloid cells with a potential role in angiogenesis. The role of functional CX3CR1 system in burn wound healing is not previously investigated.

A 2% contact burn was induced in CX3CR1$^{+/gfp}$ and CX3CR1$^{gfp/gfp}$ mice. These transgenic mice facilitate the tracking of CX3CR1 cells (CX3CR1$^{+/gfp}$) and allow evaluation of the consequence of CX3CR1 functional knockout (CX3CR1$^{gfp/gfp}$) on burn wound healing. The progression of wound healing was monitored before tissue was harvested and analyzed at day 6 and day 12 for migration of CX3CR1 cells into burn wound.

Deficiency of a functional CX3CR1 system resulted in decreased recruitment of CX3CR1 positive cells into the burn wound associated with decreased myeloid cell recruitment ($p < 0.001$) and reduced maintenance of new vessels ($p < 0.001$). Burn wound healing was prolonged ($p < 0.05$).

Our study is the first to establish a role for CX3CR1 in burn wound healing which is associated with sub-dermal angiogenesis. This chemokine receptor pathway may be attractive for therapeutic manipulation as it could increase sub-dermal angiogenesis and thereby improve time to healing.

▶ Burn injury requires skin grafting to reduce the burn surface area, reduce the incidence of sepsis, and decrease mortality. In major body surface burn injury, it is often difficult to obtain enough autologous skin for grafting, and artificial or nonautologous materials are used. Thus, it is important to be able to accelerate burn wound healing, particularly in those with superficial second-degree burns. This would lessen the need for early skin grafting in these individuals.

In this study, the role of fractalkine and CX3CR1 was evaluated in transgenic mice that were deficient in CX3CR1 compared with heterozygous controls. Results of the study showed that deficiency of CX3CR1 resulted in a significant decrease in dermal angiogenesis as well as prolonged healing of the burn wound.

These results also suggest that manipulation of this particular chemokine system would have benefit in improving dermal angiogenesis after a burn injury. It will be important for the authors to study this chemokine system in a variety of burn and full-thickness skin excisional mouse models to determine whether stimulation of this chemokine system accelerates healing, particularly in animals that may have some impairment secondary to malnutrition or other factors.

J. M. Daly, MD

A Controlled Clinical Trial With Pirfenidone in the Treatment of Pathological Skin Scarring Caused by Burns in Pediatric Patients

Armendariz-Borunda J, Lyra-Gonzalez I, Medina-Preciado D, et al (Univ of Guadalajara, Mexico; Hosp Civil de Guadalajara, Mexico; et al)
Ann Plast Surg 68:22-28, 2012

Background.—Pathologic skin scarring reversion remains a big challenge for surgeons, as disfiguring scars have a dramatic influence on patient's quality of life.

Methods.—A controlled clinical trial was conducted to evaluate 8% pirfenidone (PFD) gel administered topically 3 times a day during 6 months to 33 pediatric patients with hypertrophic scars caused by burns. A total of 30 patients with hypertrophic scars with identical Vancouver Scar Scale values were treated with pressure therapy and included as controls. Improvements were evaluated by Vancouver Scar Scale and a Visual Analog Scale. Safety parameters were determined by the presence of adverse events and monitoring laboratory and hematology parameters.

Comparison between PFD group and pressure therapy group

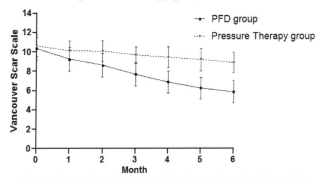

	Basal	Month 1	Month 2	Month 3	Month 4	Month 5	Month 6
Pressure therapy group	10.63 ± 1.13	10.1 ± 1.03	10.07 ± 1.05	9.67 ± 0.84	9.43 ± 1.07	9.2 ± 1.16	8.9 ± 1.03
PFD group	10.33 ± 1.16	9.24 ± 1.2	8.61 ± 1.22	7.7 ± 1.19	6.88 ± 1.11	6.24 1.12	5.88 ± 1.17

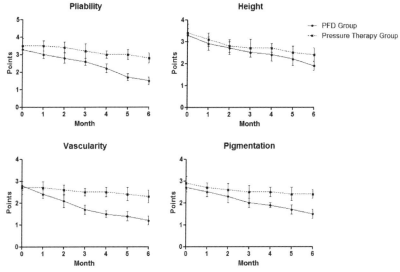

FIGURE 2.—Graphical representation comparing total and point-by-point VSS score between both the groups. We observed an improvement of 34% in PFD group than pressure therapy group at the end of the study. Comparative month versus VSS values showed statistical significance (*P* < 0.001). (Reprinted from Armendariz-Borunda J, Lyra-Gonzalez I, Medina-Preciado D, et al. A controlled clinical trial with pirfenidone in the treatment of pathological skin scarring caused by burns in pediatric patients. *Ann Plast Surg.* 2012;68:22-28.)

Results.—Patients treated with PFD during 6 months presented a continuous monthly statistically significant scar regression in comparison with the initial Vancouver measurement (*P* = <0.001). PFD group showed a higher improvement of all scar features as compared with control group treated with pressure therapy (*P* = <0.001). In the PFD group, 9 of 33 patients (27%) had their scores decreased in Vancouver classification by more than

55%, 22 patients (67%) had a 30% to 45% decrease, whereas 2 patients (6%) had a 30% decrease or less. Control group treated with pressure therapy showed a slight improvement in 16% of cases on an average. Patients did not show serious adverse effects or laboratory alterations throughout the study.

Conclusions.—Topical administration of 8% PFD gel 3 times a day is more effective and safe in the treatment of hypertrophic scars caused by burns in children, as compared with standard pressure therapy (Fig 2).

▶ Hypertrophic scar formation after burns remains a significant clinical obstacle for patients recovering from their injury. Scar compression therapy continues to be the most common, although imperfect, management strategy. Hypertrophic scars result from failure of normal wound healing. Clinically, we now understand that hypertrophic scars are influenced by the actions of a number of cytokines and growth factors, including transforming growth factor β (TGF-β), tumor necrosis factor α (TNF-α), platelet-derived growth factor, and epidermal growth factor, among others. The actions of these factors maintain the balance between degradation and biosynthesis of extracellular matrix to obtain optimal tissue repair or normal wound healing.

Pirfenidone is a broad-spectrum antifibrotic drug that modulates diverse cytokine action involving TGF-β, TNF-α, epidermal growth factor, platelet-derived growth factor, vascular endothelial growth factor, insulin-like growth factor 1, fibroblast growth factor, and others. Pirfenidone has been effective in the prevention and regression of pulmonary fibrosis, peritoneal sclerosis, hepatic cirrhosis, uterine fibromyoma, and other scarring and fibrotic conditions. It is very encouraging that a reduction in hypertrophic scarring (included as Fig 2) can be achieved by a topical gel application of a seemingly well-tolerated drug. Further trials are needed to confirm this finding.

D. W. Mozingo, MD

A Prospective Longitudinal Study of Posttraumatic Stress Disorder Symptom Trajectories After Burn Injury

Sveen J, Ekselius L, Gerdin B, et al (Uppsala Univ, Sweden)
J Trauma 71:1808-1815, 2011

Background.—Psychologic problems are common after burns, and symptoms of posttraumatic stress disorder (PTSD) are some of the most prevalent. Risk factors for PTSD have been identified, but little is known about the onset and course of these symptoms. The objective was to investigate whether there are different PTSD symptom trajectories after burns.

Methods.—Ninety-five adults with burns were enrolled in a prospective study from in-hospital treatment until 12 months after burn. Symptoms of PTSD were assessed with the Impact of Event Scale-Revised and scores at 3, 6, and 12 months after the burn were used in a cluster analysis to detect trajectories. The trajectories were compared regarding known risk factors for PTSD using non-parametric analysis of variance.

Result.—Four clusters were identified: (1) resilient, with low levels of PTSD symptoms that decreased over time; (2) recovery, with high levels of symptoms that gradually decreased; (3) delayed, with moderate symptoms that increased over time; and (4) chronic, with high levels of symptoms over time. The trajectories differed regarding several risk factors for PTSD including life events, premorbid psychiatric morbidity, personality traits, avoidant coping, in-hospital psychologic symptoms, and social support. The resilient trajectory consistently had fewer of the risk factors and differed the most from the chronic trajectory.

Conclusions.—There are subgroups among patients with burns that have different patterns of PTSD symptom development. These findings may have implications for clinical practice, such as the timing of assessment and the management of patients who present with these symptoms.

▶ Risk factors for posttraumatic stress disorder (PTSD) symptoms developing after burn injury have been identified and include female gender, psychiatric history, avoidant coping, low social support, injury severity, life threat during the trauma, and early onset of psychological symptoms. Although there is much research regarding risk factors, few studies investigate the development of PTSD symptoms over time, and few have investigated possible subgroups of patients with PTSD symptoms. When applying cluster analysis in this study, the investigators identified 4 distinct patterns of PTSD symptoms over time: resilient (40%), recovery (10%), delayed (32%), and chronic (18%) trajectories. The trajectories are similar to most findings in previous research regarding the course of PTSD symptoms. A limitation of this study is encountered following cluster analysis, in that the subgroups were small in size. However, the results are still similar with those trajectories described in previous research. Another limitation is that the study included assessments only up to 12 months after burn, even though symptom patterns may persist and evolve for a much longer time in some patients.

D. W. Mozingo, MD

Comparison of airway pressure release ventilation to conventional mechanical ventilation in the early management of smoke inhalation injury in swine

Batchinsky AI, Burkett SE, Zanders TB, et al (United States Army Inst of Surgical Res, Fort Sam Houston, TX; Brooke Army Med Ctr, Fort Sam Houston, TX)
Crit Care Med 39:2314-2321, 2011

Objective.—The role of airway pressure release ventilation in the management of early smoke inhalation injury has not been studied. We compared the effects of airway pressure release ventilation and conventional mechanical ventilation on oxygenation in a porcine model of acute respiratory distress syndrome induced by wood smoke inhalation.

Design.—Prospective animal study.

Setting.—Government laboratory animal intensive care unit.

Patients.—Thirty-three Yorkshire pigs.

Interventions.—Smoke inhalation injury.

Measurements and Main Results.—Anesthetized female Yorkshire pigs (n = 33) inhaled room-temperature pine-bark smoke. Before injury, the pigs were randomized to receive conventional mechanical ventilation (n = 15) or airway pressure release ventilation (n = 12) for 48 hrs after smoke inhalation. As acute respiratory distress syndrome developed (PaO_2/FiO_2 ratio <200), plateau pressures were limited to <35 cm H_2O. Six uninjured pigs received conventional mechanical ventilation for 48 hrs and served as time controls. Changes in PaO_2/FiO_2 ratio, tidal volume, respiratory rate, mean airway pressure, plateau pressure, and hemodynamic variables were recorded. Survival was assessed using Kaplan-Meier analysis. PaO_2/FiO_2 ratio was lower in airway pressure release ventilation vs. conventional mechanical ventilation pigs at 12, 18, and 24 hrs ($p < .05$) but not at 48 hrs. Tidal volumes were lower in conventional mechanical ventilation animals between 30 and 48 hrs post injury ($p < .05$). Respiratory rates were lower in airway pressure release ventilation at 24, 42, and 48 hrs ($p < .05$). Mean airway pressures were higher in airway pressure release ventilation animals between 6 and 48 hrs ($p < .05$). There was no difference in plateau pressures, hemodynamic variables, or survival between conventional mechanical ventilation and airway pressure release ventilation pigs.

Conclusions.—In this model of acute respiratory distress syndrome caused by severe smoke inhalation in swine, airway pressure release ventilation-treated animals developed acute respiratory distress syndrome faster than conventional mechanical ventilation-treated animals, showing a lower PaO_2/FiO_2 ratio at 12, 18, and 24 hrs after injury. At other time points, PaO_2/FiO_2 ratio was not different between conventional mechanical ventilation and airway pressure release ventilation.

▶ Airway pressure release ventilation (APRV) is a mode of ventilation that optimizes mean airway pressure by maintaining a continuous positive airway pressure interrupted by time-cycled releases of pressure to facilitate ventilation.

It has been advocated in the management of acute respiratory distress syndrome. One of the theoretical advantages of APRV is that it allows for spontaneous ventilation throughout the entire ventilation cycle, specifically during lung inflation, which may promote and maintain alveolar recruitment. Smoke inhalation injury causes complications in approximately 10% of admissions to burn centers in the United States. This injury is a unique pathophysiologic process characterized predominantly by small airway injury, and its optimal initial management may be different from that of other causes of ARDS. In this model, when compared with conventional ventilation with a target plateau pressure of 35 cm H_2O, APRV was associated with a lower P/F ratio at 12, 18, and 24 hours after injury, despite a higher peak airway pressure from 6 hours after injury until the end of the study. In this study, APRV appeared not to be of benefit when compared with conventional ventilation in management of ARDS in the first 48 hours.

D. W. Mozingo, MD

Comparison of Hospital Mortality Rates After Burn Injury in New York State: A Risk-Adjusted Population-Based Observational Study

Osler T, Glance LG, Hosmer DW (Univ of Vermont, Colchester; Univ of Rochester School of Medicine and Dentistry, NY; Univ of Massachusetts, Amherst)
J Trauma 71:1040-1047, 2011

Background.—Severity-adjusted mortality is an unequivocal measure of burn care success. Hospitals can be compared on this metric using administrative data because information required for calculating statistically adjusted risk of mortality is routinely collected on hospital admission.

Methods.—The New York State Department of Health provided information on all 13,113 thermally injured patients hospitalized at 1 of 194 hospitals between 2004 and 2008. We compared hospital survival rates using a random effects logistic model of mortality that incorporated age and several predictors that were present on admission and captured as International Classification of Diseases-9 codes: burn surface area, inhalation injury, three measures of physiologic compromise, and four medical comorbidities. Hospitals were compared on the adjusted odds of death and the number of excess deaths.

Results.—Overall mortality was 3.2%. Nine high-volume hospitals (>100 patients/year) cared for 83% of patients with burn injuries. Overall variability of the odds of mortality among these high-volume centers was modest (median odds ratio = 1.2) and we found little evidence for differences in the adjusted odds of mortality. A secondary analysis of the 185 low-volume hospitals that cared for 2,235 patients disclosed only 24 deaths. When examined in aggregate, these hospitals had better than predicted risk-adjusted mortality; a logical explanation is judicious case selection.

Conclusions.—Administrative hospital discharge data are extensive and comparably enough collected to allow comparison of the performance of burn centers. Risk-adjusted models show that patients have statistically indistinguishable risk-adjusted odds of mortality regardless of which hospital in New York State cared for them (Fig 1).

► Comparing burn injury survival rates and other measures of outcome using administrative data sets has its problems. When the UHC data sets are queried, non—burn center hospitals have much better outcomes treating burn patients than do burn centers. As in this study, there is a small, yet measurable mortality rate in burn patients treated in non—burn center hospitals. Who are these patients, and why would they not be transferred to a burn center? Maybe they had burns as a prior injury that were healed but present on admission. These details should be sorted out in future studies. Comparing survival rates among burn centers requires a risk adjustment model, and surprisingly, no such model is currently agreed upon. Although many burn mortality models were developed over the last 60 years, most are now only of historical interest, either because they were developed so long ago that they fail to reflect modern improvements in burn care or they are based on small datasets or the experience

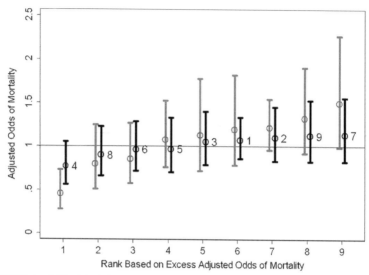

FIGURE 1.—Odds of death for nine high-volume hospitals. The gray circles and CIs are based on the model that included only TBSA, age, and inhalation as predictors, whereas the dark circles and CIs are the result of a model that contained these three predictors as well as three possible presenting physiologic derangements and four possible comorbidities. Hospitals are ranked on adjusted odds of mortality along the horizontal axis. Point estimates are labeled as in Table 2, and CIs are computed using bootstrap methods. (Reprinted from Osler T, Glance LG, Hosmer DW. Comparison of hospital mortality rates after burn injury in New York state: a risk-adjusted population-based observational study. *J Trauma.* 2011;71:1040-1047.)

of a single institution. Despite the lack of an acknowledged model, there is broad agreement that the factors important in determining survival after burn injury are namely age, total body surface area burned, and the presence of smoke inhalation injury. In this selection, the authors evaluate the outcomes of burn admission to 9 institutions in New York State admitting over 100 patients per year. These 9 burn centers had, not surprisingly, little difference in mortality rates (Fig 1). These hospitals cared for 83% of all burn admissions over the time studied.

D. W. Mozingo, MD

Emerging Gram-Negative Infections in Burn Wounds

Azzopardi EA, Azzopardi SM, Boyce DE, et al (Cardiff Univ, UK; Mater Dei Univ Hosp, Malta; The Welsh Centre for Burns and Plastic Surgery, Swansea, UK)
J Burn Care Res 32:570-576, 2011

Gram-negative infection remains a major contributor to morbidity, mortality, and cost of care. In the absence of comparative multinational epidemiological studies specific to burn patients, we sought to review literature trends in emerging Gram-negative burn wound infections within the past 60 years. Mapping trends in these organisms, although in a minority compared with the six "ESKAPE" pathogens currently being targeted by the Infectious Diseases Society of North America, would identify pathogens of increasing concern to burn physicians in the near future and develop patient profiles that may predict susceptibility to infection. *Aeromonas hydrophila* infection was identified as the emerging pathogen of note, constituting 76% of the identified publications. *A. hydrophila* constituted 96% of *Aeromonas* spp. isolates (mortality 10.7%). The following patient profile indicated predisposition to *Aeromonas* infection: mean age (mean 33.7 years, range $17 \le R \le 80$, SD = 15.6); TBSA (mean 41.1%, range $8\% \le R \le 80\%$, SD = 15.2); full-thickness skin burns (mean 27.7%, range $3\% \le R \le 60\%$, SD = 16.6); and a male predominance (81.3%). Other pathogens included *Stenotrophomonas maltophilia* *Vibrio* spp., *Chryseobacterium* spp., *Alcaligenes xylosoxidans*, and *Cedecia lapigei*. Arresting the thermal injury by untreated water was the common predisposing factor. These emerging infections clearly constitute a minority of Gram-negative bacterial infections in burn patients at present. However, these are the infections most likely to pose significant clinical challenge because of the high prevalence of multidrug resistance, rapid acquisition of multidrug resistance, high mortality, and ubiquity in the natural environment. This article therefore presents a rationale for understanding and recognizing the role of these emerging infections in burn patients.

▶ In this selection, the authors propose a rationale for the importance of understanding and recognizing the role of emerging bacterial burn wound infections, burn wound surveillance, and pharmacovigilance within this subspecialty. This review identified *Aeromonas hydrophila* as an emerging pathogen in burn wound microbiological profiles. *Stenotrophomonas maltophilia*, *Vibrio* spp, *Chryseobacterium* spp, *Cedecia lapigei*, and *Achromobacter xylosoxidans* were also identified as candidates of potential interest in burn wound infection. Clearly, these bacteria represent a minority of current infections; however, a critical review of the literature published over the past 60 years shows that these infections are significantly underreported. The propensity of these organisms, especially *A hydrophila*, to rapidly acquire multidrug resistance through antimicrobial exposure and through transference from *Pseudomonas* spp makes these organisms worthy of closer monitoring. The now common practice of "cooling the burn" by dousing the burned area with whatever water is available may also be responsible for the increased appearance of these organisms.

D. W. Mozingo, MD

Enoxaparin Dose Adjustment is Associated With Low Incidence of Venous Thromboembolic Events in Acute Burn Patients

Lin H, Faraklas I, Saffle J, et al (Univ of Utah Healthcare, Salt Lake City)
J Trauma 71:1557-1561, 2011

Background.—Inadequate antifactor Xa levels have been documented in critically ill patients given prophylactic enoxaparin and may result in increased risk of venous thromboembolic (VTE) events. The objective of this study was to examine the impact of dose adjustment of enoxaparin and associated incidence of VTE in acute burn patients.

Methods.—All acute burn patients who were treated with prophylactic enoxaparin on a burn/trauma intensive care unit were prospectively followed. Patients with subtherapeutic antifactor Xa levels had enoxaparin doses increased as per unit protocol with the goal of obtaining a therapeutic antifactor Xa level.

Results.—Eighty-four acute burn patients who were treated with enoxaparin had at least one appropriately obtained antifactor Xa level between June 2009 and October 2010. Initial antifactor Xa levels in 64 patients (76.2%) were below 0.2 U/mL, resulting in increased enoxaparin dose. Fifteen patients never achieved the target antifactor Xa level before enoxaparin was discontinued. Median final enoxaparin dose required to achieve therapeutic antifactor Xa levels was 40 mg every 12 hours (range, 20–70 mg). Using linear regression, final enoxaparin dose correlated with burn size (%total body surface area) and weight. No episodes of hemorrhage, thrombocytopenia, or heparin sensitivity were documented. Two patients (2.4%) had VTE complications despite adequate prophylaxis.

Conclusions.—Frequent occurrence of low antifactor Xa levels observed in this study demonstrated the inadequacy of standard dosing of enoxaparin for VTE prophylaxis in many patients with acute burns. Enoxaparin dose adjustment was associated with a low incidence of VTE events and no bleeding complications (Fig 1).

▶ Within 48 hours of injury, burn patients become hyperdynamic with an increased cardiac output, resulting in enhanced hepatic and renal clearance of drugs. Enoxaparin, a low-molecular-weight heparin, is metabolized primarily by the liver, and its active metabolites are cleared by renal excretion. The pathophysiologic changes that occur following burn may affect the clearance of enoxaparin and may explain the apparent inadequacy of standard dosing. Also, the agent's access to the microcirculation after subcutaneous injection may be reduced because of altered peripheral perfusion and edema formation following burn injury and fluid resuscitation. Therefore, if burn patients receive enoxaparin for venous thromboembolic (VTE) prophylaxis, it is not surprising that modification of the usual prophylactic doses might be required. The greatest limitation of this study is the small sample size. Routine duplex examinations to screen asymptomatic patients for VTE were not performed and would likely have resulted in a marked increase in detection of deep vein thrombosis as has been described

STEP ONE:	Inclusion Criteria	Exclusion Criteria:	
	All patients admitted to BTICU	Lovenox contraindicated	Intracranial bleeding/stroke
	Anticipated non-ambulatory ≥ 48 hours	Hematoma	Bleeding disorder
		HIT positive	Head injury/neurotrauma
		Cr CL≤ 30 mL/min	Serum Cr ≥ 1.6 mg/dL
		Epidural analgesia	

STEP TWO: Calculate Lovenox Dosing: Burn Admission Weight (kg)_____

Indication	Ped atric (<13 years or < 30 Kg)	Adult (30-150 Kg)	Obese adult (≥150 Kg or BMI > 35)
Prophylaxis	0.5mg/kg SQ Q12hr	30mg SQ Q12hr	0.5mg/kg SQ Q12hr
Treatment of DVT/PE	1.0mg/kg SQ Q12hr	1.0mg/kg Q12hr (round to nearest 10mg)	

INITIAL DOSE _____ mg SQ q12 hrs

STEP THREE: Assessment of Efficacy

Draw *"Anti-Xa low molecular weight heparin"* (Anti-Xa LMWH) level 4 hours after 3rd consecutive dose

Target level:

Prophylaxis: 0.2 – 0.4 IU/mL

Treatment: 0.5 – 1.0 IU/mL

Level is LOW: Increase dose by 20% to _____ mg SQ q12

Level is HIGH: Decrease dose by 20% to _____ mg SQ q12

Level is WITHIN TARGET RANGE

Dosing is interrupted for any reason: RESTART STEP 3

STEP FOUR: Check Anti-Xa level every Monday. If two consecutive levels are within therapeutic range (±)and dose is not changed, may discontinue levels.

FIGURE 1.—Burn trauma intensive care unit (BTICU) low-molecular-weight heparin (LMWH) dosing algorithm. Cr Cl, creatinine clearance; BMI, body mass index; HIT, heparin-induced thrombocytopenia. (Reprinted from Lin H, Faraklas I, Saffle J, et al. Enoxaparin dose adjustment is associated with low incidence of venous thromboembolic events in acute burn patients. *J Trauma.* 2011;71:1557-1561.)

previously. The dosing algorithm, included as Fig 1, is included in this selection to help facilitate enoxaparin dosing in clinical practice.

D. W. Mozingo, MD

Health-Related Quality of Life 2 Years to 7 Years After Burn Injury

Öster C, Willebrand M, Ekselius L (Uppsala Univ, Sweden)
J Trauma 71:1435-1441, 2011

Background.—Knowledge concerning the trajectory and predictors of health-related quality of life (HRQoL) years after burn injury is fragmentary and these factors were therefore assessed using the EQ-5D questionnaire.

Methods.—Consecutive adult burn patients were included during hospitalization and assessed at 3 months, 6 months, and 12 months. In addition, an interview was performed at 2 years to 7 years postburn. Data concerning injury characteristics, sociodemographic variables, psychiatric disorders, and HRQoL were obtained.

Results.—The EQ-5D dimension Mobility improved between hospitalization and 3 months, while Anxiety/Depression improved between 12 months and 2 years to 7 years. Other dimensions improved gradually. At 2 years to 7 years, only the dimensions Pain/Discomfort and Usual activities were lower than in the general population. In addition, overall HRQoL was lower than in the general population when measured by EQ VAS but not by EQ-5D index. EQ-5D index at 2 years to 7 years was predicted by EQ-5D index at 12 months and concurrent work status and pain. EQ VAS at 2 years to 7 years was predicted by previous assessments of work status, posttraumatic stress disorder and EQ VAS, and concurrent work status and substance abuse. Total amount of explained variance ranged between 17% and 57%.

Conclusions.—HRQoL after burn is conveniently screened by EQ VAS. Impairment after 2 years to 7 years is mainly reflected in the EQ dimensions Pain/Discomfort and Usual activities and can be predicted in part by information available before or at 12 months.

▶ Survival from major burn injury is now common and many have advocated that much more attention be directed toward assessment of functional and quality of life—related outcomes. This selection was chosen because the investigators show that former burn patients' quality of life assessment was lower than that of the general population. The regression analyses revealed that both the EQ-5D index and the EQ Visual Analog Scale at 12 months were predictors of long-term quality of life impairment, as were posttraumatic stress disorder at 12 months and an active work status when injured. In the extended model, any substance use disorder, pain, and work status were significant contributors. Improvement over time was also noted in 2 studies. In 1 of those studies, health-related quality of life had returned to near-normal levels at 12 months, although the groups with larger burn size and more in-hospital psychological distress were still functioning at lower levels relative to a general population.

D. W. Mozingo, MD

Nutrition in Burns: Galveston Contributions
Rodriguez NA, Jeschke MG, Williams FN, et al (The Univ of Texas Med Branch and Shriners Hosps for Children—Galveston; et al)
JPEN J Parenter Enteral Nutr 35:704-714, 2011

Aggressive nutrition support is recommended following severe burn injury. Initially, such injury results in a prolonged and persistent hypermetabolic response mediated by a 10- to 20-fold elevation in plasma catecholamines, cortisol, and inflammatory mediators. This response leads to twice-normal metabolic rates, whole-body catabolism, muscle wasting, and severe cachexia. Thus, it is relevant to review the literature on nutrition in burns to adjust/update treatment. Failure to meet the increased substrate requirements may result in impaired wound healing, multiorgan dysfunction, increased susceptibility to infection, and death. Therefore, aggressive nutrition support is essential to ensure adequate burn care, attenuate the hypermetabolic response, optimize wound healing, minimize devastating catabolism, and reduce morbidity and mortality. Here, the authors provide nutrition recommendations gained from prospective trials, retrospective analyses, and expert opinions based on the authors' practices in Galveston, Texas, and Vienna, Austria.

▶ Severe burn injury increases nutrition requirements because of the prolonged hypermetabolic response, which may lead to loss of lean body mass.

Although multiple treatment strategies have contributed to the improvements in morbidity and mortality of these patients, they have not proved sufficient to completely abate the response postinjury. Among these strategies, enteral nutrition is safe, widely available, and effective in decreasing loss of lean body mass. Enteral nutrition is beneficial in restoring and maintaining intestinal tract integrity and functionality. It should be initiated early after admission and followed by judicious assessment and monitoring of the patients' nutrition status. As patients recover after injury, they present multiple physiologic changes that make the task of nutrition assessment rather even more challenging. A major basic science and clinical translational research effort at the Shriners Burn Center in Galveston, Texas, has produced a great wealth of knowledge about nutritional support of burn patients. Led by David Herndon, MD, the research team has defined the nutritional programs necessary for good outcomes as well as other useful adjuncts to nutritional support. This selection is a comprehensive overview of Galveston's contributions to advancing our knowledge on nutritional support of burn injury.

D. W. Mozingo, MD

Overutilization of regional burn centers for pediatric patients—a healthcare system problem that should be corrected
Vercruysse GA, Ingram WL, Feliciano DV (Grady Memorial Hosp, Atlanta, GA)
Am J Surg 202:802-809, 2011

Background.—Minor burns represent .96% to 1.5% of emergency department visits, yet burn center referral is common. Analysis of the Grady Memorial Hospital Burn Center examined the feasibility and savings if pediatric burns were managed locally with as-needed consultation.

Methods.—Prospective data on 219 consecutive admissions to Grady Memorial Hospital Burn Center between December 2008 and September 2010 were reviewed. National and international cohorts were compared.

Results.—Sixty-six percent of patients were male, the mean age was 6.1 years, and 92% were insured. The most common mechanism of burning was liquid scalding (40%). Seventy percent had burns over <10% of the total body surface area, and 73% of all pediatric admissions healed without surgery. Thirty-six percent were discharged within 24 hours of admission. Forty-five percent of patients transferred from other facilities were discharged within 24 hours. Fifteen percent were transported by helicopter;

of those, 37% were discharged within 24 hours. Helicopter transport cost $12,500 and averaged 45 miles.

Conclusions.—Pediatric burns require assessment, debridement, and dressing changes. Grafting is rarely necessary. Patients are transferred because of a lack of training, and patients suffer economic burden and treatment delay. Savings could be realized were patients treated locally with select burn center referral.

▶ The problem of too many minor burns being treated in specialty burn centers identified by the authors of this selection stems from several sources. First, the American Burn Association burn center referral criteria are very liberal with respect to burn center referral of children. Also, these referral criteria have been, in part, the basis of litigation when poor outcomes have occurred in non—burn center hospitals. And the medical community as a whole has become less comfortable treating even minor burns over the last few decades. A potential solution has been suggested by the burn community itself. This is based on projections for a shortage of burn surgeons, as fewer burn surgeons are being trained than are retiring. A novel solution to this shortage proposes using general surgeons trained in acute care surgery to receive additional training in the assessment and care of minor burns while arranging for transfer of the more severely burned to regional burn centers. This need may become even more urgent in the coming years with an aging, more burn prone population. Training in burn assessment and care, however, is not currently a part of the curriculum of the proposed fellowship in acute care surgery. Burn management is also no longer required in general surgery residency training. By building collaboration between community practitioners and burn centers, in the future, the authors of this selection hope that community physicians would become more comfortable caring for minimally burned patients while also feeling comfortable collaborating with burn centers via video teleconference in dealing with more extensive burn patients. In this way, the decision to transfer to a burn center can become more of a joint decision, with optimal transfer of information between the local hospital and burn center in both directions, leading to better patient care and engaging the local physician in both educational and decision-making activities.

D. W. Mozingo, MD

Prospective Randomized Phase II Trial of Accelerated Reepithelialization of Superficial Second-Degree Burn Wounds Using Extracorporeal Shock Wave Therapy

Ottomann C, Stojadinovic A, Lavin PT, et al (Unfallkrankenhaus Berlin, Germany; Combat Wound Initiative Program, Rockville, MD; Boston Biostatistics Res Foundation, Framingham, MA; et al)
Ann Surg 255:23-29, 2012

Background.—As extracorporeal shock wave therapy (ESWT) can enhance healing of skin graft donor sites, this study focused on shock wave effects in burn wounds.

Methods.—A predefined cohort of 50 patients (6 with incomplete data or lost to follow-up) with acute second-degree burns from a larger study of 100 patients were randomly assigned between December 2006 and December 2007 to receive standard therapy (burn wound debridement/topical antiseptic therapy) with (n = 22) or without (n = 22) defocused ESWT (100 impulses/cm^2 at 0.1 mJ/mm^2) applied once to the study burn, after debridement. Randomization sequence was computer-generated, and patients were blinded to treatment allocation. The primary endpoint, time to complete burn wound epithelialization, was determined by independent, blinded-observer. A worst case scenario was applied to the missing cases to rule out the impact of withdrawal bias.

Results.—Patient characteristics across the 2 study groups were balanced ($P > 0.05$) except for older age (53 ± 17 vs. 38 ± 13 years, $P = 0.002$) in the ESWT group. Mean time to complete ($\geq 95\%$) epithelialization (CE) for patients that did and did not undergo ESWT was 9.6 ± 1.7 and 12.5 ± 2.2 days, respectively ($P < 0.0005$). When age (continuous variable) and treatment group (binary) were examined in a linear regression model to control the baseline age imbalance, time to CE, age was not significant ($P = 0.33$) and treatment group retained significance ($P < 0.0005$). Statistical significance ($P = 0.001$) was retained when ESWT cases with missing follow-up were assigned the longest time to CE and when controls with missing follow-up were assigned the shortest time to CE.

Conclusions.—In this randomized phase II study, application of a single defocused shock wave treatment to the superficial second-degree burn wound after debridement/topical antiseptic therapy significantly accelerated epithelialization. This finding warrants confirmation in a larger phase III trial (ClinicalTrials.gov identifier: NCT01242423) (Fig 2).

▶ In this randomized phase II clinical trial, application of a single defocused shockwave treatment to the superficial second-degree burn wound significantly

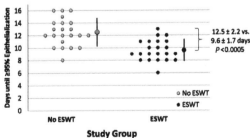

Mean number of days from burn to ≥95% epithelialization

Actual time to complete reepithelialization in patients with and without ESWT with group means and standard deviations shown to right of each group cluster.

FIGURE 2.—Mean number of days from burn to ≥95% epithelialization. (Reprinted from Ottomann C, Stojadinovic A, Lavin PT, et al. Prospective randomized phase II trial of accelerated reepithelialization of superficial second-degree burn wounds using extracorporeal shock wave therapy. *Ann Surg.* 2012;255: 23-29. © Southeastern Surgical Congress.)

accelerated reepithelialization at the treated site compared with controls. This occurred even in light of the fact that the treated patients were on average older than those in the control group. Extracorporeal shock wave therapy (ESWT) superiority warrants confirmation in a larger prospective, randomized clinical trial. ESWT may prove to be a feasible, noninvasive, safe, and cost-effective method to enhance the healing of both skin graft donor sites and superficial second-degree burns. The authors of this selection have previously reported similar findings in split thickness skin graft donor sites treated with ESWT. The positive effect of shock wave therapy on ischemic skin flap survival was demonstrated in a rat model of ischemic epigastric skin flaps where the areas of necrotic zones were reduced. This was associated with enhanced growth factor expression. Fig 2 is included in this selection demonstrating the wound healing enhancement observed with ESWT. Larger trials are warranted to confirm these findings.

D. W. Mozingo, MD

The Effect of Ketamine Administration on Nocturnal Sleep Architecture
Gottschlich MM, Mayes T, Khoury J, et al (Univ of Cincinnati College of Medicine, OH; Cincinnati Children's Hosp Med Ctr, OH)
J Burn Care Res 32:535-540, 2011

Substantial evidence exists in the acute, rehabilitative and outpatient settings demonstrating the presence of significant sleep pattern disturbances after burn injury. Although the etiology is multifactorial and includes environmental, injury, and treatment mediators, previous clinical studies have not analyzed the critically important relationship of various medications to sleep architecture. The purpose of this investigation was to describe the after-effect of ketamine on sleep patterns in seriously ill burn patients. Forty pediatric patients with a mean TBSA burn of 50.1 ± 2.9% (range, 22−89%) and full-thickness injury of 43.2 ± 3.6% (range, 24−89%) were enrolled in this sleep study. Twenty-three of the 40 patients received ketamine on the day of polysomnography testing. Standard polysomnographic sleep variables were measured from 10:00 PM until 7:00 AM. Chi-square test and t-test were used for comparison of descriptive variables between the ketamine and nonketamine groups. A logarithmic transformation was used for analysis when necessary. Ketamine administration was associated with reduced rapid eye movement (REM) sleep when compared with patients who did not receive ketamine on the day of the sleep study ($P < 0.04$). Both ketamine and nonketamine groups were clearly REM deficient when compared with nonburn norms. There was no relationship between ketamine use and effect on nocturnal total sleep time, number of awakenings, or percent of time awake or in stage 1, 2, or 3 + 4 sleep. In conclusion, ketamine was associated with altered sleep architecture as evidenced by a reduction in REM sleep. This finding does not seem to be clinically significant when considering the magnitude of overall REM sleep pattern disturbance observed in both the ketamine and nonketamine groups compared with nonburn norms. Further research is required to identify potential mechanisms of disturbed sleep so that appropriate interventions can be developed.

▶ Burn patients have severely disturbed sleep patterns manifested by decreased total sleep time; fewer stages of 3 and 4 and rapid eye movement sleep; and a predominance of light sleep with frequent awakenings. The pathophysiology underlying postburn sleep deprivation has not been fully determined but includes the inherent nature of the usual noisy and well-illuminated intensive care unit, the endogenous response to burns, concomitant pain, psychological stress, and the effect of various treatments and drugs. Poor sleep is of clinical concern because it is an added stressor and may impede recovery. High-quality restorative sleep, on the other hand, is associated with improved immune function and tissue repair and improvements in endocrine and glycemic measures. The relationship of medications to changes in sleep architecture in critically ill burn patients is largely unknown. Ketamine is widely used for procedural sedation in burn patients because it maintains blood pressure and respiratory function better than most sedative or anesthetic drugs. The authors of this selection have begun to systematically analyze those interventions that may have an impact on sleep disturbance following burn injury. The same observations and data collection could be used to study many other interventions, including environmental changes. Sleep disturbance is profound in these patients and persists well past discharge in most. Unraveling this problem will be a great challenge.

D. W. Mozingo, MD

The Results of a National Survey Regarding Nutritional Care of Obese Burn Patients
Coen JR, Carpenter AM, Shupp JW, et al (Washington Hosp Ctr, DC; et al)
J Burn Care Res 32:561-565, 2011

Little is known about the nutritional needs of obese burn patients. Given the impact of obesity on the morbidity and mortality of these patients, a uniform understanding of perceptions and practices is needed. To elucidate current practices of clinicians working with the obese burn population, the authors constructed a multidisciplinary survey designed to collect this information from practitioners in United States burn centers. An electronic approach was implemented to allow for ease of distribution and completion. A portable document format (pdf) letter was e-mailed to the members of the American Burn Association and then mailed separately to additional registered dietitians identified as working in burn centers. This letter contained a link to a 29-question survey on the SurveyMonkey.com server. Questions took the form of multiple choice and free text entry. Responses were received from physicians, mid-level practitioners, registered dietitians, and nurses. Seventy-five percent of respondents defined obesity as body mass index >30. The Harris-Benedict equation was identified as the most frequently used equation to calculate the caloric needs of burn patients (32%). Fifty-eight percent indicated that they alter their calculations for the obese patient by using adjusted body weight. Calculations for estimated protein needs varied among centers. The majority did not use hypocaloric formulas for obese patients (79%). Enteral nutrition was initiated within the first 24 hours for both obese and nonobese patients at most centers. Sixty-three percent suspend enteral nutrition during operative procedures for all patients. Oral feeding of obese patients was the most preferred route, with total parenteral nutrition being the least preferred. Longer length of stay, poor wound healing, poor graft take, and prolonged intubation were outcomes perceived to occur more in the obese burn population. In the absence of supporting research, clinicians are making adjustments to the nutritional care of obese burn patients. This indicates the need for further research to determine consistent best practices.

▶ As the national prevalence of obesity continues to climb, burn centers will experience an increase in admissions of obese patients. It is well recognized that special considerations are needed when attempting to provide appropriate nutritional therapy to this population. Preexisting metabolic derangements in these patients may contribute to their increased morbidity and mortality after thermal injury. The relationship between inflammation and obesity has been examined in many studies, and an increase in the inflammatory response in burn patients may be further enhanced in those patients who are also obese. Given the impact of obesity on the morbidity and mortality from thermal injury, a better understanding of perceptions and practices is needed. Future studies in the realm of obesity nutrition in burn patients could focus on specific interventions such as indirect calorimetry, which the investigators noted as being used rarely in their respondents. A prospective study using specific methods of nutrition adjustment is needed to determine the best nutritional approach for obese burn patients as well as to determine independent risk factors for poor outcomes in this population in a more quantitative manner.

D. W. Mozingo, MD

4   Critical Care

Acute kidney injury in patients with acute lung injury: Impact of fluid accumulation on classification of acute kidney injury and associated outcomes

Liu KD, for the National Institutes of Health National Heart, Lung, and Blood Institute Acute Respiratory Distress Syndrome Network (Univ of California San Francisco; et al)
Crit Care Med 39:2665-2671, 2011

Objective.—It has been suggested that fluid accumulation may delay recognition of acute kidney injury. We sought to determine the impact of fluid balance on the incidence of nondialysis requiring acute kidney injury in patients with acute lung injury and to describe associated outcomes, including mortality.

Design.—Analysis of the Fluid and Catheter Treatment Trial, a factorial randomized clinical trial of conservative vs. liberal fluid management and of management guided by a central venous vs. pulmonary artery catheter.

Setting.—Acute Respiratory Distress Syndrome Network hospitals.

Patients.—One thousand patients.

Interventions.—None.

Measurements and Main Results.—The incidence of acute kidney injury, defined as an absolute rise in creatinine of ≥ 0.3 mg/dL or a relative change of >50% over 48 hrs, was examined before and after adjustment of serum creatinine for fluid balance. The incidence of acute kidney injury before adjustment for fluid balance was greater in those managed with the conservative fluid protocol (57% vs. 51%, $p = .04$). After adjustment for fluid balance, the incidence of acute kidney injury was greater in those managed with the liberal fluid protocol (66% vs. 58%, $p = .007$). Patients who met acute kidney injury criteria after adjustment of creatinine for fluid balance (but not before) had a mortality rate that was significantly greater than those who did not meet acute kidney injury criteria both before and after adjustment for fluid balance (31% vs. 12%, $p < .001$) and those who had acute kidney injury before but not after adjustment for fluid balance (31% vs. 11%, $p = .005$). The mortality of those patients meeting acute kidney injury criteria after but not before adjustment for fluid balance was similar to patients with acute kidney injury both before and after adjustment for fluid balance (31% vs. 38%, $p = .18$).

Conclusions.—Fluid management influences serum creatinine and therefore the diagnosis of acute kidney injury using creatinine-based definitions.

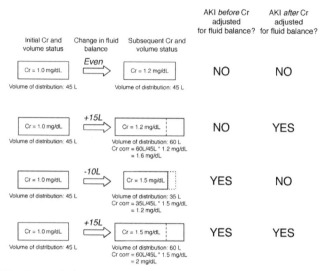

FIGURE 1.—Impact of adjustment of serum creatinine (*Cr*) for fluid balance on the ascertainment of acute kidney injury (*AKI*). (Reprinted from Liu KD, for the National Institutes of Health National Heart, Lung, and Blood Institute Acute Respiratory Distress Syndrome Network. Acute kidney injury in patients with acute lung injury: Impact of fluid accumulation on classification of acute kidney injury and associated outcomes. *Crit Care Med.* 2011;39:2665-2671, with permission from the Society of Critical Care Medicine and Lippincott Williams & Wilkins.)

Patients with "unrecognized" acute kidney injury that is identified after adjusting for positive fluid balance have higher mortality rates, and patients who have acute kidney injury before but not after adjusting for fluid balance have lower mortality rates. Future studies of acute kidney injury should consider potential differences in serum creatinine caused by changes in fluid balance and the impact of these differences on diagnosis and prognosis (Fig 1).

▶ Acute kidney injury (AKI) is a common complication in critically ill patients and is associated with a marked increase in mortality. Acute lung injury and the acute respiratory distress syndrome (ARDS) are associated with mortality rates between 25% and 40%. When patients with ARDS develop AKI, mortality rates increase to the 50% to 80% range. Over the last decade, consensus definitions have advanced the field by allowing for improved comparisons and outcome analysis. Because creatinine distributes into both the intracellular and extracellular fluid compartments, fluid accumulation may delay recognition of AKI because creatinine is diluted by the edema fluid. In conditions of negative fluid balance, creatinine may become relatively concentrated, and patients may be more likely to meet the criteria for AKI. Some argue that serum creatinine measurements should be adjusted for fluid balance and have shown that AKI is detected sooner if serum creatinine is adjusted for fluid balance in patients with AKI. The adjusted creatinine was calculated as measured serum creatinine (1 − cumulative net fluid balance/total body water). Total body water was 0.6 × patient weight. Fig 1 is included in this selection, as it shows the impact of adjustment of serum creatinine for fluid balance on the ascertainment of acute kidney injury.

D. W. Mozingo, MD

Benchmark Data From More Than 240,000 Adults That Reflect the Current Practice of Critical Care in the United States
Lilly CM, Zuckerman IH, Badawi O, et al (Univ of Massachusetts Med School, Worcester; Univ of Maryland School of Pharmacy, Baltimore; et al)
Chest 140:1232-1242, 2011

Background.—Nationwide benchmarks representing current critical care practice for the range of ICUs are lacking. This information may high-light opportunities for care improvement and allows comparison of ICU practice data.

Methods.—Data representing 243,553 adult admissions from 271 ICUs and 188 US nonfederal hospitals during 2008 were analyzed using the eICU Research Institute clinical practice database. Participating ICUs and hospitals varied widely regarding bed number, community size, academic status, geographic location, and organizational structure.

Results.—More than one-half of these critically ill adults were <65 years old, and most patients returned to their homes after hospital discharge. Most patients were admitted from an ED, had a medical admission diagnosis, and received antimicrobial therapy. Intensive treatment was common, including 27% who received mechanical ventilation, 7.5% who were supported with noninvasive ventilation, 24.3% who were treated with vasoactive infusions, > 20% who received a blood product, and 4.4% who agreed to a care limitation order during their ICU stay. Forty percent of cases had a < 10% mortality risk and did not have an intensive treatment documented.

Conclusions.—Admission to an ICU in 2008 involved active treatments that often included life support and counseling for those near the end of life and was associated with favorable outcomes for most patients.

▶ This selection provides detailed information about the current practice of critical care in the United States, including treatments provided, adherence to best practices, and acuity-adjusted outcomes. The report is based on detailed clinical practice data gathered from geographically dispersed health care systems. The data were collected and stored as part of the eICU Research Institute (eRI) data repository and included those who were discharged from the hospital during 2008 (Fig 1 in the original article). The practice patterns and acuity-adjusted outcomes provided in this selection represent benchmarks that are not available from financial or administrative databases or prior survey reports. Mortality rates, length of stay, acuity scores, treatments administered, and predicted values stratified by intensive care unit (ICU) type may be useful to monitor changes in ICU practice and to evaluate performance among the member intensive care units. The report also shows that many patients with a low mortality risk may not receive any critical care therapies during their

ICU stay. Additional studies will be needed to confirm these findings and the reliability of this extensive collection of data.

D. W. Mozingo, MD

Blood Component Ratios in Massively Transfused, Blunt Trauma Patients — A Time-Dependent Covariate Analysis

Lustenberger T, Frischknecht A, Brüesch M, et al (Goethe Univ, Frankfurt, Germany; Hosp Uster, Switzerland; Univ Hosp of Zurich, Switzerland; et al)
J Trauma 71:1144-1151, 2011

Background.—This study evaluated critical thresholds for fresh frozen plasma (FFP) and platelet (PLT) to packed red blood cell (PRBC) ratios and determined the impact of high FFP:PRBC and PLT:PRBC ratios on outcomes in patients requiring massive transfusion (MT).

Methods.—Retrospective review of a cohort of massively transfused blunt trauma patients admitted to a Level I trauma center. MT was defined as transfusion of ≥10 units of PRBC within 24 hours of admission. Critical thresholds for FFP:PRBC and PLT:PRBC ratios associated with mortality were identified using Cox regression with time-dependent variables. Impacts of high blood component ratios on 12-hour and 24-hour survival were evaluated.

Results.—During the 10-year study period, a total of 229 blunt trauma patients required a MT. At 12 hours and 24 hours after admission, a FFP:PRBC ratio threshold of 1:1.5 was found to have the strongest association with mortality. At 12 hours, 58 patients (25.4%) received a low (<1:1.5) and 171 patients (74.6%) a high (≥1:1.5) FFP:PRBC ratio. Patients in the low ratio group had a significantly higher mortality compared with those in the high ratio group (51.7% vs. 9.4%; adjusted hazard ratio [95% confidence interval] = 1.18 [1.04−1.34]; adjusted $p = 0.008$). A similar statistically significant difference was found at 24 hours after admission. For PLTs, a PLT:PRBC ratio of 1:3 was identified as the best cut-off associated with both 12-hour and 24-hour survival. At 12 hours, 79 patients (34.5%) received a low (<1:3) and 150 patients (65.5%) a high (≥1:3) PLT:PRBC ratio. After adjusting for differences between the ratio groups, no statistically significant survival advantage associated with a high PLT:PRBC ratio was found (40.5% vs. 9.3%; adjusted hazard ratio [95% confidence interval] = 1.11 [0.99−1.26]; adjusted $p = 0.082$).

Conclusion.—For massively transfused blunt trauma patients, a plasma to PRBC ratio of ≥1:1.5 was associated with improved survival at 12 hours and 24 hours after hospital admission. However, for PLTs, no statistically significant survival benefit with increasing ratio was observed. The results of this analysis highlight the need for prospective studies to evaluate the clinical significance of high blood component ratios on outcome (Table 9).

▶ Massive transfusion affects a small subset of trauma patients, ranging in incidence from 3% to 10%. Death from exsanguinating hemorrhage in this population

TABLE 9.—Clinical Outcomes in Patients Surviving 24 h Stratified by Plasma Ratio

	Total, n = 180	Low FFP: PRBC Ratio (<1:1.5), n = 21	High FFP: PRBC Ratio (≥1:1.5), n = 159	*p*	OR (95% CI)
No SIRS	3.9% (7/180)	4.8% (1/21)	3.8% (6/159)	0.587	0.78 (0.09−6.85)
SIRS 2	13.9% (25/180)	23.8% (5/21)	12.6% (20/159)	0.179	0.46 (0.15−1.40)
SIRS 3/4	41.1% (74/180)	33.3% (7/21)	42.1% (67/159)	0.441	1.46 (0.56−3.81)
Sepsis	41.1% (74/180)	38.1% (8/21)	41.5% (66/159)	0.765	1.15 (0.45−2.94)
ARDS	6.1% (11/180)	4.8% (1/21)	6.3% (10/159)	1.000	1.34 (0.16−11.05)
Infection overall	64.4% (116/180)	61.9% (13/21)	64.8% (103/159)	0.796	1.13 (0.44−2.89)
Pneumonia	38.3% (69/180)	28.6% (6/21)	39.6% (63/159)	0.328	1.64 (0.60−4.45)
Wound infection	25.6% (46/180)	28.6% (6/21)	25.2% (40/159)	0.736	0.84 (0.31−2.31)
Bacteremia	14.4% (26/180)	9.5% (2/21)	15.1% (24/159)	0.743	1.69 (0.37−7.73)
Multiple organ failure	21.1% (38/180)	23.8% (5/21)	20.8% (33/159)	0.777	0.84 (0.29−2.46)
Ventilator days, mean ± SD	12.64 ± 11.83	9.9 ± 8.7	13.0 ± 12.2	0.261	3.09 (−2.33−8.51)
Surgical ICU LOS (d), mean ± SD	18.9 ± 14.5	16.6 ± 14.3	19.2 ± 14.6	0.437	2.63 (−4.03−9.29)
Hospital LOS (d), mean ± SD	36.2 ± 25.2	38.1 ± 27.1	35.9 ± 25.0	0.704	2.23 (−9.33−13.79)
30-d mortality	15.6% (28/180)	23.8% (5/21)	14.5% (23/159)	0.332	0.54 (0.18−1.62)
In-hospital mortality	16.7% (30/180)	23.8% (5/21)	15.7% (25/159)	0.355	0.60 (0.20−1.78)

ARDS, acute respiratory distress syndrome; LOS, length of stay; SD, standard deviation; OR, odds ratio.

usually occurs early and may occur in up to 70% of patients. Most of the studies from both military and civilian trauma populations demonstrate a survival advantage from the administration of high ratios of plasma and platelets to packed red blood cells. Many institutions have implemented massive transfusion algorithms of predefined ratios of packed red blood cells, fresh frozen plasma, and platelets. The majority of studies supporting high blood component ratios during massive transfusion were performed in people injured mainly by penetrating mechanisms except where the study designs did not differentiate between injury mechanisms. In this article, the authors found no statistically significant differences in major in-hospital complications, systemic inflammatory response syndrome, or hospital or surgical ICU lengths of stay. In-hospital and 30-day mortalities were observed when the low and high fresh frozen plasma:packed red blood cell ratio groups were compared. Table 9 is included to demonstrate this point. Similarly, no differences in clinical outcomes were found when the low and high platelet:packed red blood cell ratio groups were compared. These findings conflict with many previously published reports and indicate a need for continued evaluation of this subject.

D. W. Mozingo, MD

Evaluation of Dexmedetomidine: Safety and Clinical Outcomes in Critically Ill Trauma Patients

Devabhakthuni S, Pajoumand M, Williams C, et al (Univ of Pittsburgh Med Ctr, PA; Univ of Maryland Med Ctr, Baltimore; et al)
J Trauma 71:1164-1171, 2011

Background.—To compare safety and clinical outcomes of prolonged infusions with standard-dose ($\leq$0.7 μg/kg/h) dexmedetomidine (SDD) or high-dose (>0.7 μg/kg/h) dexmedetomidine (HDD) to propofol in critically ill trauma patients.

Methods.—This was a retrospective review of 127 adult mechanically ventilated trauma patients between 2008 and 2009, who received propofol, SDD, or HDD for >24 hours. Primary outcomes were significant changes in blood pressure or heart rate. Secondary outcomes included hospital and intensive care unit (ICU) length of stay (LOS), ventilator time, and any concomitant analgesic, sedative, and antipsychotic use. Pairwise comparisons were based on Wilcoxon rank-sum test for continuous data and Pearson's chi-square test for categorical data. Statistical significance was defined as *p* value <0.05.

Results.—Patients in HDD group had higher rate of hypotension (98% vs. 78%; *p* = 0.02) but no significant differences in heart rate compared with propofol group. These patients had median longer hospital LOS (25 days vs. 12 days; *p* < 0.001), ICU LOS (20 days vs. 12 days; *p* = 0.004), and longer ventilator time (14 days vs. 7 days; *p* = 0.008). They also had increased requirements for oxycodone (74% vs. 40%; *p* = 0.003), midazolam (36% vs. 8%; *p* = 0.004), and haloperidol (50% vs. 24%; *p* = 0.02). Patients in SDD group had longer hospital LOS compared with propofol group (21 days vs. 13 days; *p* < 0.001).

Conclusion.—Higher doses of dexmedetomidine may result in higher incidence of hypotension, longer LOS, and increased concomitant analgesic, sedative, and antipsychotic use, requiring further evaluation in trauma patients (Table 7).

▶ Dexmedetomidine, a highly selective α-2-receptor agonist that acts to produce both sedative and antishivering effects, has been shown to overcome the

TABLE 7.—Clinical Outcomes

Variable*	Propofol (n = 50)	Dexmedetomidine SDD (n = 35)	HDD (n = 42)	*p*
Overall mortality	6 (12%)	1 (3%)	4 (10%)	0.35
ICU LOS (d)	12 (7–20)	17 (9–26)	20 (12–35)	0.004[†]
Hospital LOS (d)	13 (9–21)	21 (13–27)	25 (14–44)	<0.001[††]
Time on ventilator (d)	7 (4–14)	9 (5–22)	14 (8–29)	0.008[†]

*Data are presented as n (%) or median (interquartile range, 25th to 75th percentile).
[†]*p* value <0.05 indicative of significant difference when comparing HDD group to propofol group.
[‡]*p* value <0.05 indicative of significant difference when comparing SDD group to propofol group.

limitations of the γ-aminobutyric acid—mimetic sedatives. Because of its unique mechanism of action, dexmedetomidine does not significantly affect the respiratory rate and may have reduced requirements for concurrent analgesic and sedative use compared with the benzodiazepines. Currently, dexmedetomidine is approved by the Food and Drug Administration for short-term sedation, less than 24 hours, of initially intubated and mechanically ventilated patients. The differential rates of hypotension in this study, when compared with previous published reports, may also be accounted for by events independent of sedative administration, which can cause hypotension in this patient population. There are several potential reasons for the difference between this investigation and previous studies. Critically ill trauma patients are very likely to experience hemodynamic instability. Hypovolemia and hypotension from hemorrhage are compounded by vasodilatory states from systemic inflammation and sepsis. Other specific injuries, such as spinal cord injury, may also contribute to the observed differences. Some of the variance in baseline characteristics between the 3 groups in this study may explain some of the higher incidence of hypotension observed with patients in the high-dose group. Table 7 is included to summarize the major findings.

D. W. Mozingo, MD

Finding the Sweet Spot: Identification of Optimal Glucose Levels in Critically Injured Patients

Kutcher ME, Pepper MB, Morabito D, et al (Univ of California, San Francisco)
J Trauma 71:1108-1114, 2011

Background.—Conflicting data exist regarding optimal glycemic control in critically ill trauma patients. We therefore compared glucose parameters and outcomes among three different glycemic control regimens in a single trauma intensive care unit (ICU), hypothesizing that a moderate regimen would yield optimal avoidance of hyper- and hypoglycemia with equivalent outcomes when compared with a more aggressive approach.

Methods.—We retrospectively reviewed 1,422 trauma patients with at least 3-day ICU stay and five glucose measurements from May 2001 to January 2010, spanning three nonoverlapping, sequential glucose control protocols: "relaxed," "aggressive," and "moderate." For each, we extracted mean blood glucose, hypoglycemic and hyperglycemic event frequency, and glucose variability and investigated their association with outcomes.

Results.—Mortality was associated with elevated mean glucose (135.6 mg/dL vs. 126.2 mg/dL), more frequent hypoglycemic (2.67 ± 7 vs. 1.28 ± 5) and hyperglycemic (30.6 ± 28 vs. 16.0 ± 22 per 100 patient-ICU days) events, and higher glucose variability (37.1 ± 20 vs. 29.4 ± 20; all $p < 0.001$). Regression identified hyperglycemic episodes ($p < 0.05$) as an independent predictor of mortality. The "moderate" regimen had rare hyperglycemia, low glucose variability, and intermediate mean blood glucose range and frequency of hypoglycemia. Multiorgan failure and mortality did not differ between groups.

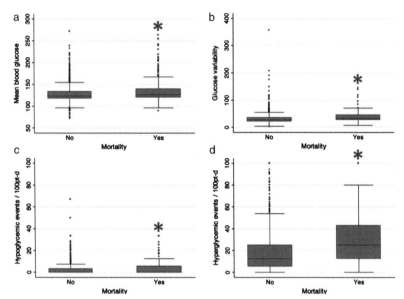

FIGURE 2.—Glycemic parameters by patient mortality. Box-whisker plots demonstrating mean blood glucose (a), glucose variability (b), and incidence of hypoglycemia (c) and hyperglycemia (d) per 100 patient-ICU days of patients who died versus those who survived. Significance by Mann-Whitney rank-sum testing with $p < 0.05$ denoted by an asterisk. (Reprinted from Kutcher ME, Pepper MB, Morabito D, et al. Finding the sweet spot: identification of optimal glucose levels in critically injured patients. *J Trauma*. 2011;71:1108-1114.)

Conclusions.—Hyperglycemic events (glucose >180 mg/dL) most strongly predicted mortality. Of glucose control protocols analyzed, the "moderate" protocol had fewest hyperglycemic events. As outcomes were otherwise equivalent between "moderate" and "aggressive" protocols, we conclude that hyperglycemia can be safely avoided using a moderate glycemic control protocol without inducing hypoglycemia (Fig 2).

▶ The association of hyperglycemia with morbidity and mortality is well documented in multiple critically ill populations. Some conflicting data and opinions exist regarding the efficacy of tight glycemic control in improving outcomes in these patient populations. A landmark prospective randomized, controlled trial of tight glycemic control published by van den Berghe et al[1] demonstrated improved outcomes in surgical intensive care unit patients with tightly controlled blood glucose. Other recent studies[2] have suggested that the increase in hypoglycemic events caused by the pursuit of tighter glycemic control regimens may be associated with increased morbidity and mortality. The authors of this article examined 3 glycemic control regimens and identified hyperglycemia as a significant predictor of mortality in the trauma patient population. Fig 2 is included as a reference to the mortality patterns. The limitations of this study include its single institution retrospective nature as well as the variability in attending trauma surgeons' practice in terms of glycemic control strategies.

The lack of criteria for mandating a standardized time period to initiate the insulin protocol makes comparison between time periods difficult.

D. W. Mozingo, MD

References

1. van den Berghe G, Wouters P, Weekers F, et al. Intensive insulin therapy in the critically ill patients. *N Engl J Med.* 2001;345:1359-1367.
2. NICE-SUGAR Study Investigators, Finfer S, Chittock DR, Su SY, et al. Intensive versus conventional glucose control in critically ill patients. *N Engl J Med.* 2009;360:1283-1297.

Gender and Acute Respiratory Distress Syndrome in Critically Injured Adults: A Prospective Study

Heffernan DS, Dossett LA, Lightfoot MA, et al (Rhode Island Hosp, Providence; et al)

J Trauma 71:878-885, 2011

Background.—The acute respiratory distress syndrome (ARDS) is a proinflammatory condition that often complicates trauma and critical illness. Animal studies have shown that both gender and sex hormones play an important role in inflammatory regulation. Human data are scant regarding the role of gender and sex hormones in developing ARDS. Our objective was to describe gender and hormonal differences in patients who develop ARDS in a large cohort of critically injured adults.

Methods.—A prospective cohort study of adult trauma patients requiring intensive care unit admission for at least 48 hours was performed. Demographic and clinical data were collected prospectively, and sex hormones were assayed at study entry (48 hours). The primary outcome was the development of ARDS. Multivariate logistic regression was used to determine the adjusted odds of death associated with differences in gender.

Results.—Six hundred forty-eight patients met entry criteria, and 180 patients developed ARDS (31%). Women were more likely to develop ARDS (35% vs. 25%, $p = 0.02$). This association remained after adjusting for age, mechanism of injury, injury severity, and blood product transfusion (odds ratio, 1.6; 95% confidence interval: 1.1−2.4; $p = 0.02$). Of patients with ARDS, there was no difference in mortality related to gender (22% mortality in women with ARDS vs. 20% in men; $p = $ not significant). A proinflammatory sex hormone profile (low testosterone and high estradiol) was associated with ARDS in both men and women.

Conclusion.—Women are more likely than men to develop ARDS after critical injury. Despite the increased incidence in ARDS, the mortality in patients with ARDS does not differ according to gender. The inflammatory properties of sex hormones may contribute to ARDS, but they do not fully explain observed gender differences (Table 1).

▶ This selection indicates that women are more likely than men to develop acute respiratory syndrome (ARDS) after critical injury. A summary of the patient

TABLE 1.—Demographic and Clinical Characteristics by Gender

	Men (n = 482)	Women (n = 166)	p
Age (yr)*	42 ± 17	45 ± 19	0.02
Body mass index (kg/m²)*	28 ± 7	28 ± 8	NS
Injury Severity Score†	29 (24–38)	34 (24–41)	NS
TRISS†	0.855	0.804	NS
AIS chest*	2.5 ± 1.7	3.0 ± 1.6	0.003
APACHE II*	17 ± 6	18 ± 5	0.03
Mechanism‡			
Blunt (%)	86	93	
Penetrating (%)	14	7	0.009
No blood product transfusion, n (%)	112 (23)	25 (15)	0.03
Mortality, n (%)	67 (14)	14 (8)	NS
ARDS, n (%)	122 (25)	58 (35)	0.02
P/F ratio 100–200	106 (87)	50 (86)	NS
Severe ARDS (P/F ratio <100)	16 (13)	8 (14)	NS

*Compared using two-sample t test.
†Compared using Wilcoxon rank sum test.
‡Compared using χ^2 test.

characteristics are included as Table 1. Despite the increased incidence of ARDS, the mortality in patients with ARDS did not differ according to gender, probably because of the relatively small number of patients developing ARDS. These findings are not fully explained by sex hormones, but there is evidence that the relationship between proinflammatory estrogens and immune-depressing testosterone and development of ARDS are important regardless of gender. The conclusions regarding sex hormones are based on a single assay at study entry. This may be misleading in that it is not clear whether the absolute values or changes in sex hormones are most important. Another limitation is that although patients are cared for according to standard practice management guidelines, the investigators did not account for differences in fluid resuscitation or ventilator management that may have influenced rates of ARDS. Interestingly, there was no difference in ventilator days between patients who did and did not develop ARDS. This also may be because of the small number of patients in each group.

D. W. Mozingo, MD

Impact of the Duration of Platelet Storage in Critically Ill Trauma Patients

Inaba K, Branco BC, Rhee P, et al (Univ of Southern California, Los Angeles, CA; Univ of Arizona, Tucson; et al)
J Trauma 71:1766-1773, 2011

Background.—There is increasing evidence that the duration of red blood cell (RBC) storage negatively impacts outcomes. Data regarding prolonged storage of other blood components, however, are lacking. The aim of this study was to evaluate how the duration of platelet storage affects trauma patient outcomes.

Methods.—Trauma patients admitted to a Level I trauma center requiring platelet transfusion (2006–2009) were retrospectively identified. Apheresis platelets (aPLT) containing $\geq 3 \times 10^{11}$ platelets/unit were used exclusively. Patients were analyzed in three groups: those who received only aPLT stored for ≤ 3 days, 4 days, and 5 days. The outcomes included mortality and complications (sepsis, acute respiratory distress syndrome, renal, and liver failure).

Result.—Three hundred eighty-one patients were available for analysis (128 received aPLT ≤ 3 days old; $109 = 4$ days old; and $144 = 5$ days old). There were no significant demographic differences between groups. Patients receiving aPLT aged $= 4$ days had significantly higher Injury Severity Score ($p = 0.022$) and were more likely to have a head Abbreviated Injury Scale ≥ 3 ($p = 0.014$). There were no differences in volumes transfused or age of RBC, plasma, cryoprecipitate, or factor VIIa. After adjusting for confounders, exposure to older aPLT did not impact mortality; however, with increasing age, complications were significantly higher. The rate of sepsis, in particular, was significantly increased (5.5% for aPLT ≤ 3 days vs. 9.2% for aPLT $= 4$ days vs. 16.7% for aPLT $= 5$ days, adjusted $p = 0.033$). For acute respiratory distress syndrome and renal and liver failure, similar trends were observed.

Conclusions.—In critically ill trauma patients, there was a stepwise increase in complications, in particular sepsis, with exposure to progressively older platelets. Further evaluation of the underlying mechanism and methods for minimizing exposure to older platelets is warranted (Table 3).

▶ Much is known about the effect of the age of packed red blood cells on their function and the detrimental effect to the patient. For platelets, the impact of the duration of storage on outcomes has not been well studied. In a single retrospective analysis of platelet transfusion in patients undergoing cardiac surgery, no association of storage age with survival or postoperative infections was

TABLE 3.—Outcomes

	aPTL Aged ≤ 3 d (n = 128)	aPTL Aged 4 d (n = 109)	aPTL Aged 5 d (n = 144)	Adjusted p
Mortality (%)	29.7% (38)	40.4% (44)	25.7% (37)	0.945
Overall complication (%)	13.3% (17)	19.3% (21)	29.2% (42)	0.005*
Sepsis (%)	5.5% (7)	9.2% (10)	16.7% (24)	0.033*
ARDS (%)	4.7% (6)	5.5% (6)	9.0% (13)	0.307
ARF (%)	5.5% (7)	5.5% (6)	8.3% (12)	0.396
Liver failure (%)	2.3% (3)	3.7% (4)	6.9% (10)	0.238
	Mean ± SD; [Median], (Range)	Mean ± SD; [Median], (Range)	Mean ± SD; [Median], (Range)	
ICU days	12.2 ± 21.6; [6], (1–181)	8.9 ± 8.7; [6], (1–52)	10.6 ± 21.6; [6], (1–181)	0.149
Hospital days	18.4 ± 25.4; [9], (1–182)	11.6 ± 12.1; [7], (1–57)	17.8 ± 23.2; [12], (1–206)	0.136

The p values were derived from multivariable analysis for ICU LOS and HLOS; and from bivariate analysis for mortality and complications. The p values were obtained after adjustment for ISS, head AIS, and platelet ABO mismatch.
*p values are significantly different ($p < 0.05$).

found. Platelets are fragile and storage requires rigorous maintenance of a tightly controlled environment, with the maximum length of storage at 5 days.

The purpose of this study was to evaluate the effect of platelet age on patient outcomes. The patients were divided into 3 cohort groups: patients who received exclusively platelets that had been stored for less than 3 days, 4 days, and 5 days. Patients who received platelets of differing age groups were excluded. The primary outcome measure examined was mortality; the secondary outcome measures were complications, intensive care unit length of stay (LOS), and hospital LOS. Table 3 is included, which summarizes the major outcome findings. Product distribution practices in which the oldest product is released first may need to be reexamined. If a medication became less effective and more harmful with storage, its release for sale would not be permitted. Why do we not have better control over our system of blood and blood-product services?

D. W. Mozingo, MD

Risk factors for positive admission surveillance cultures for methicillin-resistant *Staphylococcus aureus* and vancomycin-resistant enterococci in a neurocritical care unit

Minhas P, Perl TM, Carroll KC, et al (Johns Hopkins Univ School of Medicine, Baltimore, MD; Johns Hopkins Hosp, Baltimore, MD)
Crit Care Med 39:2322-2329, 2011

Objective.—Hospitals are under increasing pressure to perform active surveillance cultures for methicillin-resistant *Staphylococcus aureus* and vancomycin-resistant *Enterococcus*. This study aimed to identify patients at low and high risk for positive admission surveillance cultures for methicillin-resistant *Staphylococcus aureus* and vancomycin-resistant *Enterococcus* in a neurocritical care unit using readily ascertainable historical factors.

Design.—Before/after study with nested case/control study.

Setting.—Neurocritical care unit of an academic hospital.

Patients.—During the intervention period (July 2007 to June 2008), after implementation of an admission surveillance culture screening program for methicillin-resistant *Staphylococcus aureus* and vancomycin-resistant *Enterococcus*, 2,059 patients were admitted to the neurocritical care unit for a total of 5,957 patient days.

Interventions.—Cases had positive methicillin-resistant *Staphylococcus aureus* or vancomycin-resistant *Enterococcus* admission surveillance cultures within 48 hrs of hospital admission. Controls had negative cultures.

Measurements and Main Results.—Admission surveillance cultures grew methicillin-resistant *Staphylococcus aureus* and vancomycin-resistant *Enterococcus* in 35 of 823 (4.3%) and 19 of 766 (2.5%) patients, respectively. Factors significantly associated with both methicillin-resistant Staphylococcus aureus and vancomycin-resistant *Enterococcus* colonization were intravenous antibiotics and hospitalization in the past year, immunocompromised health status, intravenous drug use, long-term hemodialysis, and known prior carrier status. Transfer from an outside hospital and residence in a long-term care facility in the past year were associated with vancomycin-resistant *Enterococcus* colonization. Classification and regression tree analysis was used to identify variables that best predicted positive methicillin-resistant *Staphylococcus aureus* and vancomycin-resistant *Enterococcus* surveillance cultures. A classification and regression tree model with six of these variables yielded an overall cross-validated predictive accuracy of 87.12% to detect methicillin-resistant Staphylococcus aureus colonization. For vancomycin-resistant *Enterococcus*, a four-variable classification and regression tree model (intravenous antibiotics, hospitalization and long-term patient care in the past year, and not being "admitted same day of procedure") optimized the predictive accuracy

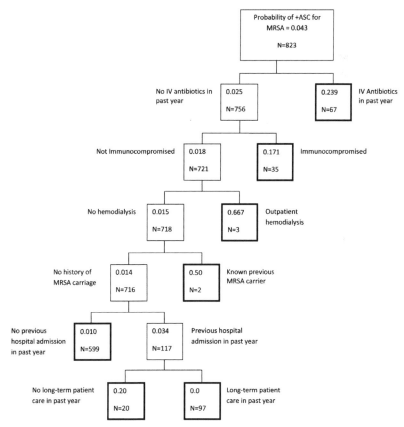

FIGURE 2.—Classification and regression tree model showing the probability of a positive active surveillance culture (+*ASC*) for methicillin-resistant *Staphylococcus aureus* (*MRSA*) (n = 823). *Unbolded boxes* represent subsets that are further split in the tree. *Bolded boxes* represent terminal nodes. Each box contains the sample size of the subset and the probability of a +ASC for MRSA. *IV,* intravenous. (Reprinted from Minhas P, Perl TM, Carroll KC, et al. Risk factors for positive admission surveillance cultures for methicillin-resistant Staphylococcus aureus and vancomycin-resistant enterococci in a neurocritical care unit. *Crit Care Med.* 2011;39:2322-2329.)

(94.91%). There were no cases of vancomycin-resistant *Enterococcus* colonization in patients admitted same day of procedure.

Conclusions.—Colonization with methicillin-resistant *Staphylococcus aureus* and vancomycin-resistant *Enterococcus* in neurocritical care patients can be predicted with a high predictive accuracy using decision trees that include four to six readily attainable risk factors. In our setting, in the absence of these risk factors and in patients admitted from home for neurosurgical procedures, routine admission surveillance cultures to the intensive care unit may not be cost-effective (Fig 2).

▶ A low but significant number of patients admitted to intensive care units are colonized with methicillin-resistant *Staphylococcus aureus* (MRSA) and vancomycin-resistant *Enterococcus* (VRE), and accurate identification of these patients is needed. A history of prior colonization only identifies a small fraction of patients at risk. In this article, the authors demonstrate that 89% of MRSA and 95% of VRE would not have been identified by prior history of MRSA or VRE colonization alone. They showed that the risk factors with the strongest predictive ability for both MRSA and VRE colonization were prior intravenous antibiotic usage and hospital admission in the past year. Other important factors for MRSA colonization were immunocompromised health status, outpatient hemodialysis, and prior MRSA carrier status. Fig 2 demonstrates this screening process for MRSA. For VRE, patients admitted from home on the same day of procedure were not likely to be colonized. These predictors need to be reevaluated in a prospective validation study, but their use may enable more cost-effective surveillance programs in the future.

D. W. Mozingo, MD

The biochemical effects of restricting chloride-rich fluids in intensive care
Yunos NM, Kim IB, Bellomo R, et al (Austin Hosp, Melbourne, Australia; et al)
Crit Care Med 39:2419-2424, 2011

Objective.—To determine the biochemical effects of restricting the use of chloride-rich intravenous fluids in critically ill patients.

Design.—Prospective, open-label, before-and-after study.

Setting.—University-affiliated intensive care unit.

Patients.—A cohort of 828 consecutive patients admitted over 6 months from February 2008 and cohort of 816 consecutive patients admitted over 6 months from February 2009.

Interventions.—We collected biochemical and fluid use data during standard practice without clinician awareness. After a 6-month period of education and preparation, we restricted the use of chloride-rich fluids (0.9% saline [Baxter, Sydney, Australia], Gelofusine [BBraun, Melsungen, Germany], and Albumex 4 [CSL Bioplasma, Melbourne, Australia]) in the intensive care unit and made them available only on specific intensive care unit specialist prescription.

Measurements and Main Results.—Saline prescription decreased from 2411 L in the control group to 52 L in the intervention group (*p* < .001), Gelofusine from 538 to 0 L (*p* < .001), and Albumex 4 from 269 to 80 L (*p* < .001). As expected, Hartmann's lactated solution prescription increased from 469 to 3205 L (*p* < .001), Plasma-Lyte from 65 to 160 L (*p* < .05), and chloride-poor Albumex 20 from 87 to 268 L (*p* < .001). After intervention, the incidence of severe metabolic acidosis (standard base excess <−5 mEq/L) decreased from 9.1% to 6.0% (*p* < .001) and severe acidemia (pH <7.3) from 6.0% to 4.9% (*p* < .001). However, the intervention also led to significantly greater incidence of severe metabolic alkalosis (standard base excess >5 mEq/L) and alkalemia (pH >7.5) with an increase from 25.4% to 32.8% and 10.5% to 14.7%, respectively (*p* < .001). The time-weighted mean

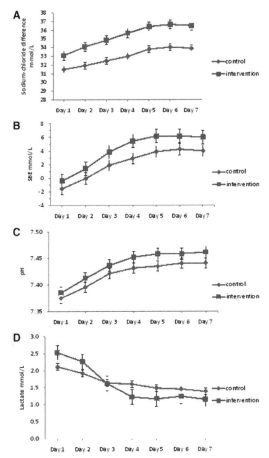

FIGURE 1.—Changes of daily means (ses) in sodium chloride difference (*A*), standard base excess (*SBE*) (*B*), pH (*C*), and lactate (*D*) for the first seven intensive care unit days. (Reprinted from Yunos NM, Kim IB, Bellomo R, et al. The biochemical effects of restricting chloride-rich fluids in intensive care. *Crit Care Med.* 2011;39:2419-2424.)

chloride level decreased from 104.9 ± 4.9 to 102.5 ± 4.6 mmol/L ($p < .001$), whereas the time-weighted mean standard base excess increased from 0.5 ± 4.5 to 1.8 ± 4.7 mmol/L ($p < .001$), mean bicarbonate from 25.3 ± 4.0 to 26.4 ± 4.1 mmol/L ($p < .001$) and mean pH from 7.40 ± 0.06 to 7.42 ± 0.06 ($p < .001$). Overall fluid costs decreased from $15,077 (U.S.) to $3,915.

Conclusions.—In a tertiary intensive care unit in Australia, restricting the use of chloride-rich fluids significantly affected electrolyte and acid-base status. The choice of fluids significantly modulates acid-base status in critically ill patients (Fig 1).

▶ The authors of this article conducted a before-and-after study to compare the biochemical and acid-base effects of restricting the use of chloride-rich fluids, namely normal saline, in critically ill patients. They demonstrated that this restriction was associated with a significant decrease in the incidence of metabolic acidosis and acidemia and significantly lower incidence of severe hyperchloremia and hypernatremia. Conversely, it increased the incidence of metabolic alkalosis and alkalemia. Fig 1 is included to outline these changes. Further studies are needed to assess the physiological and clinical impact of these biochemical and acid-base changes on patient outcomes. In many cases in critical care, a low serum sodium level is treated with additional sodium infusion in the form of normal saline solution. In many instances, what is actually needed is the reduction of free water administration. A significant cost savings was also observed in this study because of the reduction in use of normal saline.

D. W. Mozingo, MD

5 Transplantation

Introduction

Organ transplantation has now become the standard of care for many diseases. It is unfortunate that the number of people needing organs is so much greater than the number of organ donors. This inequity has led to people moving from one country to another to acquire organs. The Global Transplant Observatory has been established to follow the structure and yield from the world's systems to identify organ donors and is discussed in the article by Mahillo et al.[1] However, while organ transplantation may be the optimal form of therapy for organ failure, there are consequences from chronic immunosuppression, waiting for organs, and underlying diseases. The first series of articles addresses some of the broad issues associated with our increasing understanding of the effects of organ transplantation upon populations. Engels et al[2] describe registry cross links between transplant and cancer databases. While some cancers occur with increased frequency after transplantation, it is not uniform. There is clearly much to be learned about risks and comorbidities associated with neoplasia. Much of what we know about population risks associated with organ failure and issues described above comes from large databases. The incidence of postoperative lymphoma was compared from the UNOS/OPTN registry database as compared with the Medicare claims based data. There is as much as a 2-fold difference in the frequency of this disease.[3] This sort of analysis will ultimately allow for the placement of confidence limits around the conclusions drawn from different population databases. The article by Deshpande et al[4] uses meta-analysis of existing literature to discern outcomes of pregnancy after organ transplantation. The impact of chronic disease, the immunosuppressive drugs, and the transplant upon the likelihood and course of pregnancy is a frequent topic for men and women of child-bearing age. The finding of increased fertility after kidney transplantation is encouraging for those wanting to start a family but is sobering with respect to an increased frequency of preeclampsia, gestational diabetes, maternal hypertension, and birth weight of the child. It was interesting that the authors did not choose to analyze birth defects as one of the outcomes of pregnancy, as this is such a frequently asked question. Another group receiving special attention is children. An analysis of the USRDS database in the article by Foster et al[5] was performed to assess the long-term exposure to the "transplant milieu." The survival benefit of organ transplantation compared with dialysis was assessed after first, second, and third transplant. This important manuscript with multiple variables is muddied by the complexity of the groups. Survival benefit is demonstrated, but the cardiovascular-, infection-, and malignancy-related mortalities are all increased by the effects of chronic immunosuppression and the other factors associated with having received a kidney transplant. Safety in the system is an important variable and with the national concerns about resident work hours and physician fatigue, time of day that a procedure is performed will be the subject of concern. The study by George et al[6] addresses the questions of the time of day that a transplant is performed and outcomes. It is not at all surprising that outcomes were not influenced by the time of performance of the procedure. In fact surgical reasons for graft and patient loss do not dominate 1-year outcomes. Many other system-related issues of monitoring and follow-up far outweigh the vagaries associated with operator fatigue. There is no doubt that if a surgeon is fatigued that there will be some variances in outcomes, but as shown in this article, it is difficult to find them compared with the much more influential issues associated with transplant outcomes. The issue associated with equitable distribution of organs has been a source of discussion for decades, especially as it relates to ethnicity of the recipients. To the extent that the ethnicity of organ recipients does not look like those on the waitlist, which does not reflect the ethnic distribution of the people with disease in the country, it becomes necessary to explain the differences. Rather than discussing ethnic issues as it pertains to kidney recipients (the usual example on this topic), Liu et al[7] looks at over 20 years of lung transplantation. Prior to 2000, there was a survival difference between whites and nonwhites after lung transplantation. However, in more recent times, the percentage of nonwhites receiving lungs has increased and the survival has improved so that the white survival benefit from ethnicity has been eliminated. This analysis is encouraging. A goal in the development of an equitable organ allocation system is to preserve medical benefit while being cognizant of social goals of the population. This was part of the move towards the Lung Allocation Score (LAS) initiated in 2005. The system appears to have been initially successful. The "best" use for the recipient argument is a continual discussion and is especially applicable for the pediatric kidney recipient, where it is anticipated that the child will require more than one transplant during his or her lifetime. The role of matching histocompatibility antigens between donor organ and recipient has been hotly contested. While histocompatibility matching may represent "free" immunosuppression, the restriction of access to compatible organs may make the price too high. Vu et al[8] address some of the points of best outcomes and access to availability. This controversial subject is addressed through a single-center analysis, which unfortunately overlays local practice issues upon more broad-based policy and outcome decisions. Disease transmission through organ transplantation and the biovigilance systems that monitor and address risk assessment issues have become major points of interest in media, government and community during the past few years. The report by Ison et al[9] describes a series of events around a high-profile disease transmission that triggered the new round of discussions. This report details some of the important process issues surrounding donor assessment, informed consent, testing, and recipient follow-up. How exactly the national discussion will end remains to be seen.

With few really new agents being developed for transplant immunosuppression, there are multiple attempts to optimize existing drugs. Lymphocyte depletion has been a mainstay of many US programs after kidney transplantation. Hanaway et al[10] compare 2 regimens of lymphocyte depletion: alemtuzumab and rabbit antithymocyte polyclonal globulin for high immunologic risk patients and alemtuzumab and nondepleting IL-2 receptor blockade for low immunologic risk patients. Dose, frequency, and consequences of the administration are compared to the desired outcome of rejection-free graft function. In a controlled setting, the results demonstrate how truly successful transplant therapy has become, with greater than 95% and 90% 3-year patient survival in low immunologic risk and high risk, respectively. The 3-year kidney graft survival in low-risk patients was over 92% and in high risk grafts over 80%. If death-censored results are used, 3-year graft survival exceeded 90%. These results are not without morbidity, but the evolution of therapy over the past decade has been profound. A substantial effort is now being made to better understand the processes by which the immune system interacts with the transplanted organ. Recognition that the immune system has significant counter regulatory components has opened insights into new opportunities for graft prolongation. The Foxp3+ cell is active in modulating the immune response to specific antigens. The article by Bestard et al[11] describes the staining of these cells in 6-month protocol kidney biopsies and subsequent graft outcomes. The presence of these cells in an inflammatory infiltrate (subclinical rejection) was associated with an improved 5-year graft function contrasted with the same infiltrate but fewer Foxp3+ cells. An interesting subanalysis in this article demonstrated that mTOR-based immunosuppression regimens were more likely to have Foxp+ cells. It is clear that much work will be forthcoming in this field with a better understanding of mechanisms leading to immunologic modulations. However, before concluding that chronic kidney graft function is the consequence of alloresponses, Dzabic et al[12] raise the specter that the interaction with other immunogens contributes to altered outcomes. Analyzing biopsy material for CMV proteins, the authors demonstrated that high expression of viral proteins early after transplant was associated with increased late allograft damage and that chronic graft failure was associated with significant antigen expression. Intragraft immunologic activity is dynamic and should probably be routinely reassessed. In light of these articles, a clinical report about the use of protocol biopsy at year after transplantation was discussed in the article by Thierry et al.[13] The histology in the "stable" graft is a tool to assess the long-term function of the kidney. In this report, protocol biopsies of stable kidneys demonstrated subclinical inflammatory infiltrates in about 30% of the grafts. These kidneys were more likely to lose function with time. This group did not chronicle the types of infiltrating cells, the stimulus for the inflammation to be present, or changes in therapy that might alter subsequent outcomes. There are many variables that remain unknown about the long-term immune response to the transplanted graft. A vexing problem for the kidney transplantation community has been care for the individual with pre-existing immunity/antibodies to human alloantigens. The next two articles[14,15] discuss two aspects of this population. The first compares transplant outcomes and the techniques that identify alloantibodies. This simple idea has become quite muddy as there are now multiple techniques that identify antibodies and the different techniques possess different specificities. It is not surprising that best results still are associated when the organ antigens do not elicit a cytotoxic response. However, the observation that alloantibodies can be detected through flow cytometry or beads coated in alloantigen stresses that the immune response is not binary but is on a continuum. Montgomery et al[15] discuss the Johns Hopkins experience with attempts to reduce alloantibody levels and get patients transplanted. The controls in this study matched outcomes for what would have happened to the sensitized patient without a transplant—either stay on dialysis or wait for an "appropriately" matched kidney. In both settings, the desensitized patient fared statistically better than the continued waiting. Certainly when assessing the response adequacy to therapy, the tools used to detect alloantibody will come into play and will drive results. Optimization of transplant therapies will require new understanding of the modulation of immunologic responses. The final issue addressed in the select by Huang et al[16] is timing for organ transplantation. While preemptive kidney transplantation has been shown to result in better long-term outcomes, the role of transplantation and survival for the type 1 diabetic is a bit more uncertain. Analyzing the OPTN database, survival with either live donor kidney with or without pancreas and combined kidney/pancreas improved survival compared with preemptive deceased kidney transplantation. Discerning what specific outcome is sought is crucial for data analysis. Keeping the outcome of the individual patient is central to discussing allocation, processes, and changes.

Patients in need of liver transplantation are experiencing increasing difficulty obtaining an organ. The current MELD allocation scheme directs livers to the sickest individuals. This model by necessity directs livers away from those individuals with a lower perioperative risk and into a sicker population. Live liver transplantation has been somewhat controversial in the United States because of donor morbidities. The analysis done by the consortium from the NIH-sponsored A2ALL study[17] compares the outcomes for patients receiving either a live liver transplant or waiting for an organ from a deceased donor. The recipient of a live liver graft had a survival benefit over a similar person waiting for an organ from a deceased donor for all MELD scores. The only caveat to this conclusion was in those individuals with hepatocellular carcinoma where LDLT was not a benefit in the low-MELD patient. This is an important analysis that could be changed by a more robust deceased donor system, but given the current availability, it appears that live liver donation is markedly underused. An important question that is raised by this article relates to the relevancy of the A2ALL experience and outcomes seen across the country. Olthoff et al[18] compare live donor results from the centers participating in the A2ALL study consortium to that of the other living donor liver centers in the United States. Outcomes were markedly comparable, implying that the conclusions drawn from the study centers are transferrable to other programs across the country. This is an important message, especially as it relates to the overall survival benefit associated with early live liver transplantation. Live donation puts a healthy individual in jeopardy, and the desire for nonrisky expansion of the donor pool has led many to consider using the similar liver division techniques in deceased donor livers. Vagefi et al[19] discuss the experience of an A2ALL live liver center's experience with split liver transplantation. The in situ split has better results than an ex vivo split, but in either event there are more technical complications in the recipient than with whole grafts. However, the outcomes are satisfactory and allow for expansion of the numbers of individuals that could benefit from organ transplantation. Because of the selectivity of which donor livers are appropriate to split, the total number of available grafts is somewhat limited. However, the conclusion that the increased morbidity is acceptable because of the limited availability of organs seems sound, even without solid data. With a dearth of organs, it is hardly necessary to find new indications for liver transplantation, but the article by Mathurin et al[20] addresses outcomes for one of the more controversial indications: severe alcoholic hepatitis. There has been an aversion to transplanting people with this disease for a variety of medical and social reasons. However, the outcomes are surprisingly good with a substantial follow-up. Despite the social discussion, the medical outcomes are such that this article raises many important issues relating to indications for liver transplantation and how allocations should proceed.

Interestingly, while the biology of organ transplantation continues to evolve, the discussion about its application within the healthcare arena is becoming an increasingly important discussion with economic and resource usage endpoints. The importance of the biologic impact and new technology upon resource usage must be intertwined in the upcoming years.

Timothy L. Pruett, MD

References

1. Mahillo B, Carmona M, Álvarez M, White S, Noel L, Matesanz R. 2009 global data in organ donation and transplantation: activities, laws, and organization. *Transplantation.* 2011;92:1069-1074.
2. Engels EA, Pfeiffer RM, Fraumeni JF Jr, et al. Spectrum of cancer risk among US solid organ transplant recipients. *JAMA.* 2011;306:1891-1901.
3. Kasiske BL, Kukla A, Thomas D, et al. Lymphoproliferative disorders after adult kidney transplant: epidemiology and comparison of registry report with claims-based diagnoses. *Am J Kidney Dis.* 2011;58:971-980.
4. Deshpande NA, James NT, Kucirka LM, et al. Pregnancy outcomes in kidney transplant recipients: a systematic review and meta-analysis. *Am J Transplant.* 2011;11:2388-2404.
5. Foster BJ, Dahhou M, Zhang X, Platt RW, Hanley JA. Change in mortality risk over time in young kidney transplant recipients. *Am J Transplant.* 2011;11:2432-2442.

6. George TJ, Arnaoutakis GJ, Merlo CA, et al. Association of operative time of day with outcomes after thoracic organ transplant. *JAMA*. 2011;305:2193-2199.
7. Liu V, Weill D, Bhattacharya J. Racial disparities in survival after lung transplantation. *Arch Surg*. 2011;146:286-293.
8. Vu LT, Baxter-Lowe LA, Garcia J, et al. HLA-DR matching in organ allocation: balance between waiting time and rejection in pediatric kidney transplantation. *Arch Surg*. 2011;146:824-829.
9. Ison MG, Llata E, Conover CS, et al. Transmission of human immunodeficiency virus and hepatitis C virus from an organ donor to four transplant recipients. *Am J Transplant*. 2011;11:1218-1225.
10. Hanaway MJ, Woodle ES, Mulgaonkar S, et al. Alemtuzumab induction in renal transplantation. *N Engl J Med*. 2011;364:1909-1919.
11. Bestard O, Cuñetti L, Cruzado JM, et al. Intragraft regulatory T cells in protocol biopsies retain Foxp3 demethylation and are protective biomarkers for kidney graft outcome. *Am J Transplant*. 2011;11:2162-2172.
12. Dzabic M, Rahbar A, Yaiw KC, et al. Intragraft cytomegalovirus protein expression is associated with reduced renal allograft survival. *Clin Infect Dis*. 2011;53:969-976.
13. Thierry A, Thervet E, Vuiblet V, et al. Long-term impact of subclinical inflammation diagnosed by protocol biopsy one year after renal transplantation. *Am J Transplant*. 2011;11:2153-2161.
14. Higgins R, Lowe D, Hathaway M, et al. Human leukocyte antigen antibody-incompatible renal transplantation: excellent medium-term outcomes with negative cytotoxic crossmatch. *Transplantation*. 2011;92:900-906.
15. Montgomery RA, Lonze BE, King KE, et al. Desensitization in HLA-incompatible kidney recipients and survival. *N Engl J Med*. 2011;365:318-326.
16. Huang E, Wiseman A, Okumura S, Kuo HT, Bunnapradist S. Outcomes of preemptive kidney with or without subsequent pancreas transplant compared with pre-emptive simultaneous pancreas/kidney transplantation. *Transplantation*. 2011;92:1115-1122.
17. Berg CL, Merion RM, Shearon TH, et al. Liver transplant recipient survival benefit with living donation in the model for endstage liver disease allocation era. *Hepatology*. 2011;54:1313-1321.
18. Olthoff KM, Abecassis MM, Emond JC, et al. Outcomes of adult living donor liver transplantation: comparison of the Adult-to-adult Living Donor Liver Transplantation Cohort Study and the national experience. *Liver Transpl*. 2011;17:789-797.
19. Vagefi PA, Parekh J, Ascher NL, Roberts JP, Freise CE. Outcomes with split liver transplantation in 106 recipients: the University of California, San Francisco, experience from 1993 to 2010. *Arch Surg*. 2011;146:1052-1059.
20. Mathurin P, Moreno C, Samuel D, et al. Early liver transplantation for severe alcoholic hepatitis. *N Engl J Med*. 2011;365:1790-1800.

2009 Global Data in Organ Donation and Transplantation: Activities, Laws, and Organization

Mahillo B, Carmona M, Álvarez M, et al (Organización Nacional de Trasplantes, Madrid, Spain; World Health Organization, Geneva, Switzerland; et al)
Transplantation 92:1069-1074, 2011

The Global Observatory on Donation and Transplantation represents the most comprehensive source of worldwide data concerning activities in organ donation and transplantation and information on legal and organizational aspects. Of the countries reporting information, 84.7% have a national structure supervising or coordinating donation and transplantation and

91% have specific legislation. Worldwide approximately 104,065 solid organ transplants are performed each year. There is a vast difference in rates of kidney and liver transplantation, especially from deceased donor depending on the level of development. This analysis provides an overview of existing organizational structures, related legislation, and activities.

▶ Organ transplantation and donation is performed/overseen differently around the world. Significant attention has been to the need for organs and the lengths that people will go to obtain them. The need for more information about organ retrieval and allocation is necessary for improvements within national systems and to address issues relating to transplant tourism. The Global Observatory on Transplantation and Donation that is run through the World Health Organization is an important step toward improving such information. It demonstrates the tremendous heterogeneity in practice, efficiency, and organ availability for people in need of organ transplantation around the world.

T. Pruett, MD

Spectrum of Cancer Risk Among US Solid Organ Transplant Recipients
Engels EA, Pfeiffer RM, Fraumeni JF Jr, et al (Natl Cancer Inst, Rockville, MD; et al)
JAMA 306:1891-1901, 2011

Context.—Solid organ transplant recipients have elevated cancer risk due to immunosuppression and oncogenic viral infections. Because most prior research has concerned kidney recipients, large studies that include recipients of differing organs can inform cancer etiology.

Objective.—To describe the overall pattern of cancer following solid organ transplantion.

Design, Setting, and Participants.—Cohort study using linked data on solid organ transplant recipients from the US Scientific Registry of Transplant Recipients (1987- 2008) and 13 state and regional cancer registries.

Main Outcome Measures.—Standardized incidence ratios (SIRs) and excess absolute risks (EARs) assessing relative and absolute cancer risk in transplant recipients compared with the general population.

Results.—The registry linkages yielded data on 175 732 solid organ transplants (58.4% for kidney, 21.6% for liver, 10.0% for heart, and 4.0% for lung). The overall cancer risk was elevated with 10 656 cases and an incidence of 1375 per 100 000 person-years (SIR, 2.10 [95% CI, 2.06-2.14]; EAR, 719.3 [95% CI, 693.3-745.6] per 100 000 person-years). Risk was increased for 32 different malignancies, some related to known infections (eg, anal cancer, Kaposi sarcoma) and others unrelated (eg, melanoma, thyroid and lip cancers). The most common malignancies with elevated risk were non-Hodgkin lymphoma (n = 1504; incidence: 194.0 per 100 000 person-years; SIR, 7.54 [95% CI, 7.17-7.93]; EAR, 168.3 [95% CI, 158.6-178.4] per 100 000 person-years) and cancers of the lung (n = 1344; incidence: 173.4 per 100 000 person-years; SIR, 1.97 [95% CI, 1.86-2.08]; EAR, 85.3 [95% CI, 76.2-94.8] per 100 000 person-years), liver (n = 930; incidence: 120.0 per 100 000 person-years; SIR, 11.56 [95% CI, 10.83-12.33]; EAR, 109.6 [95% CI, 102.0-117.6] per 100 000 person-years), and kidney (n = 752; incidence: 97.0 per 100 000 person-years; SIR, 4.65 [95% CI, 4.32-4.99]; EAR, 76.1 [95% CI, 69.3-83.3] per 100 000 person-years). Lung cancer risk was most elevated in lung recipients (SIR, 6.13 [95% CI, 5.18-7.21]) but also increased among other recipients (kidney: SIR, 1.46 [95% CI, 1.34-1.59]; liver: SIR, 1.95 [95% CI, 1.74-2.19]; and heart: SIR, 2.67 [95% CI, 2.40-2.95]). Liver cancer risk was elevated only among liver recipients (SIR, 43.83 [95% CI, 40.90-46.91]), who manifested exceptional risk in the first 6 months (SIR, 508.97 [95% CI, 474.16-545.66]) and a 2-fold excess risk for 10 to 15 years thereafter (SIR, 2.22 [95% CI, 1.57-3.04]). Among kidney recipients, kidney cancer risk was elevated (SIR, 6.66 [95% CI, 6.12-7.23]) and bimodal in onset time. Kidney cancer risk also was increased in liver recipients (SIR, 1.80 [95% CI, 1.40-2.29]) and heart recipients (SIR, 2.90 [95% CI, 2.32-3.59]).

Conclusion.—Compared with the general population, recipients of a kidney, liver, heart, or lung transplant have an increased risk for diverse infection-related and unrelated cancers.

▶ Long-term survival of organ transplant recipients results in questions about the risk for the development of cancer after chronic immunosuppression. The authors merged large cancer and transplant databases to assess the risk of cancer in the transplant population. The conclusions were not unexpected: about a 2-fold higher incidence of cancer after transplantation, an increased incidence of tumors likely to be present in the recipient at the time of transplant (liver and lung recipients), and viral infection—associated tumors (Epstein-Barr virus, human herpesvirus 8). The risk of cancer development appears to be increased but cannot be adjusted for transplant-specific variables (possible donor derived transmission, class of immunosuppressive agents used, and number of rejection episodes) from an increased frequency caused solely by chronic immunosuppression. This is a tremendously complex field but one that recipients are entitled to understand.

T. Pruett, MD

Lymphoproliferative Disorders After Adult Kidney Transplant: Epidemiology and Comparison of Registry Report With Claims-Based Diagnoses
Kasiske BL, Kukla A, Thomas D, et al (Minneapolis Med Res Foundation, MN; Univ of Minnesota, Minneapolis; Bristol-Myers Squibb Pharmaceuticals, Plainsboro, NJ; et al)
Am J Kidney Dis 58:971-980, 2011

Background.—Posttransplant lymphoproliferative disorder (PTLD) is a major complication of kidney transplant.

Study Design.—Retrospective cohort study comparing PTLD incidence rates using US Medicare claims and Organ Procurement and Transplantation Network (OPTN) data, examining risk factors for PTLD in OPTN data, and studying recipient and graft survival after PTLD diagnosis.

Setting & Participants.—All adult first-transplant patients who underwent deceased or living donor kidney-only transplants in 2000-2006 (n = 89,485) followed up through 3 years posttransplant.

Predictors.—Recipient and donor characteristics, HLA mismatches, viral serologic test results, and initial immunosuppression.

Outcomes.—OPTN-reported or Medicare claims—based PTLD diagnosis, recipient and graft survival after OPTN-reported PTLD diagnosis.

Measurements.—Adjusted HRs for PTLD diagnosis estimated using a Cox proportional hazards model; probability of survival free of all-cause graft failure estimated using the Kaplan-Meier method.

Results.—The incidence rate of PTLD during the first posttransplant year was 2-fold higher in Medicare claims (0.46/100 patient-years; 95% CI, 0.39-0.53) than in OPTN data (0.22/100 patient-years; 95% CI, 0.17-0.27). Factors associated with increased rates of PTLD included older age, white race (vs African American), induction with T-cell—depleting antibodies, Epstein-Barr virus seronegativity at the time of transplant, and cytomegalovirus seronegativity at the time of transplant. The adjusted risk of death with graft function was 17.5 (95% CI, 14.3-21.4) times higher after a report of PTLD, and the risk of death-censored graft failure was 5.5 (95% CI, 3.9-7.7) times higher.

Limitations.—Shortcomings inherent in large databases, including inconsistencies in patient follow-up, reporting, and coding practices by transplant centers; insufficient registry data to analyze acute rejection episodes and antirejection treatment; no available data for potential effects of different types of PTLD treatment on patient outcomes.

Conclusions.—Despite the limitations of data collected by registries, PTLD clearly is an important complication; both mortality and death-censored graft failure increase after PTLD.

▶ Much of the knowledge that is used in transplantation comes from analyses of the data that are mandatorily submitted to the Organ Procurement and Transplantation Network (OPTN)/United Network for Organ Sharing (UNOS). This has proven to be extremely useful in understanding the implication of outcomes of transplantation. Because many of the analyses are predicated upon the data being reliable, a head-to-head comparative study of 2 large databases on the same population of people would serve to test the relative reliability of the system. A contrast of transplant recipients that were reported to develop posttransplant lymphoproliferative disease (PTLD) served to test the comparability of 2 large databases. The OPTN registry and the Centers for Medicare & Medicaid Services claims data demonstrated that the frequency of PTLD differed by a factor of 2 when the 2 were analyzed. While this raises some significant issues relating to data reliability, the trending analysis was still reflective of the population at risk. While confidence intervals may be of significance, the important component of this study is to stress the importance of which data are useful to assess.

T. Pruett, MD

Pregnancy Outcomes in Kidney Transplant Recipients: A Systematic Review and Meta-Analysis
Deshpande NA, James NT, Kucirka LM, et al (Johns Hopkins School of Medicine, Baltimore, MD)
Am J Transplant 11:2388-2404, 2011

Approximately 50 000 women of reproductive age in the United States are currently living after kidney transplantation (KT), and another 2800 undergo KT each year. Although KT improves reproductive function in women with ESRD, studies of post-KT pregnancies are limited to a few voluntary registry analyses and numerous single-center reports. To obtain more generalizable inferences, we performed a systematic review and meta-analysis of articles published between 2000 and 2010 that reported pregnancy-related outcomes among KT recipients. Of 1343 unique studies, 50 met inclusion criteria, representing 4706 pregnancies in 3570 KT recipients. The overall post-KT live birth rate of 73.5% (95% CI 72.1−74.9) was higher than the general US population (66.7%); similarly, the overall post-KT miscarriage rate of 14.0% (95% CI 12.9−15.1) was lower (17.1%). However, complications of preeclampsia (27.0%, 95% CI 25.2−28.9), gestational diabetes (8.0%, 95% CI 6.7−9.4), Cesarean section (56.9%, 95% CI 54.9−58.9) and preterm delivery (45.6%, 95% CI 43.7−47.5) were higher than the general US population (3.8%, 3.9%, 31.9% and 12.5%, respectively). Pregnancy outcomes were more favorable in studies with lower mean maternal ages; obstetrical complications were higher in studies with shorter mean interval between KT and pregnancy. Although post-KT pregnancy is feasible, complications are relatively high and should be considered in patient counseling and clinical decision making.

▶ A return to as normal of lifestyle as feasible is a major goal of organ transplantation. The desire to have a family is common among young adults that are markedly thwarted by end-stage kidney disease. A meta-analysis found that after kidney transplantation, an increased birth rate and decreased miscarriage rate compared with the general US population occurred. This benefit was offset by a higher rate of preeclampsia, preterm labor, gestational diabetes, lower birth weights, and rates of cesarean section. While kidney transplantation goes a long way toward restoring normal reproductive capacity, pregnancy and transplantation are still complex enough to maintain the designation as high risk.

T. Pruett, MD

Change in Mortality Risk Over Time in Young Kidney Transplant Recipients
Foster BJ, Dahhou M, Zhang X, et al (McGill Univ Faculty of Medicine, Montreal, Quebec, Canada)
Am J Transplant 11:2432-2442, 2011

Mortality risk for kidney transplant recipients may change with increasing accumulated exposure to the "transplantation milieu." We sought to characterize changes over time in mortality rate and in age-, sex- and race-standardized mortality ratios (SMR) relative to the general population, and to estimate the association between increasing time since first transplant and mortality risk. A total of 18 911 patients who received a first transplant at <21 years old (1983—2006), and whose data were recorded in the USRDS, were studied. There were 2713 deaths over a median follow-up of 8.9 (interquartile range 4.0—14.5; maximum 23) years. Among those with graft function, mortality was highest in the first post transplant year; beyond the first year of the first transplant, age-adjusted mortality rates and SMRs decreased slightly over follow-up. Cause of death was cardiovascular for 34.6%, infection for 19.5%, malignancy for 5.8%, other for 21.4% and unknown for 18.7%. For every 1-year time increment after the end of the first post transplant year, age-adjusted all-cause and cardiovascular mortality rates fell by 1% (p = 0.06) and 16% (p = 0.007), respectively; infection-related mortality rate did not change over time (p = 0.5). These results suggest that exposure to the transplantation milieu has no cumulative negative effects on cardiovascular health over the long term.

▶ Children represent a special category as transplant recipients. The benefit of a successful kidney transplant for growth and mental development has long been recognized. An analysis of the USRDS database assessed the effect of the "transplant milieu" on survival after kidney transplantation/retransplantation/dialysis. Kidney failure in children is a serious risk for life. While transplantation improves survival compared with dialysis, it is not surprising that when undergoing a major surgical procedure and being administered immunosuppression, overall survival is less likely than in the general population. Cardiovascular disease is a significant cause of mortality in the pediatric age group, and understanding and managing the variables of this risk is important. However, there are infection and malignancy issues that need to be reassessed under retransplant circumstances. As kids often require multiple transplants, anticipating probable complications in advance is important.

T. Pruett, MD

Association of Operative Time of Day With Outcomes After Thoracic Organ Transplant

George TJ, Arnaoutakis GJ, Merlo CA, et al (Johns Hopkins Med Institutions, Baltimore, MD)
JAMA 305:2193-2199, 2011

Context.—Recent emphasis on systems-based approaches to patient safety has led to several studies demonstrating worse outcomes associated with surgery at night.

Objective.—To evaluate whether operative time of day was associated with thoracic organ transplant outcomes, hypothesizing that it would not be associated with increased morbidity or mortality.

Design, Setting, and Participants.—We conducted a retrospective cohort study of adult heart and lung transplant recipients in the United Network for Organ Sharing database from January 2000 through June 2010. Primary stratification was by operative time of day (night, 7 PM-7 AM; day, 7 AM-7 PM).

Main Outcome Measures.—Primary end points were short-term survival, assessed by the Kaplan-Meier method at 30, 90, and 365 days. Secondary end points encompassed common postoperative complications. Risk-adjusted multivariable Cox proportional hazards regression examined mortality.

Results.—A total of 27 118 patients were included in the study population. Of the 16 573 who underwent a heart transplant, 8346 (50.36%) did so during the day and 8227 (49.64%) during the night. Of the 10 545 who underwent a lung transplant, 5179 (49.11%) did so during the day and 5366 (50.89%) during the night. During a median follow-up of 32.2 months (interquartile range, 11.2-61.1 months), 8061 patients (28.99%) died. Survival was similar for organ transplants performed during the day and night. Survival rates at 30 days for heart transplants during the day were 95.0% vs 95.2% during the night (hazard ratio [HR], 1.05; 95% confidence interval, 0.83-1.32; *P* =.67) and for lung transplants during the day were 96.0% vs 95.5% during the night (HR, 1.22; 95% CI, 0.97-1.55; *P* =.09). At 90 days, survival rates for heart transplants were 92.6% during the day vs 92.7% during the night (HR, 1.05; 95% CI, 0.88-1.26; *P* =.59) and for lung transplants during the day were 92.7% vs 91.7% during the night (HR, 1.23; 95% CI, 1.04-1.47; *P* =.02). At 1 year, survival rates for heart transplants during the day were 88.0% vs 87.7% during the night (HR, 1.05; 95% CI, 0.91-1.21; *P* =.47) and for lung transplants during the day were 83.8% vs 82.6% during the night (HR, 1.08; 95% CI, 0.96-1.22; *P* =.19). Among lung transplant recipients, there was a slightly higher rate of airway dehiscence associated with nighttime transplants (57 of 5022 [1.1%] vs 87 of 5224 [1.7%], *P* =.02).

Conclusion.—Among patients who underwent thoracic organ transplants, there was no significant association between operative time of day and survival up to 1 year after organ transplant.

▶ Transplantation is performed when organs are available and not by routine operating room schedules. The increasing national concern with operator fatigue and work hours led to the study that assessed heart transplant outcomes as a function of the time of day the procedure was performed. The finding that outcomes were similar whether a transplant was performed during day or night is reassuring but only reemphasizes that organ transplant results are heavily influenced by nonsurgical decision making. The typical reasons for graft failure and patient death are only partially explained by surgical decision making. In this sort of analysis, variances in surgical decision-making induced by the cycle of the day will be minimized in the more dominant variables.

T. Pruett, MD

Racial Disparities in Survival After Lung Transplantation
Liu V, Weill D, Bhattacharya J (Stanford Univ, CA)
Arch Surg 146:286-293, 2011

Context.—Racial disparities have not been comprehensively evaluated among recipients of lung transplantation.

Objectives.—To describe the association between race and lung transplant survival and to determine whether racial disparities have changed in the modern (2001-2009) compared with the historical (1987-2000) transplant eras.

Design, Setting, and Patients.—A retrospective cohort study of 16 875 adults who received primary lung transplants from October 16, 1987, to February 19, 2009, was conducted using data from the United Network of Organ Sharing.

Main Outcome Measures.—We measured the risk of death after lung transplant for nonwhites compared with whites using time-to-event analysis.

Results.—During the study period, 14 858 white and 2017 nonwhite patients underwent a lung transplant; they differed significantly at baseline. The percentage of nonwhite transplant recipients increased from 8.8% (before 1996) to 15.0% (2005-2009). In the historical era, 5-year survival was lower for nonwhites than whites (40.9% vs 46.9%). Nonwhites were at an increased risk of death independent of age, health and socioeconomic status, diagnosis, geographic region, donor organ characteristics, and operative factors (hazard ratio, 1.15; 95% confidence interval, 1.01-1.30). In subgroup analysis of the historical era, blacks had worsened 5-year survival compared with whites (39.0% vs 46.9%) and black women had worsened survival compared with white women (36.9% vs 48.9%). In the modern transplant era, survival improved for all patients. However, a greater improvement among nonwhites has eliminated the disparities in survival between the races (5-year survival, 52.5% vs 51.6%).

Conclusion.—In contrast to the historical era, there was no significant difference in lung transplant survival in the modern era between whites and nonwhites.

▶ Racial disparities in organ transplant outcomes have been repetitively discussed after kidney transplantation. These significant differences have been observed and attributed to a plethora of social, immune, and concomitant disease conditions. The contributing factors that explain the observations, however, remain to be fully elucidated. A study of the US experience (Organ Procurement and Transplantation Network database) has yielded an interesting twist on ethnic description and its effect on lung transplant survival. By analyzing 30 years of lung transplants, a variety of observations could be made. First, differences in survival observed early in the transplant experience have recently disappeared. The diseases that afflict ethnic groups are not equally distributed across the waitlist, and the ethnic distribution of those waiting and those receiving transplantable organs is not identical. The balance between optimizing outcomes and maintaining equal access for all citizens, irrespective of race or creed, is one that requires continual observation.

T. Pruett, MD

HLA-DR Matching in Organ Allocation: Balance Between Waiting Time and Rejection in Pediatric Kidney Transplantation
Vu LT, Baxter-Lowe LA, Garcia J, et al (Univ of California at San Francisco)
Arch Surg 146:824-829, 2011

Objectives.—To determine the impact of HLA-DR mismatching on rejection, graft survival, and sensitization in a local allocation system that emphasizes donor quality rather than HLA antigen matching for pediatric patients and to determine the likelihood of finding an appropriate donor based on HLA-DR mismatch.

Design.—Retrospective cohort study.

Setting.—A single institution.

Patients.—A total of 178 patients younger than 21 years who underwent kidney transplantation with daclizumab induction between 1997 and 2006.

Main Outcome Measures.—The association between HLA-DR mismatching and rejection or graft survival was determined using survival analysis. Sensitization was defined as a posttransplantation panel reactive antibody level greater than 0% in patients with a pretransplantation level of 0%.

Results.—Median follow-up was 4.1 years (interquartile range, 2.1-6.1 years). One- and 5-year graft survival rates were 97% and 82%, respectively. HLA-DRB1 mismatches were a significant risk factor for rejection; patients with 1- or 2-HLA-DRB1 mismatches had 1.7 times greater odds of rejection than those with 0-HLA-DR mismatches ($P=.006$). HLA-DRB1 mismatching was not a significant risk factor for either graft failure or sensitization, but history of rejection was an independent predictor of graft failure (hazard ratio, 7.7; $P=.01$) and sensitization (odds ratio, 9.7; $P=.001$). Although avoiding HLA-DRB1 mismatching reduces rejection, the probability of finding ABO-matched local donors younger than 35 years without DR mismatches was extremely low.

Conclusion.—Although avoiding HLA-DRB1 mismatching is beneficial, the likelihood of finding an HLA-DRB1—matched donor should also be considered in donor selection.

▶ The determination of who gets a kidney is fraught with medical vagaries and ethical conundrums. The University of California-San Francisco experience with pediatric kidney transplantation assessed the impact of HLA matching on kidney loss or becoming sensitized to other alloantigens. The authors demonstrated that HLA matching decreased the likelihood of subsequent sensitization but decreased the frequency of becoming a high priority recipient for a kidney. A rejection episode has a high risk for the generation of sensitization. This observation raises questions about patient treatment that are not addressed within the article, such as treatment with lymphocyte-depleting antibody versus corticosteroids, outcome differences between live donation and deceased donor kidneys, and time to development of acute rejection. Policy goals designed to benefit kidney children must incorporate a wide variety of variables and not be limited to univariate analyses.

T. Pruett, MD

Transmission of Human Immunodeficiency Virus and Hepatitis C Virus From an Organ Donor to Four Transplant Recipients

Ison MG, the HIV-HCV Transplantation Transmission Investigation Team (Northwestern Univ Feinberg School of Medicine, Chicago, IL; et al)
Am J Transplant 11:1218-1225, 2011

In 2007, a previously uninfected kidney transplant recipient tested positive for human immunodeficiency virus type 1 (HIV) and hepatitis C virus (HCV) infection. Clinical information of the organ donor and the recipients was collected by medical record review. Sera from recipients and donor were tested for serologic and nucleic acid-based markers of HIV and HCV infection, and isolates were compared for genetic relatedness. Routine donor serologic screening for HIV and HCV infection was negative; the donor's only known risk factor for HIV was having sex with another man. Four organs (two kidneys, liver and heart) were transplanted to four recipients. Nucleic acid testing (NAT) of donor sera and posttransplant sera from all recipients were positive for HIV and HCV. HIV nucleotide sequences were indistinguishable between the donor and four recipients, and HCV subgenomic sequences clustered closely together. Two patients subsequently died and the transplanted organs failed in the other two patients. This is the first recognized cotransmission of HIV and HCV from an organ donor to transplant recipients. Routine posttransplant HIV and HCV serological testing and NAT of recipients of organs from donors with suspected risk factors should be considered as routine practice.

▶ Human immunodeficiency virus and hepatitis C virus transmission to multiple organ recipients sparked a broad discussion within the media, transplant community, and oversight community about the relative risks of disease transmission through organ transplantation. This report describes a specific event that has been an impetus to generate new guidelines for donor and recipient assessments for disease transmission. The authors discuss limitations of current testing techniques and other facets of risk assessment. The discussion regarding individual risk assessments and system responsibility to assess those risks is increasing and will continue until there are some modifications of the existing processes.

T. Pruett, MD

Alemtuzumab Induction in Renal Transplantation

Hanaway MJ, for the INTAC Study Group (Univ of Alabama at Birmingham; et al)

N Engl J Med 364:1909-1919, 2011

Background.—There are few comparisons of antibody induction therapy allowing early glucocorticoid withdrawal in renal-transplant recipients. The purpose of the present study was to compare induction therapy involving alemtuzumab with the most commonly used induction regimens in patient populations at either high immunologic risk or low immunologic risk.

Methods.—In this prospective study, we randomly assigned patients to receive alemtuzumab or conventional induction therapy (basiliximab or rabbit antithymocyte globulin). Patients were stratified according to acute rejection risk, with a high risk defined by a repeat transplant, a peak or current value of panel-reactive antibodies of 20% or more, or black race. The 139 high-risk patients received alemtuzumab (one dose of 30 mg, in 70 patients) or rabbit antithymocyte globulin (a total of 6 mg per kilogram of body weight given over 4 days, in 69 patients). The 335 low-risk patients received alemtuzumab (one dose of 30 mg, in 164 patients) or basiliximab (a total of 40 mg over 4 days, in 171 patients). All patients received tacrolimus and mycophenolate mofetil and underwent a 5-day glucocorticoid taper in a regimen of early steroid withdrawal. The primary end point was biopsy-confirmed acute rejection at 6 months and 12 months. Patients were followed for 3 years for safety and efficacy end points.

Results.—The rate of biopsy-confirmed acute rejection was significantly lower in the alemtuzumab group than in the conventional-therapy group at both 6 months (3% vs. 15%, P<0.001) and 12 months (5% vs. 17%, P<0.001). At 3 years, the rate of biopsy confirmed acute rejection in low-risk patients was lower with alemtuzumab than with basiliximab (10% vs. 22%, P = 0.003), but among high-risk patients, no significant difference was seen between alemtuzumab and rabbit antithymocyte globulin (18% vs. 15%, P = 0.63). Adverse-event rates were similar among all four treatment groups.

Conclusions.—By the first year after transplantation, biopsy-confirmed acute rejection was less frequent with alemtuzumab than with conventional therapy. The apparent superiority of alemtuzumab with respect to early biopsy-confirmed acute rejection was restricted to patients at low risk for transplant rejection; among high-risk patients, alemtuzumab and rabbit antithymocyte globulin had similar efficacy. (Funded by Astellas Pharma Global Development; INTAC ClinicalTrials.gov number, NCT00113269.)

▶ Therapies for immunosuppression have become quite varied. This article assesses kidney transplant steroid withdrawal outcomes as a function of type of antibody induction therapy. The comparison of alemtuzumab with either thymoglobulin (antithymocyte globulin) or basiliximab (anti-IL-2R) demonstrated how successful the current regimens have become. Conventional therapies result in 1-year rejection rates of less than 20%, but with alemtuzumab, low-risk patients had a yearly rejection rate of only 5%. There are a plethora of concerns about the use of such a long depletion duration, but studies such as this reduce the concerns about routine use.

T. Pruett, MD

Intragraft Regulatory T Cells in Protocol Biopsies Retain Foxp3 Demethylation and Are Protective Biomarkers for Kidney Graft Outcome

Bestard O, Cuñetti L, Cruzado JM, et al (Hosp Universitari de Bellvitge, Barcelona, Spain; et al)
Am J Transplant 11:2162-2172, 2011

Presence of subclinical rejection (SCR) with IF/TA in protocol biopsies of renal allografts has been shown to be an independent predictor factor of graft loss. Also, intragraft Foxp3+ T_{reg} cells in patients with SCR has been suggested to differentiate harmful from potentially protective infiltrates. Nonetheless, whether presence of Foxp3 T_{reg} cells in patients with SCR and IF/TA may potentially protect from a deleterious graft outcome has not yet been evaluated. This is a case-control study in which 37 patients with the diagnosis of SCR and 68 control patients with no cellular infiltrates at 6-month protocol biopsies matched for age and time of transplantation were evaluated. We first confirmed that numbers of intragraft Foxp3-expressing T cells in patients with SCR positively correlates with Foxp3 demethylation at the T_{reg}-specific demethylation region. Patients with SCR without Foxp3+ T_{reg} cells within graft infiltrates showed significantly worse 5-year graft function evolution than patients with SCR and Foxp3+ T_{reg} cells and those without SCR. When presence of SCR and IF/TA were assessed together, presence of Foxp3+ T_{reg} could discriminate a subgroup of patients showing the same graft outcome as patients with a normal biopsy. Thus, presence of Foxp3+ T_{reg} cells in patients with SCR even with IF/TA is associated with a favorable long-term allograft outcome.

▶ Our understanding of the immunological response to the transplanted organ is undergoing a transformation. Histology has been the primary way through which we identify organ rejection. Infiltrating cells from a transplanted organ may look the same under the microscope, but they are now proving to be made up of different lymphocyte phenotypes. Regulatory T cells modify the immune response to a host of antigens and are increasingly thought to be important in the allores-ponse. This study found that cells that infiltrate the kidneys demonstrated a variety of phenotypes and that even Foxp3[+] cells within the kidney have different levels of protein expression. Our knowledge about the immunologic cellular dialogue is rapidly changing, and many more studies such as this one will help change our understanding of the response to the transplanted organ.

T. Pruett, MD

Intragraft Cytomegalovirus Protein Expression Is Associated With Reduced Renal Allograft Survival

Dzabic M, Rahbar A, Yaiw K-C, et al (Karolinska Univ Hosp, Stockholm, Sweden; et al)
Clin Infect Dis 53:969-976, 2011

Background.—Cytomegalovirus (CMV) infection is a risk factor for acute and chronic rejection of transplanted organs and is thought to mediate rejection indirectly.

Methods.—In this retrospective observational cohort study, early- and end-stage biopsies from renal allografts lost because of chronic allograft dysfunction (n = 29) were examined for CMV antigens and DNA using immunohistochemistry, in situ hybridization, and real-time polymerase chain reaction.

Results.—CMV immediate-early and late proteins were present in 27 (93%) of 29 of the end-stage chronic allograft dysfunction biopsies and in 64% of the corresponding early biopsies but not in pretransplant biopsies from CMV-seronegative donors (n = 3). Graft survival time was reduced in patients with moderate or high CMV levels in the graft soon after transplantation compared with that in patients with no or low CMV levels in the graft. No significant difference was observed in serum creatinine obtained at the time of early biopsies.

Conclusions.—We provide evidence that intragraft CMV protein expression is associated with end-stage chronic renal allograft dysfunction, that intragraft CMV levels increase as graft function deteriorates, and that CMV protein expression in the grafts soon after transplant is associated with reduced graft survival. Thus, CMV may have a pathological role in chronic renal allograft dysfunction.

▶ While the immune response to alloantigens is thought to be a major cause in the failure of kidney transplants, there are many other biologic variables active after transplantation. The report from Uppsala suggests that viral antigen expression serves as a significant immune stimulus in the progressive renal dysfunction. While a direct causative effect is not shown, there is the sugges-tion that more viral protein is associated with greater renal dysfunction. Whether chemoprophylaxis would effectively diminish viral antigen expression remains to be shown. It would have been helpful if the authors had demonstrated that a concomitant cytomegalovirus-specific immune response accompanied the expression of viral antigens, but the importance of a multifaceted biologic response within the transplanted kidney is an important and intriguing observation.

T. Pruett, MD

Long-term Impact of Subclinical Inflammation Diagnosed by Protocol Biopsy One Year After Renal Transplantation

Thierry A, Thervet E, Vuiblet V, et al (Univ Hosp, Poitiers, France; Necker Hosp, Paris, France; Univ Hosp of "Maison Blanche", Reims, France; et al)
Am J Transplant 11:2153-2161, 2011

The long-term impact of subclinical acute rejection (SCAR) on renal graft function remains poorly understood. Furthermore, the interpretation of borderline lesions is difficult and their incidence is variable. The aim of this study was to analyze the characteristics of subclinical inflammation (SCI) in protocol biopsies performed 1-year after renal transplantation. SCI was defined as the presence of borderline lesions or SCAR according to the Banff 2005 classification. The patients included were a subpopulation of the CONCEPT study in which patients were randomized 3 months after transplantation to receive either sirolimus (SRL) or cyclosporine A (CsA) in combination with mycophenolate mofetil. At 1 year, we observed SCI in 37 of the 121 patients observed with an evaluable biopsy. The incidence was more frequent in the SRL group (SRL 45.2% vs. CsA 15.3%). At 30 months, SCI was associated with a significantly lower level of estimated glomerular filtration rate (mean MDRD 50.8 [$\pm$13.3] vs. 57.7 [$\pm$16.3] mL/min/1.73 m^2, p = 0.035). In conclusion, SCI at 1-year posttransplantation is associated with worsening renal function and is more frequent in SRL-treated patients. Therefore, evaluation of SCI may be a valuable tool to allow the optimization of immunosuppressive regimens.

▶ Kidney transplantation has experienced a markedly reduced frequency of acute rejection. However, the long-term results have demonstrated a persistent loss of organs. The presence of inflammation within the "stable" kidney is proving to be a predictor of kidneys that are at risk for the more aggressive tubular atrophy and interstitial fibrosis. The report by Thierry et al found inflammation in a subset of kidneys with stable function 1 year after transplant. Those grafts with inflammation were at increased risk for damage and progressive loss of function. There is much to be discerned about immunologic processes and the long-term function of transplanted kidneys. Increasing investigation into cell trafficking, immune stimulation, and modulation will be necessary if kidneys are to extend long-term function.

T. Pruett, MD

Human Leukocyte Antigen Antibody-Incompatible Renal Transplantation: Excellent Medium-Term Outcomes With Negative Cytotoxic Crossmatch

Higgins R, Lowe D, Hathaway M, et al (Univ Hosps Coventry and Warwickshire, West Midlands, UK; Natl Blood and Transplant, Birmingham, West Midlands, UK)

Transplantation 92:900-906, 2011

Background.—Human leukocyte antigen (HLA) antibody-incompatible renal transplantation has been increasingly performed since 2000 but with few data on the medium-term outcomes.

Methods.—Between 2003 and 2011, 84 patients received renal transplants with a pretreatment donor-specific antibody (DSA) level of more than 500 in a microbead assay. Seventeen patients had positive complement-dependent cytotoxic (CDC) crossmatch (XM), 44 had negative CDC XM and positive flow cytometric XM, and 23 had DSA detectable by microbead only. We also reviewed 28 patients with HLA antibodies but no DSA at transplant. DSAs were removed with plasmapheresis pretransplant, and patients did not routinely receive antithymocyte globulin posttransplant.

Results.—Mean follow-up posttransplantation was 39.6 (range 2—91) months. Patient survival after the first year was 93.8%. Death-censored graft survival at 1, 3, and 5 years was 97.5%, 94.2%, and 80.4%, respectively, in all DSA+ve patients, worse at 5 years in the CDC+ve than in the CDC—ve/DSA+ve group at 45.6% and 88.6%, respectively (*P*<0.03). Five-year graft survival in the DSA—ve group was 82.1%. Rejection occurred in 53.1% of DSA+ve patients in the first year compared with 22% in the DSA—ve patients (*P*<0.003).

Conclusions.—HLA antibody-incompatible renal transplantation had a high success rate if the CDC XM was negative. Further work is required to predict which CDC+ve XM grafts will be successful and to treat slowly progressive graft damage because of DSA in the first few years after transplantation.

▶ Technology has altered the ability to discern preexisting immunologic conditions in kidney recipients. Having an antibody against donor human leukocyte antigen has been associated with hyperacute rejection and markedly inferior outcomes in contrast to a recipient without alloantibody. However, the ability to find antibodies has made many wonder whether each test for them is similar and how clinicians should respond to antibodies' presence. This article from the United Kingdom examined 84 patients identified over an 8-year period with alloantibody, being discerned either by binding to antigen beads, flow cytometry with donor cells, or complement-dependent cytotoxicity assay and treatments with plasma exchange, intravenous immunoglobulin, and transplantation. The results were acceptable but confirmed that each test has a different sensitivity of antibody detection and meaning. However, with an increasing percentage of those waiting for kidney transplants being sensitized to alloantigens, the importance of prompt identification and treatment is key.

T. Pruett, MD

Desensitization in HLA-Incompatible Kidney Recipients and Survival

Montgomery RA, Lonze BE, King KE, et al (Johns Hopkins Med Institutions, Baltimore, MD)
N Engl J Med 365:318-326, 2011

Background.—More than 20,000 candidates for kidney transplantation in the United States are sensitized to HLA and may have a prolonged wait for a transplant, with a reduced transplantation rate and an increased rate of death. One solution is to perform live-donor renal transplantation after the depletion of donor-specific anti-HLA antibodies. Whether such antibody depletion results in a survival benefit as compared with waiting for an HLA-compatible kidney is unknown.

Methods.—We used a protocol that included plasmapheresis and the administration of low-dose intravenous immune globulin to desensitize 211 HLA-sensitized patients who subsequently underwent renal transplantation (treatment group). We compared rates of death between the group undergoing desensitization treatment and two carefully matched control groups of patients on a waiting list for kidney transplantation who continued to undergo dialysis (dialysis-only group) or who underwent either dialysis or HLA-compatible transplantation (dialysis-or-transplantation group).

Results.—In the treatment group, Kaplan–Meier estimates of patient survival were 90.6% at 1 year, 85.7% at 3 years, 80.6% at 5 years, and 80.6% at 8 years, as compared with rates of 91.1%, 67.2%, 51.5%, and 30.5%, respectively, for patients in the dialysisonly group and rates of 93.1%, 77.0%, 65.6%, and 49.1%, respectively, for patients in the dialysis-or-transplantation group (P<0.001 for both comparisons).

Conclusions.—Live-donor transplantation after desensitization provided a significant survival benefit for patients with HLA sensitization, as compared with waiting for a compatible organ. By 8 years, this survival advantage more than doubled. These data provide evidence that desensitization protocols may help overcome incompatibility barriers in live-donor renal transplantation. (Funded by the National Institute of Diabetes and Digestive and Kidney Diseases and the Charles T. Bauer Foundation.)

▶ People with alloantibodies have difficulties with transplantation. A positive crossmatch with donor cells has precluded organ transplants for thousands of individuals. Over the last several years, a variety of techniques have been described with the intent of making the nontransplantable patient a viable candidate. This report describes the Hopkins experience with their desensitization techniques. The survival outcomes associated with receiving a kidney transplant are quite remarkable for durability and results. However, other options, such as paired kidney exchange, are available to obtain kidney transplants for the difficult-to-transplant patient. The challenge for the community is to find the most durable, cost-effective measures that will benefit the patient with end-stage renal disease.

T. Pruett, MD

Outcomes of Preemptive Kidney With or Without Subsequent Pancreas Transplant Compared With Preemptive Simultaneous Pancreas/Kidney Transplantation

Huang E, Wiseman A, Okumura S, et al (Univ of California at Los Angeles; Univ of Colorado Health Sciences Ctr, Aurora)
Transplantation 92:1115-1122, 2011

Background.—Prior studies have indicated that type 1 diabetic (T1DM) recipients of a simultaneous pancreas-kidney (SPK) transplant have greater short-term mortality compared with living donor kidney (LDK) transplantation. Whether this association remains and how outcomes compare to deceased donor kidney (DDK) transplantation in the preemptive setting are unknown.

Methods.—Using data on recipients transplanted between 2000 and 2010 from the Organ Procurement and Transplantation Network/United Network of Organ Sharing, patient and graft survival (calculated from the time of kidney transplant) of pancreas after preemptive LDK (PALK, n=389), preemptive LDK not receiving a pancreas transplant (LDK/noP, n=289), preemptive DDK (n=112), and preemptive SPK transplantations (n=1402) were compared.

Results.—At 6 years, patient survival was excellent (PALK=89.4%, LDK/noP=84.9%, DDK=81.2%, and SPK=91.1%) and not different between PALK, LDK/noP, and SPK (*P* value vs. PALK: LDK/noP=0.08; SPK=0.85) but was lower with preemptive DDK versus preemptive PALK (*P*=0.03). When both LDK groups were considered together, there was higher mortality in the first 180 days after transplant with preemptive DDK (3.7% vs. 1.1%; *P*=0.03) and similar mortality with preemptive SPK (2.3%; *P*=0.07). After multivariate adjustment, there was a trend toward increased risk of death with preemptive DDK compared with preemptive PALK (hazard ratio: 1.91; 95% confidence interval: 0.95–3.84).

Conclusions.—Patient survival associated with preemptive transplantation among T1DM recipients was excellent at 6 years, with the greatest survival favoring PALK, LDK/noP, and SPK rather than DDK. In contrast with prior studies reporting greater short-term mortality with SPK among the general T1DM population, short-term mortality after preemptive transplant is similar between LDK and SPK.

▶ Treatment of patients with end-stage renal disease in the United States is variable. Patients with type 1 diabetes are a population with substantial dialysis-associated morbidity and mortality. Despite the limitations of registry data, this report shows a remarkable survival benefit associated with preemptive kidney transplantation. The benefit of preemptive living donor kidney transplantation tends to exceed that of deceased donation, but the addition of a pancreas transplant with either a deceased kidney or after live kidney transplant improves outcomes compared with deceased kidney transplantation. This sort of analysis emphasizes the benefit associated with preemptive transplantation and should stimulate therapies to optimize patient survival.

T. Pruett, MD

Liver Transplant Recipient Survival Benefit with Living Donation in the Model for Endstage Liver Disease Allocation Era
Berg CL, Merion RM, Shearon TH, et al (Univ of Virginia Health System, Charlottesville; Univ of Michigan and Arbor Res Collaborative for Health, Ann Arbor; Univ of Michigan, Ann Arbor; et al)
Hepatology 54:1313-1321, 2011

Receipt of a living donor liver transplant (LDLT) has been associated with improved survival compared with waiting for a deceased donor liver transplant (DDLT). However, the survival benefit of liver transplant has been questioned for candidates with Model for Endstage Liver Disease (MELD) scores <15, and the survival advantage of LDLT has not been demonstrated during the MELD allocation era, especially for low MELD patients. Transplant candidates enrolled in the Adult-to-Adult Living Donor Liver Transplantation Cohort Study after February 28, 2002 were followed for a median of 4.6 years. Starting at the time of presentation of the first potential living donor, mortality for LDLT recipients was compared to mortality for patients who remained on the waiting list or received DDLT (no LDLT group) according to categories of MELD score (<15 or ≥15) and diagnosis of hepatocellular carcinoma (HCC). Of 868 potential LDLT recipients (453 with MELD <15; 415 with MELD ≥15 at entry), 712 underwent transplantation (406 LDLT; 306 DDLT), 83 died without transplant, and 73 were alive without transplant at last follow-up. Overall, LDLT recipients had 56% lower mortality (hazard ratio [HR] = 0.44, 95% confidence interval [CI] 0.32-0.60; $P < 0.0001$). Among candidates without HCC, mortality benefit was seen both with MELD <15 (HR = 0.39; $P = 0.0003$) and MELD ≥15 (HR = 0.42; $P = 0.0006$). Among candidates with HCC, a benefit of LDLT was not seen for MELD <15 (HR = 0.82, $P = 0.65$) but was seen for MELD ≥15 (HR = 0.29, $P = 0.043$).

Conclusion.—Across the range of MELD scores, patients without HCC derived a significant survival benefit when undergoing LDLT rather than waiting for DDLT in the MELD liver allocation era. Low MELD candidates with HCC may not benefit from LDLT.

▶ Living donation puts a healthy person at risk for the benefit of someone sick. This fact is especially evident in the setting of liver transplantation. The benefit for the potential recipient has been known for the more ill, but the wisdom of pursuing adult live liver transplantation in individuals less ill has been questioned. The National Institutes of Health—sponsored study focusing on adult living liver transplantation found a survival benefit for liver recipients under a Model for Endstage Liver Disease score of 15 compared with waiting for a liver from a deceased donor. While factors associated with observation are dependent on deceased organ availability and quality, it reemphasizes that liver failure, even in those that appear less ill, represents a significant life risk that has an amenable therapy.

T. Pruett, MD

Outcomes of Adult Living Donor Liver Transplantation: Comparison of the Adult-to-Adult Living Donor Liver Transplantation Cohort Study and the National Experience

Olthoff KM, the Adult-to-Adult Living Donor Liver Transplantation Cohort Study Group (Univ of Pennsylvania, Philadelphia; et al)
Liver Transpl 17:789-797, 2011

The study objectives were to determine whether the findings of the Adult-to-Adult Living Donor Liver Transplantation Cohort Study (A2ALL) reflect the U.S. national experience and to define risk factors for patient mortality and graft loss in living donor liver transplantation (LDLT). A2ALL previously identified risk factors for mortality after LDLT, which included early center experience, older recipient age, and longer cold ischemia time. LDLT procedures at 9 A2ALL centers ($n = 702$) and 67 non-A2ALL centers ($n = 1664$) from January 1998 through December 2007 in the Scientific Registry of Transplant Recipients database were analyzed. Potential predictors of time from transplantation to death or graft failure were tested using Cox regression. No significant difference in overall mortality between A2ALL and non-A2ALL centers was found. Higher hazard ratios (HRs) were associated with donor age (HR $= 1.13$ per 10 years, $P = 0.0002$), recipient age (HR $= 1.20$ per 10 years, $P = 0.0003$), serum creatinine levels (HR $= 1.52$ per loge unit increase, $P < 0.0001$), hepatocellular carcinoma (HR $= 2.12$, $P < 0.0001$) or hepatitis C virus (HR $= 1.18$, $P = 0.026$), intensive care unit stay (HR $= 2.52$, $P < 0.0001$) or hospitalization (HR $= 1.62$, $P < 0.0001$) versus home, earlier center experience (LDLT case number 15: HR $= 1.61$, $P < 0.0001$, and a cold ischemia time >4.5 hours (HR $= 1.79$, $P = 0.0006$). Except for center experience, risk factor effects between A2ALL and non-A2ALL centers were not significantly different. Variables associated with graft loss were identified and showed similar trends. In conclusion, mortality and graft loss risk factors were similar in A2ALL and non-A2ALL centers. These analyses demonstrate that findings from the A2ALL consortium are relevant to other centers in the U.S. performing LDLT, and conclusions and recommendations from A2ALL may help to guide clinical decision making.

▶ Live donors have been a source of organs since kidney transplantation became a clinical reality. Expansion of live donation to be routinely available for liver transplantation has been controversial but necessary. The Adult-to-Adult Living Donor Liver Transplantation Cohort Study consortium has been useful in describing the outcomes and risks associated with this source of organs, but the applicability to the general population has not been demonstrated. An analysis of the national database confirmed the basic similarity of the consortium observations with the experience from other centers. The observations of increased donor age, diagnosis of hepatocellular carcinoma, higher serum creatinine, and intensive care unit admission were associated with increased risk of graft loss in the broader national experience. Whether these observations will result in limited access to care or in trials to demonstrate solutions will be a challenge to the community.

T. Pruett, MD

Outcomes With Split Liver Transplantation in 106 Recipients: The University of California, San Francisco, Experience From 1993 to 2010

Vagefi PA, Parekh J, Ascher NL, et al (Univ of California, San Francisco)
Arch Surg 146:1052-1059, 2011

Background.—Split liver transplantation (SLT) allows for expansion of the deceased donor pool.

Objectives.—To assess outcomes and the impact of splitting technique (in situ vs ex vivo) in SLT recipients.

Design.—Single-center retrospective review (September 18, 1993, to July 1, 2010).

Setting.—University medical center.

Patients.—One hundred six SLT recipients.

Main Outcome Measures.—Postoperative graft and patient survival and postoperative complications.

Results.—In adults, 1-, 5-, and 10-year overall patient survival was 93%, 77%, and 73%, respectively; overall graft survival was 89%, 76%, and 65%, respectively; ex vivo split patient survival was 93%, 85%, and 74%, respectively; and ex vivo graft survival was 86%, 77%, and 63%, respectively. In situ split patient and graft survival was 94% at 1 year and 75% at 5 years. Postoperative complications included biliary (29%), vascular (11%), unplanned reexploratory surgery (11%), incisional hernia (8%), small-for-size syndrome (n=1), need for shunt at the time of SLT (n=1), and primary nonfunction (n=1). In children, 1-, 5-, and 10-year overall patient survival was 84%, 75%, and 69%, respectively; overall graft survival was 77%, 63%, and 57%, respectively; ex vivo split patient survival was 83%, 73%, and 73%, respectively; and ex vivo graft survival was 75%, 59%, and 59%, respectively. In situ split patient and graft survival was 86% at 1 and 5 years. Postoperative complications included biliary (40%), vascular (26%), and primary nonfunction (n=1).

Conclusions.—Split liver transplantation remains an excellent option for expansion of the deceased donor pool for adult and pediatric populations. Postoperative morbidity remains high; however, this is justifiable owing to limited resources.

▶ Limited availability of organs has led to the development of techniques that will allow increased numbers of people access to life-saving organs. The techniques used during live liver donation have been applied to deceased organs, with the hope of obtaining 2 transplantable livers from a single donor. The University of California—San Francisco has had significant experience with live donation but still found a higher rate of biliary and vascular complications in the split liver group. Their conclusion may be understandable that organ need and the potential benefit warranted the increased morbidity, but any recipient must still balance the difference in what is "best" against what is available. This is the dilemma of organ transplantation.

T. Pruett, MD

Early Liver Transplantation for Severe Alcoholic Hepatitis

Mathurin P, Moreno C, Samuel D, et al (Centre Hospitalier Universitaire (CHU) de Lille and Université Nord de France, Lille; Université Libre de Bruxelles, Brussels; Université Paris-Sud, Villejuif, France; et al)

N Engl J Med 365:1790-1800, 2011

Background.—A 6-month abstinence from alcohol is usually required before patients with severe alcoholic hepatitis are considered for liver transplantation. Patients whose hepatitis is not responding to medical therapy have a 6-month survival rate of approximately 30%. Since most alcoholic hepatitis deaths occur within 2 months, early liver transplantation is attractive but controversial.

Methods.—We selected patients from seven centers for early liver transplantation. The patients had no prior episodes of alcoholic hepatitis and had scores of 0.45 or higher according to the Lille model (which calculates scores ranging from 0 to 1, with a score ≥ 0.45 indicating nonresponse to medical therapy and an increased risk of death in the absence of transplantation) or rapid worsening of liver function despite medical therapy. Selected patients also had supportive family members, no severe coexisting conditions, and a commitment to alcohol abstinence. Survival was compared between patients who underwent early liver transplantation and matched patients who did not.

Results.—In all, 26 patients with severe alcoholic hepatitis at high risk of death (median Lille score, 0.88) were selected and placed on the list for a liver transplant within a median of 13 days after nonresponse to medical therapy. Fewer than 2% of patients admitted for an episode of severe alcoholic hepatitis were selected. The centers used 2.9% of available grafts for this indication. The cumulative 6-month survival rate ($\pm SE$) was higher among patients who received early transplantation than among those who did not ($77 \pm 8\%$ vs. $23 \pm 8\%$, P<0.001). This benefit of early transplantation was maintained through 2 years of follow-up (hazard ratio, 6.08; P=0.004). Three patients resumed drinking alcohol: one at 720 days, one at 740 days, and one at 1140 days after transplantation.

Conclusions.—Early liver transplantation can improve survival in patients with a first episode of severe alcoholic hepatitis not responding to medical therapy. (Funded by Société Nationale Française de Gastroentérologie.)

▶ When there are too few organs for those in need, self abuse by the recipient becomes a very controversial topic. This experience from France probably could not have been done in the United States given our current allocation climate. However, the survival benefit associated with liver transplantation for severe alcoholic hepatitis is substantial. Only 1.8% of patients with the diagnosis qualified for transplantation, with the majority excluded for predisposition to addiction or unfavorable social/family profiles. Clearer definition of appropriate thresholds and specific tests used to discern such exclusion criteria would be necessary to avoid the appearance of capricious selection within the US system. The profound survival benefit and relatively low rate of recidivism (3 of 26 patients) supports a revisiting of the rigid time of sobriety.

T. Pruett, MD

6 Surgical Infections

Introduction

Infection after surgery is a major complication that is costly in terms of lives and money. It is now a major effort by the Center for Medicare and Medicaid Services to reduce the morbidity associated with surgical infections. The first selection[1] is an assessment from Switzerland assessing the impact of surgery upon the acquisition of healthcare associated infections (HAI). Roughly 10% of surgical patients had HAI and roughly half the infections were directly associated with the surgical site. Surgical patients were healthier, but had more extrinsic breaks in normal barriers of infection (ventilator, urinary catheter, central venous catheters, ICU stay, etc). Infectious morbidity has been measured and known to be significant, but the costs of infection are now becoming the focus of study. Vaughan-Sarrazin et al[2] evaluated the cost of postoperative sepsis from within the Veteran's Administration. In those patients with postoperative sepsis, the cost of care was doubled compared with those without infection. This was especially true in those patients with prolonged mechanical ventilation, requiring reintubation, and those with heart failure. Sepsis is not the same as surgical site infection, but HAI and SSI are interrelated. The cost, in terms of mortality and dollars, identified within this study is profound. The knowledge of factors that contribute to surgical infections has grown over the years. The article by Alexander et al[3] is a comprehensive compendium of existing knowledge. Many of the factors reviewed and identified have been incorporated into current "best practice" within our healthcare systems. Variables such as operating room etiquette, patient preparation, reduction of bacteria within the wound, postoperative patient oxygenation, glucose control, temperature, and smoking all affect outcomes. These variables continue to be a source of discussion pertaining to their relative contribution for the clinical outcome.

The next series of articles addresses many of the known variables in context of variations and nuance. The article Piessen et al[4] describes outcomes of a standardized procedure (left colon resection) as a function of the indication for surgery. Left colectomy for either diverticular disease or carcinoma has different risk factors for infection development. The surgical site complications and morbidities differ, apparently from the differential patient factors associated with the specific disease conditions. This selection stresses that clinical conditions can significantly impact the consequences associated with specific surgical procedures. The study by

Neal et al[5] is even more nuanced in that complications after the same procedure for the same indication were stratified by presence or absence of an underlying inflammatory response. Those individuals with an increased risk score described within the paper had on multivariate analysis, impaired survival and infectious complications. Risk stratification is not as simple as formerly thought. Morowitz et al[6] describe the revolution that is occurring in the understanding of how external and internal environmental factors influence the phenotype of bacteria residing in humans. The authors give a more basic science foundation for the findings observed within the preceding clinical studies. Of growing importance is the understanding of the effects that the environment has on the human microbiome. This plays out in one of the major debates within the field of infection prevention: duration of antimicrobial prophylaxis after the operative procedure. A typical recommendation is that antibiotics should be stopped when the wound is closed. After cardiac procedures, many cardiac surgeons have felt that the healing bone has more risk for infection and therefore would benefit from a protracted antibiotic course. The meta-analysis conducted by Mertz et al[7] concludes that the literature supports the continuation of prophylactic antibiotics for more than 24 hours, but the authors also note that there are many weaknesses within the prophylaxis literature. Their conclusion certainly does not support the notion that shorter courses of antibiotics will improve outcomes or reduce sternal and deep wound infections. Recognition of disease and access to care is an important variable in the outcomes associated with infection. Paquette et al[8] compared the outcomes of rural versus urban patients with appendicitis and found that the rate of perforation was significantly increased in those from rural areas. This was especially true for those individuals who were transferred from a rural to urban setting. The benefit of access to care and prompt therapy for an urgent condition is shown in this article and should be a factor in policy decisions regarding the upcoming surgeon shortage. The study by Bickel et al[9] readdresses the premise that hyperoxia can reduce the risk of clinical surgical site infection. In this randomized study, the benefit of oxygen was noted, but only in those wounds created to treat phlegmonous or perforated appendicitis. Risk reduction was not noted in either the wounds to remove a normal or acute appendicitis. The rationale of therapeutic interventions may only be for certain infection risk thresholds. Another variant therapy for the heavily contaminated wound is to leave the skin open. This tactic has been proven over time; however, the inconvenience and cosmetic outcome for the patient is often not satisfactory. To achieve the same end without many of the untoward effects, the authors of article 10[10] describe the effective use of loose primary skin closure with daily probing of the skin apposition to affect egress of subcutaneous fluid after appendectomy for perforation. The reduction in SSI was impressive: 3% versus 19%. These articles suggest that there are multiple methods that can be used to reduce the wound risks associated with heavily contaminated surgical wounds. Another variable in the generation of SSI that is not commonly addressed is that of obesity. In a large retrospective analysis[11] of an insurance claims database (over 7000 patients), patients undergoing total or segmental colectomy were found to have a 60% increase in risk for SSI when the BMI >30. As this variable is rarely included in risk stratification for complication development, the authors have begun the necessary process of risk stratification refinement if we are to use SSI frequency in national standards. There are many unaddressed issues with this analysis, as the infection risk with increased weight is more likely a continuous rather than a dichotomous variable. The data were not presented as a continuum, and an assessment of risk as a function of obesity severity was not assessed nor was the degree of risk from malnutrition assessed from the other perspective.

It is common practice in this "evidence-based medicine" era to try and effect change by bundling together a group of interventions shown to be associated with a desired outcome. The study by Jain et al[12] assessed the bundle of active surveillance, contact precautions, hand hygiene, and culture change to decrease MRSA colonization and subsequent infection in the VA system. The authors demonstrated that by decreasing MRSA carriage among the patients in the VA system, the percentage of MRSA infections decreased. This finding would be very important if either the total number of HAI was decreased or if there was an associated outcome difference in patients with MRSA line infections, pneumonia, etc, when contrasted with the more "usual" organisms. The authors did not address either of these issues. Anthony et al[13] describe a study to assess bundled therapies intended to decrease surgical site infections. In a single institution (VA), randomized study, 5 evidence-based practices were bundled together with the intent to decrease SSI over conventional practice. Almost 200 patients were included in this intent-to-treat study of colorectal procedures. The practices had all been shown to be associated with decreased SSI and included absence of bowel preparation, patient warming before and during surgery, supplemental oxygen during and after surgery, intra-operative fluid limits, and use of a surgical wound protector. The study was stopped early because the results did not support that the bundled therapies did not decrease SSI; rather the bundle was associated with a 45% rate of SSI compared with 24% in the conventional therapy group. This finding of a 2.49-fold increased risk of SSI must make one pause. The rate of SSI is too high and one must query the overall validity of the process, but the bundled treatments were statistically shown by univariate analysis to be associated with SSI reduction. Combining these multiple modalities resulted in the opposite outcome. The authors' discussion makes many cogent points about vagaries of the studies or techniques not completely understood or controlled. However, the importance of this study is in assessing outcomes. The typical process improvements used in hospital systems are used upon a diverse population of people. This study stresses the point that process metrics must be used to assess efficacy. Had this process been done outside of a study context, the adverse quality outcome that was observed would have been missed and many people would have suffered for the application of a good thought.

Finally, the final 3 articles are intended to highlight several factors in the application of surgical therapy for infections known to require surgery for cure. The study by Kiefer et al[14] seeks to address the role of surgical intervention for infective endocarditis. The traditional indications have been changing/worsening valvular insufficiency and recurrent embolic disease. The current study addressed the population with NYHA grades of heart failure and demonstrated a significant survival benefit from surgical intervention, but most strikingly in class III-IV. The absence of discussion regarding the type of procedure performed, rate of infectious complications, or reinfection of prosthetic material was troublesome. The study clearly demonstrated the benefit of surgical intervention as therapy for infectious endocarditis; it just did not aid in stratifying the relative efficacy of the varied surgical techniques. Rahman et al[15] describe the injection of intrapleural enzymes in the treatment of the infected pleural space. It had previously been shown that intrapleural injection of tissue plasminogen (t-PA) alone into an empyema after tube thoracotomy did not result in improved outcomes as compared to tube drainage alone. The authors hypothesized that persistence of bacterial DNA within the infected fluid either modified the immune response or made the fluid inherently more viscous and less amenable to tube drainage. The described study included assignment to one of 4 arms of tube drainage with instillation of (1) t-PA alone, (2) DNase alone, (3) t-PA + DNase, or (4) placebo treatment. The goal of therapy was to resolve the infection and avoid the need for surgical decortication. The analysis demonstrated that single enzyme therapy was not effective in treatment of empyema beyond the benefit of tube drainage, but the combination of t-PA and DNase did reduce the odd ratio for surgical referral (decortication). The study demonstrated the benefit of adjunct therapies as effective in reducing the need for more invasive therapies. The final selection by Duron et al[16] addresses one of the dilemmas that every practicing surgeon confronts: what to do with an abnormality found by a newer technology. In this report, chart reviews were performed of those CT scan reports with a diagnosis of pneumatosis intestinalis, the finding of gas within the wall of the intestine. In the days before CT, pneumatosis was associated with intestinal ischemia and typically was an indication for urgent surgical exploration. Forty-seven percent of patients either improved spontaneously or had an unrevealing laparotomy. Of the individuals chosen by the surgical team for a procedure, 87% had an intervention and 13% found no pathology. Sixteen percent of all patients were deemed unsalvageable and given palliative care. Discrimination of clinical variables was difficult. Multivariate analysis confirmed that the usual findings of intraabdominal pathology still were predictive (abdominal distention, rebound tenderness and lactic academia were all associated with intraoperative pathology). The importance of findings that are out of context with clinical findings remains to be discerned. Studies such as this will help put radiographic findings in appropriate clinical context.

Surgical infections are regaining attention because of the association with regulatory consequences. The development of appropriate risk stratification to discern organizations and providers that fall outside the acceptable range will be difficult. The literature speaks to the interrelated nature of physiologic conditions within the host, infectious agents, surgical technique, and extrinsic pharmaceutical agents. The continued attention paid to surgical infections will certainly lead to newer appreciation of this all-too-common outcome.

Timothy L. Pruett, MD

References

1. Sax H, Uçkay I, Balmelli C, et al. Overall burden of healthcare-associated infections among surgical patients. Results of a national study. *Ann Surg.* 2011;253: 365-370.
2. Vaughan-Sarrazin MS, Bayman L, Cullen JJ. Costs of postoperative sepsis: The business case for quality improvement to reduce postoperative sepsis in Veterans Affairs Hospitals. *Arch Surg.* 2011;146:944-951.
3. Alexander JW, Solomkin JS, Edwards MJ. Updated recommendations for control of surgical site infections. *Ann Surg.* 2011;253:1082-1093.
4. Piessen G, Muscari F, Rivkine E, et al. Prevalence of and risk factors for morbidity after elective left colectomy: cancer vs noncomplicated diverticular disease. *Arch Surg.* 2011;146:1149-1155.
5. Neal CP, Mann CD, Garcea G, Briggs CD, Dennison AR, Berry DP. Preoperative systemic inflammation and infectious complications after resection of colorectal liver metastases. *Arch Surg.* 2011;146:471-478.
6. Morowitz MJ, Babrowski T, Carlisle EM, et al. The human microbiome and surgical disease. *Ann Surg.* 2011;253:1094-1101.
7. Mertz D, Johnstone J, Loeb M. Does duration of perioperative antibiotic prophylaxis matter in cardiac surgery? A systematic review and meta-analysis. *Ann Surg.* 2011;254:48-54.
8. Paquette IM, Zuckerman R, Finlayson SR. Perforated appendicitis among rural and urban patients: implications of access to care. *Ann Surg.* 2011;253:534-538.
9. Bickel A, Gurevits M, Vamos R, Ivry S, Eitan A. Perioperative hyperoxygenation and wound site infection following surgery for acute appendicitis: a randomized, prospective, controlled trial. *Arch Surg.* 2011;146:464-470.
10. Towfigh S, Clarke T, Yacoub W, et al. Significant reduction of wound infections with daily probing of contaminated wounds: a prospective randomized clinical trial. *Arch Surg.* 2011;146:448-452.
11. Wick EC, Hirose K, Shore AD, et al. Surgical site infections and cost in obese patients undergoing colorectal surgery. *Arch Surg.* 2011;146:1068-1072.
12. Jain R, Kralovic SM, Evans ME, et al. Veterans Affairs initiative to prevent methicillin-resistant *Staphylococcus aureus* infections. *N Engl J Med.* 2011;364: 1419-1430.
13. Anthony T, Murray BW, Sum-Ping JT, et al. Evaluating an evidence-based bundle for preventing surgical site infection: a randomized trial. *Arch Surg.* 2011;146: 263-269.
14. Kiefer T, Park L, Tribouilloy C, et al. Association between valvular surgery and mortality among patients with infective endocarditis complicated by heart failure. *JAMA.* 2011;306:2239-2247.
15. Rahman NM, Maskell NA, West A, et al. Intrapleural use of tissue plasminogen activator and DNase in pleural infection. *N Engl J Med.* 2011;365:518-526.
16. Duron VP, Rutigliano S, Machan JT, Dupuy DE, Mazzaglia PJ. Computed tomographic diagnosis of pneumatosis intestinalis: clinical measures predictive of the need for surgical intervention. *Arch Surg.* 2011;146:506-510.

Overall Burden of Healthcare-Associated Infections Among Surgical Patients: Results of a National Study

Sax H, Uçkay I, Balmelli C, et al (Univ of Geneva Hosps and Faculty of Medicine, Switzerland; Regional Hosp of Lugano, Switzerland; et al)
Ann Surg 253:365-370, 2011

Objective.—To assess the overall burden of healthcare-associated infections (HAIs) in patients exposed and nonexposed to surgery.

Background.—Targeted HAI surveillance is common in healthcare institutions, but may underestimate the overall burden of disease.

Methods.—Prevalence study among patients hospitalized in 50 acute care hospitals participating in the Swiss Nosocomial Infection Prevalence surveillance program.

Results.—Of 8273 patients, 3377 (40.8%) had recent surgery. Overall, HAI was present in 358 (10.6%) patients exposed to surgery, but only in 206 (4.2%) of 4896 nonexposed ($P < 0.001$). Prevalence of surgical site infection (SSI) was 5.4%. Healthcare-associated infections prevalence excluding SSI was 6.5% in patients with surgery and 4.7% in those without ($P < 0.0001$). Patients exposed to surgery carried less intrinsic risk factors for infection (age >60 years, 55.6% vs 63.0%; American Society of Anesthesiologists score >3, 5.9% vs 9.3%; McCabe for rapidly fatal disease, 3.9% vs 6.6%; Charlson comorbidity index >2, 12.3% vs 20.9%, respectively; all $P < 0.001$) than those nonexposed, but more extrinsic risk factors (urinary catheters, 39.6% vs 14.1%; central venous catheters, 17.8% vs 7.1%; mechanical ventilation, 4.7% vs 1.3%; intensive care stay, 18.3% vs 8.8%, respectively; all $P<0.001$). Exposure to surgery independently predicted an increased risk of HAI (odds ratio 2.43; 95% CI 2.0–3.0).

Conclusions.—Despite a lower intrinsic risk, patients exposed to surgery carried more than twice the overall HAI burden than those nonexposed; almost half was accountable to SSI. Extending infection control efforts beyond SSI prevention in these patients might be rewarding, especially because of the extrinsic nature of risk factors.

▶ This study from Switzerland assessed the impact of surgery on health care—associated infections (HAIs). This survey of a national, voluntary database gives an important perspective on costs associated with HAIs and surgical interventions. By definition, nonsurgical patients will not have surgical site infections (SSIs), but surgical patients can have infections that are not immediately associated with the surgical site. This truism was borne out in this study, where surgical patients (about 40% of the total hospital patient volumes) had HAIs about twice as often as nonsurgical patients. In surgical patients, the overall SSI rate was 5.4% and the non-SSI HAIs was 6.5%, compared with 4.7% of HAIs in the nonsurgical population. The added infection costs associated with surgery do not always revolve around the prevention of SSIs, and efforts should be made to address other HAIs in addition to SSI prevention.

T. Pruett, MD

Costs of Postoperative Sepsis: The Business Case for Quality Improvement to Reduce Postoperative Sepsis in Veterans Affairs Hospitals

Vaughan-Sarrazin MS, Bayman L, Cullen JJ (Univ of Iowa College of Medicine)
Arch Surg 146:944-951, 2011

Objective.—To estimate the incremental costs associated with sepsis as a complication of general surgery, controlling for patient risk factors that may affect costs (eg, surgical complexity and comorbidity) and hospital-level variation in costs.

Design.—Database analysis.

Setting.—One hundred eighteen Veterans Health Affairs hospitals.

Patients.—A total of 13 878 patients undergoing general surgery during fiscal year 2006 (October 1, 2005, through September 30, 2006).

Main Outcome Measures.—Incremental costs associated with sepsis as a complication of general surgery (controlling for patient risk factors and hospital-level variation of costs), as well as the increase in costs associated with complications that co-occur with sepsis. Costs were estimated using the Veterans Health Affairs Decision Support System, and patient risk factors and postoperative complications were identified in the Veterans Affairs Surgical Quality Improvement Program database.

Results.—Overall, 564 of 13 878 patients undergoing general surgery developed postoperative sepsis, for a rate of 4.1%. The average unadjusted cost for patients with no sepsis was $24 923, whereas the average cost for patients with sepsis was 3.6 times higher at $88 747. In risk-adjusted analyses, the relative costs were 2.28 times greater for patients with sepsis relative to patients without sepsis (95% confidence interval, 2.19-2.38), with the difference in risk-adjusted costs estimated at $26 972 (ie, $21 045 vs $48 017). Sepsis often co-occurred with other types of complications, most frequently with failure to wean the patient from mechanical ventilation after 48 hours (36%), postoperative pneumonia (31%), and reintubation for respiratory or cardiac failure (29%). Costs were highest when sepsis occurred with pneumonia or failure to wean the patient from mechanical ventilation after 48 hours.

Conclusion.—Given the high cost of treating sepsis, a business case can be made for quality improvement initiatives that reduce the likelihood of postoperative sepsis.

▶ In general, as a person becomes sicker, they will require more resources to monitor and care for them. That is not an earth-shattering observation. The study from the Veterans Affairs system assessed the cost of caring for an individual with postoperative sepsis or severe sepsis with the postoperative course of one not becoming so sick. Not surprisingly, those with sepsis cost more to treat (a bit more than 2×) and had a higher rate of death than the cohort. This analysis was performed on all general surgery patients operated on in the fiscal year 2006. With more than 13 000 eligible procedures, the power of analysis was robust. The authors note that surgical site infection (SSI) is not directly associated with sepsis and that the models addressing SSI reduction will probably not affect this outcome. There remains much to do with appropriate risk stratification and timely interventions outside the operating theater to reduce the risks associated with sepsis.

T. Pruett, MD

Updated Recommendations for Control of Surgical Site Infections
Alexander JW, Solomkin JS, Edwards MJ (Univ of Cincinnati College of Medicine, OH)
Ann Surg 253:1082-1093, 2011

Objective.—The objective of this study is to provide updated guidelines for the prevention of surgical wound infections based upon review and interpretation of the current and past literature.

Background.—The development and treatment of surgical wound infections has always been a limiting factor to the success of surgical treatment. Although continuous improvements have been made, surgical site infections continue to occur at an unacceptable rate, annually costing billions of dollars in economic loss caused by associated morbidity and mortality.

Methods.—The Centers for Disease Control (CDC) provided extensive recommendations for the control of surgical infections in 1999. Review of the current literature with interpretation of the findings has been done to update the recommendations.

Results.—New and sometimes conflicting studies indicate that coordination and application of techniques and procedures to decrease wound infections will be highly successful, even in patients with very high risks.

Conclusions.—This review suggests that uniform adherence to the proposed guidelines for the prevention of surgical infections could reduce wound infections significantly; namely to a target of less than 0.5% in clean wounds, less than 1% in clean contaminated wounds and less than 2% in highly contaminated wounds and decrease related costs to less than one-half of the current amount.

▶ Surgical site infection (SSI) has been an untoward consequence for as long as surgeons have made an incision. Much is known about techniques to diminish the rate and risk for the development of SSI. The authors give a broad perspective on the current knowledge of the variables in surgical technique and preparation, contamination of the operative wound, and management strategies as they influence the infectious consequences from performing operations. This review is an excellent summary of 2011 knowledge of SSI prevention/causation by some of the prominent leaders in surgical infections.

T. Pruett, MD

Prevalence of and Risk Factors for Morbidity After Elective Left Colectomy: Cancer vs Noncomplicated Diverticular Disease

Piessen G, for FRENCH (Fédération de Recherche EN CHirurgie) (Hôpital Huriez, Lille, France; et al)
Arch Surg 146:1149-1155, 2011

Hypothesis.—Independent risk factors for postoperative morbidity after colectomy are most likely linked to disease characteristics.

Design.—Retrospective analysis.

Setting.—Twenty-eight centers of the French Federation for Surgical Research.

Patients.—In total, 1721 patients (1230 with colon cancer [CC] and 491 with diverticular disease [DD]) from a databank of 7 prospective, multisite, randomized trials on colorectal resection.

Intervention.—Elective left colectomy via laparotomy.

Main Outcome Measures.—Preoperative and intraoperative risk factors for postoperative morbidity.

Results.—Overall postoperative morbidity was higher in CC than in DD (32.4% vs 30.3%) but the difference was not statistically significant ($P = .40$). Two independent risk factors for morbidity in CC were antecedent heart failure (odds ratio [OR], 3.00; 95% confidence interval [CI], 1.42-6.32) ($P = .003$) and bothersome intraluminal fecal matter (2.08; 1.42-3.06) ($P = .001$). Three independent risk factors for morbidity in DD were at least 10% weight loss (OR, 2.06; 95% CI, 1.25-3.40) ($P = .004$), body mass index (calculated as weight in kilograms divided by height in meters squared) exceeding 30 (2.05; 1.15-3.66) ($P = .02$), and left hemicolectomy (vs left segmental colectomy) (2.01; 1.19-3.40) ($P = .009$).

Conclusions.—Patients undergoing elective left colectomy for CC or for DD constitute 2 distinct populations with completely different risk factors for morbidity, which should be addressed differently. Improving colonic cleanliness (by antiseptic enema) may reduce morbidity in CC. In DD, morbidity may be reduced by appropriate preoperative nutritive support (by immunonutrition), even in patients with obesity, and by preference of left segmental colectomy over left hemicolectomy. By decreasing morbidity, mortality should be lowered as well, especially when reoperation becomes necessary.

▶ Colonic surgery is associated with significant risk of surgical infection. This study further subdivided the indication for left colon resection into the 2 common indications: carcinoma and diverticular disease. Interestingly, the infectious morbidity differed by the indication. In part, this should not be too surprising, as the pathology and physiology associated with the conditions differ. The need for diminution of bacterial numbers to optimize outcomes after carcinoma and nutrition and limitation of the resection for diverticular disease is intriguing. Surgical infections are influenced by many factors, and optimal outcomes will only be achieved by controlling the operative variables.

T. Pruett, MD

Preoperative Systemic Inflammation and Infectious Complications After Resection of Colorectal Liver Metastases

Neal CP, Mann CD, Garcea G, et al (Leicester General Hosp, UK)

Arch Surg 146:471-478, 2011

Background.—Postoperative complications are associated with a poor long-term prognosis after resection of colorectal liver metastases via an undetermined mechanism. The preoperative systemic inflammatory response, itself a predictor of poor survival, was recently shown to independently predict postoperative infectious complications after primary colorectal cancer resection.

Objective.—To examine the association of postoperative infectious complications with preoperative systemic inflammation and survival in patients undergoing resection of colorectal liver metastases.

Design.—Retrospective study based on a prospectively updated database.

Setting.—A United Kingdom tertiary referral hepatobiliary unit.

Patients.—A total of 202 consecutive patients with colorectal liver metastases undergoing hepatectomy between January 1, 2000, and April 30, 2006.

Main Outcome Measures.—Multivariable analyses were performed to correlate preoperative and operative variables with postoperative complications and to correlate complications with long-term survival after metastasectomy.

Results.—Ninety-day mortality and morbidity were 2.0% and 25.7%, respectively. The preoperative systemic inflammatory response independently predicted the development of infectious complications ($P = .009$) and major infectious complications ($P = .005$) after hepatectomy, along with performance of trisectionectomy. Infectious complications were associated with poor long-term survival after metastasectomy but lost independent significance when systemic inflammatory variables were included in multivariable analyses.

Conclusions.—The preoperative systemic inflammatory response independently predicts the development of infectious complications after colorectal liver metastases resection. Although infectious complications are associated with adverse long-term prognosis after hepatectomy, they lacked independent prognostic value when systemic inflammatory variables were also considered, suggesting that much of their prognostic value arises from their association with the preoperative systemic inflammatory response.

▶ People have differing physiologic and immune responses to diseases amenable to surgical intervention. This study assesses the outcomes of individuals undergoing hepatic resection for colorectal metastases. Multivariate analysis highlighted that extended liver resection and neutrophilia were the elements associated with increased infectious morbidity. However, preoperative measures of the inflammatory response, such as C reactive protein, neutrophilia, hypoalbuminemia, and concomitant clinical risk score, were found to be associated with decreased survival from tumors and increased risk for infectious complications.

This is important for the preoperative assessment, manipulation, and risk assessment for an individual patient. The concept that there are significant differences in the nutrition underlying cardiopulmonary reserve that will significantly affect clinical outcomes is not new to the surgical community. The notion that subtle laboratory differences in immunologic responsiveness can modify clinical outcomes has not yet gained acceptance within the community. How significantly the postoperative infectious morbidities modify the immune responses remains uncertain in these groups.

T. Pruett, MD

The Human Microbiome and Surgical Disease

Morowitz MJ, Babrowski T, Carlisle EM, et al (The Univ of Chicago Pritzker School of Medicine, IL)
Ann Surg 253:1094-1101, 2011

Objective.—The purpose of this review article is to summarize what is currently known about microbes associated with the human body and to provide examples of how this knowledge impacts the care of surgical patients.

Background.—Pioneering research over the past decade has demonstrated that human beings live in close, constant contact with dynamic communities of microbial organisms. This new reality has wide-ranging implications for the care of surgical patients.

Methods and Results.—Recent advances in the culture-independent study of the human microbiome are reviewed. To illustrate the translational relevance of these studies to surgical disease, we discuss in detail what is known about the role of microbes in the pathogenesis of obesity, gastrointestinal malignancies, Crohn disease, and perioperative complications including surgical site infections and sepsis. The topics of mechanical bowel preparation and perioperative antibiotics are also discussed.

Conclusions.—Heightened understanding of the microbiome in coming years will likely offer opportunities to refine the prevention and treatment of a wide variety of surgical conditions.

▶ Pasteur demonstrated that "spontaneous generation of the species" does not occur. The logical consequence of that premise is that infections of the surgical wound or devices come from somewhere. The current explosion in nucleic acid probes of the human microbiome has allowed for many new insights that should change the way that we approach minimization of risk of surgical site infection. This review underscores how little we currently know about the influences the human microenvironment places on the diversity of gene expression within the human microbial population. It is probable that a number of the discordant outcomes observed from clinical trials relating to surgical infections are dependent on unanticipated bacterial modifications. The studies and techniques described in this review add a crucial and underexplored component of surgical infections.

T. Pruett, MD

Does Duration of Perioperative Antibiotic Prophylaxis Matter in Cardiac Surgery? A Systematic Review and Meta-Analysis

Mertz D, Johnstone J, Loeb M (McMaster Univ, Hamilton, Ontario, Canada)
Ann Surg 254:48-54, 2011

Objective.—We aimed to compare the efficacy of short-term (<24 hours) versus longer-term antibiotic prophylaxis (≥24 hours) in open heart surgery.

Background.—The optimal duration of antibiotic prophylaxis for adults undergoing cardiac surgery is unknown and guideline recommendations are inconsistent.

Methods.—We searched MEDLINE, EMBASE, CINAHL, and CENTRAL for parallel-group randomized trials comparing any antibiotic prophylaxis administered for <24 hours to any antibiotic prophylaxis for ≥24 hours in adult patients undergoing open heart surgery. Reference lists of selected articles, clinical practice guidelines, review articles, and congress abstracts were searched. Study selection, data extraction and assessment of risk of bias were performed independently by 2 reviewers.

Results.—Of the 1338 citations identified by our search strategy, 12 studies involving 7893 patients were selected. Compared with short-term antibiotic prophylaxis, longer-term antibiotic prophylaxis reduced the risk of sternal surgical site infection (SSI) by 38% (risk ratio 1.38, 95% confidence interval (CI) 1.13–1.69, $P = 0.002$) and deep sternal SSI by 68% (risk ratio 1.68, 95% CI 1.12–2.53, $P = 0.01$). There were no statistically significant differences in mortality, infections overall and adverse events. Eleven of the trials were at high risk for bias due to limitations in study design.

Conclusions.—Perioperative antibiotic prophylaxis of ≥24 hours may be more efficacious in preventing sternal SSIs in patients undergoing cardiac surgery compared to shorter regimens. The findings however are limited by the heterogeneity of antibiotic regimens used and the risk of bias in the published studies.

▶ Duration of preventive/prophylactic antibacterial agents has been a source of controversy within the surgical community. With increasing numbers of bacteria resistant to the available antibacterial agents, there has been a drive to minimize pressure on hospital bacterial flora by diminishing prolonged prophylactic use. Should the goal of prophylactic therapy be to obtain the lowest rate of surgical site infection (SSI) and deep wound infection, shortest length of stay, and fewest readmissions? This study does a meta-analysis of 12 studies and almost 7900 patients for duration of prophylactic antibiotics in cardiac surgery patients. The outcomes assessed were SSI, sternal infections, deep chest infections, and mortality. Antibiotic therapy for less than 24 hours was associated with a higher risk of sternal and deep wound infections. The authors noted many weaknesses of the existing literature (differences in effectiveness of various regimens against contaminating bacteria and changes in flora that modify efficacy of certain classes of drugs) and the relative limitations associated with the analysis. However, the existing literature does suggest that if one wants to minimize the risk of sternal wound infection development after cardiac surgery, prophylactic antibiotics should be continued for more than 24 hours.

T. Pruett, MD

Perforated Appendicitis Among Rural and Urban Patients: Implications of Access to Care
Paquette IM, Zuckerman R, Finlayson SRG (Dartmouth Hitchcock Med Ctr, Lebanon, NH; Hosp of Saint Raphael, New Haven, CT)
Ann Surg 253:534-538, 2011

Objective.—To determine whether rural patients are more likely to present with perforated appendicitis compared with urban patients.

Background.—Appendiceal perforation has been associated with increased morbidity, length of hospital stay, and overall health care costs. Recent arguments suggest that high rates of appendiceal rupture may be unrelated to the quality of hospital care, and rather associated with inadequate access to surgical care.

Methods.—We performed a retrospective cohort study of 122,990 patients with acute appendicitis from the Nationwide Inpatient Sample from 2003 to 2004. International Classification of Diseases diagnosis 9 (ICD-9) codes were used to determine appendiceal perforation. Urban influence codes from the US Department of Agriculture were used to determine rural versus urban status. Univariate and multivariate analyses were used to determine patient and hospital factors associated with perforation.

Results.—Overall, 32.07% of patients presented with perforation. Rural patients were more likely than urban patients to present with perforation (35.76% vs. 31.48%). Factors associated with perforation in multivariate analysis were age more than 40 years, male gender, transfer from another facility, black race, poorest 25th percentile, Charlson score of 3 or higher, and rural residence. Thirty percent of rural patients were treated in urban hospitals. Rural patients treated at urban hospitals were more likely to present with perforation compared with rural patients treated at rural hospitals (OR = 1.23).

Conclusions.—Patients from rural areas have higher rates of perforation with acute appendicitis than urban patients. This difference persists when accounting for other factors associated with perforation. These differences in perforation rates suggest disparities in access to timely surgical care.

▶ Clinical outcomes are mixed among medical diagnostic and therapeutic decisions and a plethora of socioeconomic access issues. Where one lives turns out to affect the kind of care received. This article demonstrates that people treated for appendicitis in a rural setting are more likely to have a perforation compared with those in an urban setting. The authors explore a variety of reasons and demonstrate some salient differences in the populations but postulate that variable access to care is the operative differential. Those individuals surgically treated in a rural hospital (surgical care locally available) had similar risk for perforation as those individuals in an urban setting. However, it was not possible to state whether the increased risk noted in the other population was the consequence of surgical care being unavailable, necessitating a transfer to an urban hospital, or that the individual lived in a remote spot and a delay in presentation increased the likelihood of perforation. Irrespective of the issue, the differences in populations are important and suggest that variable strategies of care may be required for urban and rural settings.

T. Pruett, MD

Perioperative Hyperoxygenation and Wound Site Infection Following Surgery for Acute Appendicitis: A Randomized, Prospective, Controlled Trial

Bickel A, Gurevits M, Vamos R, et al (Western Galilee Hosp, Nahariya, Israel)
Arch Surg 146:464-470, 2011

Objective.—To assess the influence of hyperoxygenation on surgical site infection by using the most homogeneous study population.

Design.—A randomized, prospective, controlled trial.

Setting.—Department of surgery in a government hospital.

Patients.—A total of 210 patients who underwent open surgery for acute appendicitis. In the study group, patients received 80% oxygen during anesthesia, followed by high-flow oxygen for 2 hours in the recovery room. The control group received 30% oxygen, as usual.

Intervention.—Open appendectomy via incision in the right lower quadrant of the abdomen.

Main Outcome Measures.—Surgical site infection, mainly assessed by the ASEPSIS (additional treatment, serous discharge, erythema, purulent discharge, separation of deep tissues, isolation of bacteria, and stay in hospital prolonged >14 days) system score.

Results.—Surgical site infections were recorded in 6 of 107 patients (5.6%) in the study group vs 14 of 103 patients (13.6%) in the control group ($P = .04$). Significant differences in the ASEPSIS score were also found. The mean hospital stay was longer in the control group (2.92 days) compared with the study group (2.51 days) ($P = .01$).

Conclusion.—The use of supplemental oxygen is advantageous in operations for acute appendicitis by reducing surgical site infection rate and hospital stay.

Trial Registration.—clinicaltrials.gov Identifier: NCT01002365.

▶ The role of supplemental oxygen in the management strategy to prevent surgical site infection (SSI) remains unsettled. This study took a new twist and applied hyperoxia to patients undergoing open appendectomy. Other treatments between the groups were identical. All wounds were closed primarily, irrespective of the degree of wound contamination. The findings for use of hyperoxia were overall statistically significant ($P = .04$), but the only single statistically significant group was in the use for the phlegmonous appendix ($P = .049$), although perforation was close to statistical significance with smaller numbers. The true role of hyperoxia is not yet clear, but the ease of administration and relative low risk make it an easy adjunct in the SSI minimization strategy.

T. Pruett, MD

Significant Reduction of Wound Infections With Daily Probing of Contaminated Wounds: A Prospective Randomized Clinical Trial

Towfigh S, Clarke T, Yacoub W, et al (Cedars-Sinai Med Ctr, Los Angeles, CA; Univ of Southern California, Los Angeles, CA; Washington Univ, St Louis, MO)
Arch Surg 146:448-452, 2011

Hypothesis.—Local wound management using a simple wound-probing protocol (WPP) reduces surgical site infection (SSI) in contaminated wounds, with less postoperative pain, shorter hospital stay, and improved patient satisfaction.

Design.—Prospective randomized clinical trial.

Setting.—Academic medical center.

Patients.—Adult patients undergoing open appendectomy for perforated appendicitis were enrolled from January 1, 2007, through December 31, 2009.

Interventions.—Study patients were randomized to the control arm (loose wound closure with staples every 2 cm) or the WPP arm (loosely stapled closure with daily probing between staples with a cotton-tipped applicator until the wound is impenetrable). Intravenous antibiotic therapy was initiated preoperatively and continued until resolution of fever and normalization of the white blood cell count. Follow-up was at 2 weeks and at 3 months.

Outcome Measures.—Wound pain, SSI, length of hospital stay, other complications, and patient satisfaction.

Results.—Seventy-six patients were enrolled (38 in the WPP arm and 38 in the control arm), and 49 (64%) completed the 3-month follow-up. The patients in the WPP arm had a significantly lower SSI rate (3% vs 19%; $P= .03$) and shorter hospital stays (5 vs 7 days; $P= .049$) with no increase in pain ($P= .63$). Other complications were similar ($P= .63$). On regression analysis, only WPP significantly affected SSI rates ($P= .02$). Age, wound length, body mass index, abdominal circumference, and diabetes mellitus had no effect on SSI. Patient satisfaction at 3 months was similar ($P= .69$).

Conclusions.—Surgical site infection in contaminated wounds can be dramatically reduced by a simple daily WPP. This technique is not painful and can shorten the hospital stay. Its positive effect is independent of age, diabetes, body mass index, abdominal girth, and wound length. We recommend wound probing for management of contaminated abdominal wounds.

▶ Management of the contaminated/purulent wound has not been standardized within the surgical literature. Perforated appendicitis remains one of the common diseases treated by surgeons and is often treated using open techniques. Surgical site infection (SSI) in this setting can be significant. This study appears to be the offshoot of the practice of a single surgeon. Placing a cotton swab into the surgical wound attempts to approximate the condition of an open wound allowing for the egress of infected fluid. While there may be many practical reasons that this technique varies from that of an open wound, the results of this randomized study spoke to the efficacy of having skilled study nurses perform daily interventions on the surgical wound. The authors noted that the wound infection rate in the probed wounds was only 3%, whereas the SSI in conventional closure and antibiotics was a more traditional 19%. One can query whether a wound vac would have accomplished a similar outcome in a shorter period; however, the point remains that probing of the wound and evacuation of fluid from the wound is associated with an improved outcome.

T. Pruett, MD

Surgical Site Infections and Cost in Obese Patients Undergoing Colorectal Surgery

Wick EC, Hirose K, Shore AD, et al (Johns Hopkins Univ School of Medicine, Baltimore, MD; et al)
Arch Surg 146:1068-1072, 2011

Objectives.—To measure the effect of obesity on surgical site infection (SSI) rates and to define the cost of SSIs in patients undergoing colorectal surgery.

Design, Setting, and Patients.—This is a retrospective cohort study of 7020 colectomy patients using administrative claims data from 8 Blue Cross and Blue Shield insurance plans. Patients who had a total or segmental colectomy for colon cancer, diverticulitis, or inflammatory bowel disease between January 1, 2002, and December 31, 2008, were included.

Main Outcome Measures.—We compared 30-day SSI rates among obese and nonobese patients and calculated total costs from all health care claims for 90 days following surgery. Multivariate logistic regression was performed to identify risk factors for SSIs.

Results.—Obese patients had an increased rate of SSI compared with nonobese patients (14.5% vs 9.5%, respectively; $P < .001$). Independent risk factors for these infections were obesity (odds ratio=1.59; 95% confidence interval, 1.32-1.91) and open operation as compared with a laparoscopic procedure (odds ratio=1.57; 95% confidence interval, 1.25-1.97).

The mean total cost was $31 933 in patients with infection vs $14 608 in patients without infection (*P* < .001). Total length of stay was longer in patients with infection than in those without infection (mean, 9.5 vs 8.1 days, respectively; *P* < .001), as was the probability of hospital readmission (27.8% vs 6.8%, respectively; *P* < .001).

Conclusions.—Obesity increases the risk of an SSI after colectomy by 60%, and the presence of infection increases the colectomy cost by a mean of $17 324. Payfor-performance policies that do not account for this increased rate of SSI and cost of caring for obese patients may lead to perverse incentives that could penalize surgeons who care for this population.

▶ Surgical site infection (SSI) will become a quality measure released to the public and as such must be followed by providers and be appropriately adjusted for risk. The discussion around appropriate risk adjustment will prove interesting. Irrespective of the broad applicability of the methods used in this article, the conclusion is illuminating. In general, the risk of SSI increases about 60% when a colorectal operation is performed on an obese person. The authors used a binary definition of obese: body mass index (BMI) ≥30. One would, of course, presume that the risk associated with obesity would be similar if the BMI was 29 or 31, but such an analysis was not performed in this study. If we are to incorporate such simple metrics into risk adjustment stratification, it will be necessary to discern risks predicated on the continuum of risk factors and not binary elements. One could also envision a risk associated with heart disease or diabetes. The impact of these diagnoses cannot be effectively assessed just by stating its presence. There is much to be learned from other communities about the public release of information.

T. Pruett, MD

Veterans Affairs Initiative to Prevent Methicillin-Resistant *Staphylococcus aureus* Infections

Jain R, Kralovic SM, Evans ME, et al (VA Pittsburgh Healthcare System, PA; Univ of Cincinnati College of Medicine, OH; et al)
N Engl J Med 364:1419-1430, 2011

Background.—Health care—associated infections with methicillin-resistant *Staphylococcus aureus* (MRSA) have been an increasing concern in Veterans Affairs (VA) hospitals.

Methods.—A "MRSA bundle" was implemented in 2007 in acute care VA hospitals nationwide in an effort to decrease health care—associated infections with MRSA. The bundle consisted of universal nasal surveillance for MRSA, contact precautions for patients colonized or infected with MRSA, hand hygiene, and a change in the institutional culture whereby infection control would become the responsibility of everyone who had contact with patients. Each month, personnel at each facility entered into a central database aggregate data on adherence to surveillance practice, the prevalence of MRSA colonization or infection, and health care—associated transmissions of and infections with MRSA. We assessed the effect of the MRSA bundle on health care—associated MRSA infections.

Results.—From October 2007, when the bundle was fully implemented, through June 2010, there were 1,934,598 admissions to or transfers or discharges from intensive care units (ICUs) and non-ICUs (ICUs, 365,139; non-ICUs, 1,569,459) and 8,318,675 patient-days (ICUs, 1,312,840; and non-ICUs, 7,005,835). During this period, the percentage of patients who were screened at admission increased from 82% to 96%, and the percentage who were screened at transfer or discharge increased from 72% to 93%. The mean ($\pm$SD) prevalence of MRSA colonization or infection at the time of hospital admission was $13.6 \pm 3.7\%$. The rates of health care—associated MRSA infections in ICUs had not changed in the 2 years before October 2007 (P=0.50 for trend) but declined with implementation of the bundle, from 1.64 infections per 1000 patient-days in October 2007 to 0.62 per 1000 patient-days in June 2010, a decrease of 62% (P<0.001 for trend). During this same period, the rates of health care—associated MRSA infections in non-ICUs fell from 0.47 per 1000 patient-days to 0.26 per 1000 patient-days, a decrease of 45% (P<0.001 for trend).

Conclusions.—A program of universal surveillance, contact precautions, hand hygiene, and institutional culture change was associated with a decrease in health care—associated transmissions of and infections with MRSA in a large health care system.

▶ Bacteria causing surgical infections either come from the flora that resides on the patient or from the health care environment. In this context, hospital infection control attempts to identify vectors associated with the spread of antibiotic-resistant organisms. This includes methicillin-resistant *Staphylococcus aureus*, vancomycin-resistant enterococcus, and the resistant enterobacteriacae. *Staphylococcus* is a particularly common isolate from surgical site infections and hospital controls for the acquisition and spread of methicillin-resistant *S aureus* (MRSA) has been the focus of many infections. The Veterans Affairs process improvement tactic of bundling techniques designed to limit the spread of MRSA ultimately demonstrated significant benefit. The authors were not clear which (if any) tactic was the dominant variable associated with the desired outcome and diminished rates of MRSA infections. What would have been interesting to know, but was not reported, was whether the incidence of health care—associated infections also decreased or stayed the same, but only the percentage of pneumonia, line infections, etc, associated with MRSA declined. Depending on which organism fills the void, total risk/benefit for the patient may be reduced or increased. Finding the appropriate endpoint in any of these studies is of paramount importance.

T. Pruett, MD

Evaluating an Evidence-Based Bundle for Preventing Surgical Site Infection: A Randomized Trial

Anthony T, Murray BW, Sum-Ping JT, et al (Univ of Texas Southwestern Med School, Dallas)

Arch Surg 146:263-269, 2011

Objective.—To determine if an evidence-based practice bundle would result in a significantly lower rate of surgical site infections (SSIs) when compared with standard practice.

Design.—Single-institution, randomized controlled trial with blinded assessment of main outcome. The trial opened in April 2007 and was closed in January 2010.

Setting.—Veterans Administration teaching hospital.

Patients.—Patients who required elective transabdominal colorectal surgery were eligible. A total of 241 subjects were approached, 211 subjects were randomly allocated to 1 of 2 interventions, and 197 were included in an intention-to-treat analysis.

Interventions.—Subjects received either a combination of 5 evidence-based practices (extended arm) or were treated according to our current practice (standard arm). The interventions in the extended arm included (1) omission of mechanical bowel preparation; (2) preoperative and intraoperative warming; (3) supplemental oxygen during and immediately after surgery; (4) intraoperative intravenous fluid restriction; and (5) use of a surgical wound protector.

Main Outcome Measure.—Overall SSI rate at 30 days assessed by blinded infection control coordinators using standardized definitions.

Results.—The overall rate of SSI was 45% in the extended arm of the study and 24% in the standard arm ($P = .003$). Most of the increased number of infections in the extended arm were superficial incisional SSIs (36% extended arm vs 19% standard arm; $P = .004$). Multivariate analysis suggested that allocation to the extended arm of the trial conferred a 2.49-fold risk (95% confidence interval, 1.36-4.56; $P = .003$) independent of other factors traditionally associated with SSI.

Conclusions.—An evidence-based intervention bundle did not reduce SSIs. The bundling of interventions, even when the constituent interventions have been individually tested, does not have a predictable effect on outcome. Formal testing of bundled approaches should occur prior to implementation.

Trial Registration.—clinicaltrials.gov Identifier: NCT00953784.

▶ Many process improvement projects in the US health care system are based on evidence-based medicine. This article underscores the importance of clinical assessment and reporting before leaping to broad system changes. The authors bundled 5 well-recognized, evidence-based techniques to diminish surgical site infections into a control package and compared outcomes of surgical site infections resulting after randomization with conventional care. The outcome was that the bundled best practice group had an increased risk of developing surgical site infections. Although the authors went to considerable lengths to discuss the possible reasons that utilization of a bundled best practice might result in worsened outcomes, their conclusion included the following: "The assumption that single measures identified by randomized controlled trials can be grouped into a bundle and effect an outcome in a predictable and positive fashion is not supported by the findings of this study." This study underscores the importance of continuing to explore not only univariate factors on outcomes, but also the possibility that clinical interactions and procedures may result in diverse interactions.

T. Pruett, MD

Association Between Valvular Surgery and Mortality Among Patients With Infective Endocarditis Complicated by Heart Failure
Kiefer T, Park L, Tribouilloy C, et al (Duke Univ Med Ctr, Durham, NC; South Hosp Amiens, France; et al)
JAMA 306:2239-2247, 2011

Context.—Heart failure (HF) is the most common complication of infective endocarditis. However, clinical characteristics of HF in patients with infective endocarditis, use of surgical therapy, and their associations with patient outcome are not well described.

Objectives.—To determine the clinical, echocardiographic, and microbiological variables associated with HF in patients with definite infective endocarditis and to examine variables independently associated with in-hospital and 1-year mortality for patients with infective endocarditis and HF, including the use and association of surgery with outcome.

Design, Setting, and Patients.—The International Collaboration on Endocarditis–Prospective Cohort Study, a prospective, multicenter study enrolling 4166 patients with definite native- or prosthetic-valve infective endocarditis from 61 centers in 28 countries between June 2000 and December 2006.

Main Outcome Measures.—In-hospital and 1-year mortality.

Results.—Of 4075 patients with infective endocarditis and known HF status enrolled, 1359 (33.4% [95% CI, 31.9%-34.8%]) had HF, and 906 (66.7% [95% CI, 64.2%-69.2%]) were classified as having New York Heart Association class III or IV symptom status. Within the subset with HF, 839 (61.7% [95% CI, 59.2%-64.3%]) underwent valvular surgery during the index hospitalization. In-hospital mortality was 29.7% (95% CI, 27.2%-32.1%) for the entire HF cohort, with lower mortality observed in patients undergoing valvular surgery compared with medical therapy alone (20.6% [95% CI, 17.9%-23.4%] vs 44.8% [95% CI, 40.4%-49.0%], respectively; $P < .001$). One-year mortality was 29.1% (95% CI, 26.0%-32.2%) in patients undergoing valvular surgery vs 58.4% (95% CI, 54.1%-62.6%) in those not undergoing surgery ($P < .001$). Cox proportional hazards modeling with propensity score adjustment for surgery showed that advanced age, diabetes mellitus, health care–associated infection, causative microorganism (*Staphylococcus aureus* or fungi), severe HF

(New York Heart Association class III or IV), stroke, and paravalvular complications were independently associated with 1-year mortality, whereas valvular surgery during the initial hospitalization was associated with lower mortality.

Conclusion.—In this cohort of patients with infective endocarditis complicated by HF, severity of HF was strongly associated with surgical therapy and subsequent mortality, whereas valvular surgery was associated with lower in-hospital and 1-year mortality.

▶ Surgical repair of the infected cardiac valve is life saving. This report confirms that the greater the valvular damage, the greater the likelihood of survival. What was intriguing in this report was the lack of microbiologic information. Other than noting worse results from infective endocarditis with *Staphylococcus aureus* or fungus as the causative pathogens, the authors do little to delineate preoperative and postoperative management strategies. What percentage of patients with repair eventually either reinfected a prosthetic valve or ring? Did it matter how long the infective endocarditis was treated prior to surgery? Was there a difference in outcome if the patient received single or multiple agents against the infecting organism? The authors confirmed the teaching in the text books: an indication for surgical intervention in people with infective endocarditis includes worsening cardiac function and embolic phenomena. Judgment is still an important and unquantified aspect of surgical intervention.

T. Pruett, MD

Intrapleural Use of Tissue Plasminogen Activator and DNase in Pleural Infection

Rahman NM, Maskell NA, West A, et al (Churchill Hosp, Oxford, UK; Univ of Bristol, UK; Medway Maritime Hosp, Gillingham, UK; et al)
N Engl J Med 365:518-526, 2011

Background.—More than 30% of patients with pleural infection either die or require surgery. Drainage of infected fluid is key to successful treatment, but intrapleural fibrinolytic therapy did not improve outcomes in an earlier, large, randomized trial.

Methods.—We conducted a blinded, 2-by-2 factorial trial in which 210 patients with pleural infection were randomly assigned to receive one of four study treatments for 3 days: double placebo, intrapleural tissue plasminogen activator (t-PA) and DNase, t-PA and placebo, or DNase and placebo. The primary outcome was the change in pleural opacity, measured as the percentage of the hemithorax occupied by effusion, on chest radiography on day 7 as compared with day 1. Secondary outcomes included referral for surgery, duration of hospital stay, and adverse events.

Results.—The mean (± SD) change in pleural opacity was greater in the t-PA—DNase group than in the placebo group ($-29.5 \pm 23.3\%$ vs. $-17.2 \pm 19.6\%$; difference, -7.9%; 95% confidence interval [CI], -13.4

to −2.4; P=0.005); the change observed with t-PA alone and with DNase alone (−17.2±24.3 and −14.7±16.4%, respectively) was not significantly different from that observed with placebo. The frequency of surgical referral at 3 months was lower in the t-PA—DNase group than in the placebo group (2 of 48 patients [4%] vs. 8 of 51 patients [16%]; odds ratio for surgical referral, 0.17; 95% CI, 0.03 to 0.87; P=0.03) but was greater in the DNase group (18 of 46 patients [39%]) than in the placebo group (odds ratio, 3.56; 95% CI, 1.30 to 9.75; P=0.01). Combined t-PA—DNase therapy was associated with a reduction in the hospital stay, as compared with placebo (difference, −6.7 days; 95% CI, −12.0 to −1.9; P=0.006); the hospital stay with either agent alone was not significantly different from that with placebo. The frequency of adverse events did not differ significantly among the groups.

Conclusions.—Intrapleural t-PA—DNase therapy improved fluid drainage in patients with pleural infection and reduced the frequency of surgical referral and the duration of the hospital stay. Treatment with DNase alone or t-PA alone was ineffective. (Funded by an unrestricted educational grant to the University of Oxford from Roche UK and by others; Current Controlled Trials number, ISRCTN57454527.)

▶ The management of the infected pleural space (empyema) has traditionally proven quite morbid. The routine use of video-assisted thoracoscopic surgery has diminished but has not eliminated the morbidity. The role of tube drainage plus antibiotics has not proven to be a reliable therapy. The sequela of pleural infection has been infection embedded in a thick fibrous rind; the prospect of fibrinolytic agents is attractive. While original studies did not show benefit, this article describes a large multicenter study comparing 4 different therapies. When t-PA and DNAse are added together into the infected chest cavity, outcomes are improved. Neither enzyme resulted in benefit by itself; it was only the combination of enzymes that demonstrated statistical improvement in opacity clearance and diminished need for subsequent surgical debridement. Whether this combination of enzymes is optimal is not clear but speaks to the need of refinement in the pursuit of a less morbid, successful treatment of infections that often required surgical debridement for successful resolution.

T. Pruett, MD

Computed Tomographic Diagnosis of Pneumatosis Intestinalis: Clinical Measures Predictive of the Need for Surgical Intervention
Duron VP, Rutigliano S, Machan JT, et al (Warren Alpert Med School of Brown Univ, Providence, RI; Thomas Jefferson Univ, Philadelphia, PA)
Arch Surg 146:506-510, 2011

Objective.—To determine which clinical, laboratory, and radiographic parameters predict positive operative findings in patients with pneumatosis intestinalis on computed tomography (CT).

Design.—Retrospective record review.

Setting.—Tertiary care hospital and affiliated community hospital.

Patients.—One hundred fifty consecutive patients diagnosed as having pneumatosis intestinalis on CT.

Main Outcome Measures.—Presence or absence of abdominal pathological findings at laparotomy and mortality rates.

Results.—Of the 150 patients studied, 54 (36%) were managed nonoperatively, 72 (48%) were managed operatively, and 24 (16%) were considered unsalvageable and given comfort measures only. Sixty patients (47%) improved with nonoperative management or had negative intraoperative findings. In the nonoperative group, 50 (93%) improved (n=50) and 3 (5%) crossed over to surgery. One patient (2%) died. In the operative group, 63 patients (87%) had operative findings requiring intervention and 9 (13%) had negative results on exploration. Twenty-one patients (28%) died. Univariate analysis identified numerous predictors of positive intraoperative findings, including history of coronary artery disease, tachycardia, tachypnea, hypotension, peritonitis, abdominal distention, and lactic acidemia. The significant radiographic findings included dilated loops of bowel, portal venous gas, and atherosclerosis on CT. On multivariate analysis, only abdominal distention (odds ratio=13.19; $P = .001$), peritonitis (odds ratio=9.35; $P = .007$), and lactic acidemia (odds ratio= 2.29; $P = .02$) were predictive of positive intraoperative findings.

Conclusions.—Many patients with pneumatosis intestinalis on CT can be successfully treated nonoperatively. In determining a management strategy, abnormal physical examination findings were more predictive of the need for surgical intervention than laboratory values or radiographic findings.

▶ Technology continues to change, and findings with newer techniques may not mean the same as a similar diagnosis with an older technique. Air in the intestinal wall has traditionally been associated with intestinal ischemia and intraperitoneal infection and is an indication for operative intervention. However, pneumatosis is sometimes identified in people without severe symptoms. These findings led to the analysis. More than a third of the patients were treated successfully without an operation. Interestingly, the predictive identification of people with positive operative findings rested more with traditional clinical findings (distention, peritoneal signs, lactic acidemia) than with radiographic findings. This article reemphasizes that all abnormalities identified by modern radiographic techniques have pathology that would be best treated by surgical intervention. The need for good clinical judgment continues to be the core of best outcomes.

T. Pruett, MD

7   Endocrine

Utility and Interobserver Agreement of Ultrasound Elastography in the Detection of Malignant Thyroid Nodules in Clinical Care

Merino S, Arrazola J, Cárdenas A, et al (Hospital Clínico San Carlos, Madrid, Spain)

AJNR Am J Neuroradiol 32:2142-2148, 2011

Background and Purpose.—Malignancy correlates with hardness of tissues and US elastography can potentially analyze the stiffness of lesions. Our aim was to evaluate the utility of US elastography in the detection of malignant nodules and to investigate interobserver agreement with this technique.

Materials and Methods.—One-hundred three consecutive patients with 106 thyroid nodules were examined prospectively with conventional B-mode sonography and real-time US elastography. All patients were referred for FNAB. Conventional B-mode sonography and US elastographic examinations were performed, and images were separated and independently interpreted by 2 radiologists blinded to pathologic results. US elastogram evaluation was based on a simplified classification of stiffness based on gray-scale patterns, tumor size compared with B-mode, and margins. Interobserver agreement was studied. FNAB was used as the reference standard for the diagnosis of benign nodules, but histopathologic evaluations were performed when results suspicious for malignancy or malignant results were obtained on FNAB as well as in indeterminate lesions.

Results.—In our study, pattern of stiffness based on gray-scale and classification proposed were statistically significant and predicted malignancy with 100% sensitivity and 40.6% specificity. Tumor size when compared with B-mode images or margins was not statistically significant in our study. No false-negatives were found, and an NPV of 100% was seen. Interobserver agreement for US elastography was excellent in our study, with a κ index of 0.82 (95% CI).

Conclusions.—We believe that US elastography is a promising technique that can assist in the evaluation of thyroid nodules and can potentially diminish the number of FNAB procedures needed. We believe that it may be useful to introduce US elastography into routine clinical practice.

▶ Real-time elastography is an adjunct to routine ultrasound that measures the stiffness or elasticity of tissue, in this case specifically the thyroid nodule. It has slowly gained proponents in Europe as a useful assessment that could even be a potential replacement for fine-needle aspiration (FNA) in the classification of

151

thyroid nodules. The stiffness of a thyroid nodule is usually scored on a 4-point scale, where scores of 1 and 2 are considered firm and suggestive of a malignant nodule and scores of 3 and 4 are considered softer and suggestive of a benign nodule. In a standard determination of the elasticity of a nodule, the radiologist applies a gentle force to the neck over the nodule and then a value is determined based on the distortion of the nodule.

In this series 106 nodules were evaluated, all of which had both cytologic and histopathologic controls. The authors categorized nodules on the basis of elastography into 3 groups similar to standard cytology categorization: benign, indeterminate, and suspicious. All nodules classified as benign were benign on final pathology (100% negative predictive value), and only nodules in the indeterminate and suspicious groups were malignant (which they classified as 100% sensitivity for malignancy). The major limitation of the study is that 88 of the 106 nodules were benign on cytology, and so the utility of this technique in indeterminate nodules on FNA, the ones for which additional information would be most useful, cannot be assessed in this article. While it seems unlikely that elastography will replace FNA, the technology could be very useful in the follow-up of nodules previously classified as benign on FNA.

T. J. Fahey, MD

Is Elastography Actually Useful in the Presurgical Selection of Thyroid Nodules with Indeterminate Cytology?
Lippolis PV, Tognini S, Materazzi G, et al (Univ of Pisa, Italy)
J Clin Endocrinol Metab 96:E1826-E1830, 2011

Background.—Although fine-needle aspiration cytology remains the mainstay of the preoperative workup of thyroid nodules, those with follicular proliferation still represent a diagnostic challenge. Real-time elastography (RTE) estimates the stiffness/elasticity of lesions and is regarded as a promising technique for the presurgical selection of thyroid nodules (including those with indeterminate cytology).

Aim.—Our aim was to verify the potential role of RTE in the presurgical diagnosis of cancer in a large cohort of consecutive patients with follicular thyroid nodules.

Patients and Methods.—One hundred two patients were submitted to conventional ultrasonography and RTE evaluation before being operated on for thyroid nodule with indeterminate cytology (54% single nodules). Tissue stiffness on RTE was scored from 1 (greatest elasticity) to 4 (no elasticity).

Results.—At conventional ultrasonography examination, the nodules (median diameter 2.2 cm) were solid (cystic areas <10%); microcalcifications were detected in 56% of them and a hypoechoic pattern in 64%. Elasticity was high in eight cases only (score 1–2) although low in 94 (score 3–4). Cancer was diagnosed in 36 nodules (35%), being associated with microcalcifications ($P < 0.0001$) and inversely related to nodule diameter ($P < 0.01$). Malignancy was detected in 50% of the nodules with RTE score 1—2 and in 34% of those with score 3—4. Therefore, either the positive (34%) or the negative predictive value (50%) was clinically negligible.

Conclusions.—The current study does not confirm the recently reported usefulness of RTE in presurgical selection of nodules with indeterminate cytology and suggest the need for quantitative analytical assessment of nodule stiffness to improve RTE efficacy.

▶ This study, from the well-known group in Pisa, highlights the potential difficulty of applying real-time elastography to indeterminate lesions. Here the authors document that there are several other ultrasonographic features of thyroid nodules that may more reliably discriminate between benign and malignant follicular lesions, including the presence of microcalcifications. Elastography, like ultrasound in general, is a highly user-dependent imaging modality. Although the authors did try to introduce a rough estimate of the pressure being applied to the neck over the nodule to try to generate some consistency in the technique, they concluded that a more quantitative calculation of the nodule elasticity may lead to more reliable results. As noted, it may be that the most useful application of elastography in the future will be as an adjunct to standard ultrasound in the follow-up of nodules previously determined to be benign by fine needle aspiration.

T. J. Fahey, MD

The Use of Preoperative Routine Measurement of Basal Serum Thyrocalcitonin in Candidates for Thyroidectomy due to Nodular Thyroid Disorders: Results from 2733 Consecutive Patients

Chambon G, Alovisetti C, Idoux-Louche C, et al (Centre Hospitalier Universitaire de Nîmes, France; Hôpital Privéles Franciscaines, Nîmes Cedex 1, France)
J Clin Endocrinol Metab 96:75-81, 2011

Context.—The preoperative routine measurement of basal serum thyrocalcitonin (CT) in candidates for thyroidectomy due to thyroid nodules is currently a subject of debate.

Objective.—The objective of this study was to evaluate the role of systematic basal serum CT measurement in improving the diagnosis and surgical treatment of medullary thyroid carcinoma (MTC) in patients undergoing thyroidectomy for nodular thyroid disorders, regardless of preoperative CT levels.

Design.—We determined basal serum CT levels in 2733 consecutive patients before thyroid surgery and performed a pentagastrin test in patients with hypercalcitoninemia. We correlated basal and stimulated CT levels with intraoperative and definitive histopathological findings, and we analyzed the impact of these results on surgical procedures.

Results.—Twelve MTCs were found among the 43 patients with basal serum CT level of 10 pg/ml or greater. Two MTCs were present among the

TABLE 1.—Basal CT Levels, Stimulated CT Levels, Histological Findings, and Characteristics of MTC in the 43 Patients Referred for Surgical Treatment of Nodular Thyroid Diseases and for whom Preoperative Basal Serum CT Levels were Greater than 10 pg/ml

Patient No.	Sex	Age (yr)	Basal Serum CT Level (pg/ml)	Stimulated Serum CT Peak (pg/ml)	MTC TN Stage/Size	CCH	Other Histopathologicals Findings
1	F	45	12	—	pT1 pN0/1.5 mm	No	Benign nodular goiter
2	F	54	14	53	pT1 pNX/5 mm	No	No Benign nodular goiter, lymphocytic thyroiditis foci
3	H	66	17	—	pT1 pNx/3 mm	No	Benign nodular goiter
4	F	54	45	—	pT1 pN0/6 mm	Yes	Papillary carcinoma
5	F	58	85	—	pT1 pN1b/6 mm	Yes	Toxic benign nodular goiter
6	H	54	206	7,510	pT1 pN0/16 mm	No	None
7	F	81	580	—	pT1 pN0/11 mm	No	None
8	F	83	655	14,000	pT1 pN0/19 mm	No	None
9	H	63	1,900	—	pT2 pN1b/22 mm	No	None
10	F	82	4,419	—	pT3 pN1b/39 mm	No	Papillary microcarcinoma
11	F	61	5,654	—	pT2 pN0/30 mm	No	None
12	F	81	13,000	—	pT3 pN1b/27 mm	No	Lymphocytic thyroiditis foci
13	F	61	12	53	No	Yes	Solitary benign adenoma
14	H	51	12	126	No	Yes	Multifocal papillary microcarcinoma
15	H	67	13	63	No	No	Benign nodular goiter
16	H	57	13	74	No	Yes	Solitary benign adenoma
17	F	45	13	80	No	Yes	Benign nodular goiter
18	H	55	13	203	No	No	Papillary microcarcinoma
19	F	45	14	40	No	Yes	Solitary benign adenoma
20	H	30	14	213	No	Yes	Benign nodular goiter
21	F	70	15	38	No	Yes	Benign nodular goiter
22	H	70	15	38	No	Yes	Thyroiditis, papillary microcarcinoma
23	F	33	15	60	No	Yes	Benign nodular goiter
24	H	59	16	159	No	Yes	Benign nodular goiter
25	H	53	16	159	No	Yes	Solitary benign adenoma
26	F	30	17	38	No	Yes	Benign nodular goiter
27	H	50	18	163	No	Yes	Benign nodular goiter, lymphocytic thyroiditis foci
28	F	43	20	45	No	Yes	Benign nodular goiter
29	H	47	20	56	No	Yes	Benign nodular goiter, lymphocytic thyroiditis foci
30	F	28	20	59	No	Yes	Benign nodular goiter
31	H	64	20	70	No	Yes	Solitary benign adenoma
32	H	52	20	112	No	Yes	Benign nodular goiter
33	H	62	20	161	No	Yes	Solitary benign adenoma
34	H	50	21	450	No	Yes	Benign nodular goiter
35	H	52	22	79	No	Yes	Benign nodular goiter
36	H	64	25	244	No	Yes	Benign nodular goiter
37	H	48	26	100	No	Yes	Solitary benign adenoma
38	H	54	27	249	No	Yes	Benign nodular goiter
39	H	50	28	112	No	Yes	Solitary benign adenoma
40	H	52	34	—	No	Yes	Solitary benign adenoma
41	H	54	35	268	No	Yes	Benign nodular goiter
42	H	61	36	—	No	Yes	Benign nodular goiter
43	F	58	59	—	No	Yes	Benign nodular goiter

F, Female; —, no data available.

2690 patients with normal CT levels. MTC was always present in patients with a basal CT of 60 pg/ml or greater. For CT levels ranging from 10 to 59 pg/ml, MTC was diagnosed in 11% of patients. When preoperative hypercalcitoninemia was present, total thyroidectomy associated with comprehensive intraoperative histopathological analysis allowed the intraoperative diagnosis of five latent, subclinical MTCs. The pentagastrin test gave no additional diagnostic information for the management of patients with elevated preoperative basal serum CT level.

Conclusion.—Routine measurement of CT in the preoperative work-up of nodular thyroid disorders is useful. This procedure improves intraoperative diagnosis of MTC and enables adapted initial surgery, the most determinant factor of treatment success (Table 1).

▶ Routine measurement of serum calcitonin (CT) level in all patients who present with nodular thyroid disease is still advocated by some, despite a specificity that is so low that many consider it to be unwarranted, if not contraindicated, by many. In this article, the authors measured serum CT level only in patients who were scheduled to undergo thyroid surgery for another indication; they used a value of 10 pg/mL as the threshold to alter the preoperative and surgical management of these patients. Prior to 2008, all patients with a basal CT level of > 10 pg/mL underwent pentagastrin stimulation and then total thyroidectomy. Pentagastrin became unavailable in 2008, and so subsequent patients just underwent total thyroidectomy. The results are all contained in Table 1. It can be seen that although the overall detection rate in patients with a CT value greater than 10 pg/mL was approximately 28%, for patients who had a CT value < 60 pg/mL, the detection rate was only 11%, and only one of these would not have been adequately treated by hemithyroidectomy alone (1 of the 4 medullary thyroid carcinomas [MTCs] was found in the contralateral lobe and would not have been included in the initially planned operation).

The question remains as to whether the use of CT measurement as a part of the preoperative workup will prove to be cost effective. The authors do not help us guide the use of preoperative CT measurement; there must be some patients for whom it did not matter, such as those who had a cytologic diagnosis of papillary thyroid carcinoma. It is suggested in the discussion that those tumors that were macro-MTCs would have been evaluated for possible MTC as part of the routine evaluation, but further information is not given. So the issue is really whether the prognosis and outcome of the 5 patients with micro-MTC would really have been changed by the knowledge of a mild CT level elevation. It would seem the answer is "No," and in an era of increased cost consciousness, even restricting CT testing to preoperative patients may still not provide enough yield to recommend it routinely.

T. J. Fahey, MD

The Predictive Value of the Fine-Needle Aspiration Diagnosis "Suspicious for a Follicular Neoplasm, Hürthle Cell Type" in Patients With Hashimoto Thyroiditis

Roh MH, Jo VY, Stelow EB, et al (Univ of Michigan Med School, Ann Arbor; Univ of Virginia Health System, Charlottesville; et al)
Am J Clin Pathol 135:139-145, 2011

A fine-needle aspiration sample composed exclusively of Hürthle cells is interpreted as "suspicious for a follicular neoplasm, Hürthle cell type" (SFNHCT). Because some nonneoplastic Hürthle cell proliferations in Hashimoto thyroiditis (HT) mimic this cytologic pattern, we examined the positive predictive value (PPV) for malignancy of SFNHCT in patients with HT. Between 1992 and 2007, 401 patients with cytologic findings of SFNHCT were identified at 3 institutions. Histologic follow-up was available for 287 (71.6%), and malignancy was diagnosed in 69 (24.0%). Malignancy was present in 2 (PPV = 9.5%) of 21 patients with HT compared with 67 (PPV = 25.2%) of 266 patients without HT ($P = .081$). Although the difference in the rate of malignancy between the HT and non-HT cohorts did not reach statistical significance, the lower risk of malignancy in the HT cohort more closely approximates the risk of cases interpreted as "atypia of undetermined significance." For this reason, it might be appropriate for Hürthle cell—only aspirates from patients with HT to be categorized as either atypia of undetermined significance or SFNHCT (Table 2).

▶ The finding of Hürthle cells on fine-needle aspiration (FNA) typically raises the level of concern among physicians, as Hürthle cell carcinomas have become to be more feared than other differentiated thyroid carcinomas. The authors here have examined the effect of Hürthle cell findings in nodules with and without a background of Hashimoto thyroiditis (HT). This article demonstrates that the risk of malignancy in the presence of HT is lower than that for Hürthle cell lesions in the absence of HT (Table 2). Given the lower risk of malignancy

TABLE 2.—Corresponding Histologic Findings for the Aspirated Nodules in Patients With and Without HT

	UVA	BWH	MGH	Total
Patients with HT	7	10	4	21
Neoplastic nodules*	1	6	2	9 (PPV = 42.9%)[†]
Carcinomas	0	2	0	2 (PPV = 9.5%)[‡]
Patients without HT	48	155	63	266
Neoplastic nodules*	33	93	57	183 (PPV = 68.8%)[†]
Carcinomas	15	39	13	67 (PPV = 25.2%)[‡]
No. of FNAs interpreted as SFNHCT	55	165	67	287

BWH, Brigham and Women's Hospital, Boston, MA; FNAs, fine-needle aspiration samples; HT, Hashimoto thyroiditis; MGH, Massachusetts General Hospital, Boston; PPV, positive predictive value; SFNHCT, "suspicious for a follicular neoplasm, Hürthle cell type"; UVA, University of Virginia Health System, Charlottesville.
*Represents the sum of adenomas and carcinomas.
[†]$P = .016$.
[‡]$P = .081$.

in the group with HT versus the group without HT (9.5% vs 25.2%), the authors conclude that perhaps these nodules should be placed in the cytologic category of atypia of undetermined significance and be relegated to observation and repeat FNA. An alternative approach would be to more confidently recommend hemithyroidectomy in these patients. The fact is that more than 40% of these nodules proved to be neoplastic on final pathology (Table 2), and the adenoma to carcinoma sequence is well established for Hürthle cell nodules. Regardless of how the data are interpreted, it does highlight the need for further study of Hürthle cell nodules on a molecular basis to assist in the characterization of Hürthle cell lesions so that more informed decisions can be made by doctors and patients.

T. J. Fahey, MD

Cost-Effectiveness of a Novel Molecular Test for Cytologically Indeterminate Thyroid Nodules
Li H, Robinson KA, Anton B, et al (Johns Hopkins Univ School of Medicine, Baltimore, MD)
J Clin Endocrinol Metab 96:E1719-E1726, 2011

Context.—Determining which patients with thyroid nodules require surgery is limited by cytologically indeterminate findings. A new approach for preoperative molecular classification of cytologically indeterminate thyroid nodules has a reported sensitivity of 91% and specificity of 75%; however, its cost-effectiveness has yet to be assessed.

Objective.—Our objective was to evaluate the 5-yr cost-effectiveness of routine use of a molecular test in adult patients with indeterminate fine-needle aspiration biopsy results from a societal perspective.

Design.—A 16-state Markov decision model was developed. Probabilities, costs, and quality-adjusted life years (QALY) were estimated from literature review, U.S. Department of Health and Human Services data, Medicare reimbursement schedules, and expert opinion.

Setting and Subjects.—Decision analysis of a hypothetical group of adult patients with cytologically indeterminate thyroid nodules was conducted.

Main Outcome Measures.—Incremental cost-effectiveness ratio was calculated as incremental cost (measured in U.S. dollars) divided by incremental effectiveness (measured in QALY).

Results.—Modifying current practice with use of the molecular test resulted in 74% fewer surgeries for benign nodules with no greater number of untreated cancers. Over 5 yr, mean discounted cost estimates were $12,172 for current practice and $10,719 with the molecular test. Current practice and molecular test use produced 4.50 and 4.57 QALY, respectively.

Conclusions.—Use of this novel molecular test for differential diagnosis of cytologically indeterminate thyroid nodules can potentially avoid almost three fourths of currently performed surgeries in patients with benign nodules. Compared with current practice based on cytological findings alone, use of this test may result in lower overall costs and modestly improved quality of life for patients with indeterminate thyroid nodules.

▶ Molecular assays of thyroid nodule fine-needle aspirations (FNAs) will be part of routine clinical testing for indeterminate thyroid nodules. How the results are used remains to be determined. This article argues that a benign classification on a gene expression assay will allow patients to avoid surgery and show that this is cost effective over a 5-year period. As one of the investigators that have contributed to this literature over the last 10+ years, I applaud the introduction of a molecular test into clinical practice. However, the conclusions reached in this article are severely flawed. Cost savings over 5 years is based on using the test just once over this period. Because the test costs $3200, and because it is likely—as with any indeterminate FNA—that each patient will have more than 1 additional FNA in a 5-year period if they opt for observation, with an additional cost of a subsequent molecular test, the cost savings in this model quickly becomes extra expense and a cost burden of more than $1500. Additional observation time will inevitably drive up the cost substantially. While it may (and should) spare some very elderly patients from hemithyroidectomy, most patients with follicular lesions are young and otherwise healthy; follow-up of these lesions will become very costly but will benefit Veracyte and its shareholders (including one of the authors) substantially. A molecular test like this, without the ability to discriminate between neoplastic and hyperplastic nodules (if such a difference exists), will be best used for identifying patients who have malignancy and who therefore will be treated appropriately from the time of diagnosis.

T. J. Fahey, MD

Impact of Mutational Testing on the Diagnosis and Management of Patients with Cytologically Indeterminate Thyroid Nodules: A Prospective Analysis of 1056 FNA Samples

Nikiforov YE, Ohori NP, Hodak SP, et al (Univ of Pittsburgh School of Medicine, PA)
J Clin Endocrinol Metab 96:3390-3397, 2011

Context.—Thyroid nodules are common in adults, but only a small fraction of them is malignant. Fine-needle aspiration (FNA) cytology provides a definitive diagnosis of benign or malignant disease in many cases, whereas about 25% of nodules are indeterminate, hindering most appropriate management.

Objective.—The objective of the investigation was to study the clinical utility of molecular testing of thyroid FNA samples with indeterminate cytology.

Design.—Residual material from 1056 consecutive thyroid FNA samples with indeterminate cytology was used for prospective molecular analysis that included the assessment of cell adequacy by a newly developed PCR assay and testing for a panel of mutations consisted of *BRAF V600E, NRAS* codon 61, *HRAS* codon 61, and *KRAS* codons 12/13 point mutations and *RET/PTC1, RET/PTC3,* and *PAX8/PPAR*γ rearrangements.

Results.—The collected material was adequate for molecular analysis in 967 samples (92%), which yielded 87 mutations including 19 *BRAF,* 62 *RAS,* 1 *RET/PTC,* and five *PAX8/PPAR*γ. Four hundred seventy-nine patients who contributed 513 samples underwent surgery. In specific categories of indeterminate cytology, *i.e.* atypia of undetermined significance/follicular lesion of undetermined significance, follicular neoplasm/suspicious for a follicular neoplasm, and suspicious for malignant cells, the detection of any mutation conferred the risk of histologic malignancy of 88, 87, and 95%, respectively. The risk of cancer in mutation-negative nodules was 6, 14, and 28%, respectively. Of 6% of cancers in mutation-negative nodules with atypia of undetermined significance/follicular lesion of undetermined significance cytology, only 2.3% were invasive and 0.5% had extrathyroidal extension.

Conclusion.—Molecular analysis for a panel of mutations has significant diagnostic value for all categories of indeterminate cytology and can be helpful for more effective clinical management of these patients.

▶ The group from Pittsburgh has looked at mutation analysis in a large number of samples with indeterminate cytology. This extensive analysis demonstrates that mutation analysis is highly accurate in predicting the presence of cancer when a mutation is detected, and the mutation detection by fine-needle aspiration was 95% of the rate in the final histopathologic sample. While there is a very high positive predictive value if a mutation is detected for nodules in the 3 indeterminate classes, the sensitivity for malignancy is substantially less. This number is a little harder to determine from the article, since only approximately half of the patients who had mutation analysis underwent surgery and had a definitive diagnosis. Overall, *BRAF* mutations were detected in only 19 of 967 nodules (2%). Since this is the most useful of the mutations to determine (given that virtually 100% of *BRAF*-positive nodules will be malignant), the use of determining just *BRAF* status in indeterminate nodules is questionable. Fig 2 from the original article demonstrates that the majority of *BRAF*-positive tumors are in the "suspicious" category, a group of patients who would probably undergo total thyroidectomy as the initial operation without additional testing given the high incidence of cancer in this group.

In sum, the role of mutation analysis as compared with other upcoming more sensitive methods of detection of malignancy in indeterminate nodules will probably mean that mutation analysis will be unnecessary in the future.

T. J. Fahey, MD

A multicenter cohort study of total thyroidectomy and routine central lymph node dissection for cN0 papillary thyroid cancer

Popadich A, Levin O, Lee JC, et al (Univ of Sydney Endocrine Surgical Unit, New South Wales, Australia; UCLA David Geffen School of Medicine; et al)

Surgery 150:1048-1057, 2011

Background.—The role of routine central lymph node dissection (CLND) for papillary thyroid cancer (PTC) remains controversial. The aim of this study was to evaluate the impact of routine CLND after total thyroidectomy (TTx) in the management of patients with PTC who were clinically node negative at presentation with emphasis on stimulated thyroglobulin (Tg) levels and reoperation rates.

Methods.—This retrospective, multicenter, cohort study used pooled data from 3 international Endocrine Surgery units in Australia, the United States, and England. All study participants had PTC >1 cm without preoperative evidence of lymph node disease (cN0). Group A patients had TTx alone and group B had TTx with the addition of CLND.

Results.—There were 606 patients included in the study. Group A had 347 patients and group B 259 patients. Stimulated Tg values were lower in group B before initial radioiodine ablation (15.0 vs 6.6 ng/mL; $P = .025$). There was a trend toward a lower Tg at final follow-up in group B (1.9 vs 7.2 ng/mL; $P = .11$). The rate of reoperation in the central compartment was lower in group B (1.5 vs 6.1%; $P = .004$). The number of CLND procedures required to prevent 1 central compartment reoperation was calculated at 20.

Conclusion.—The addition of routine CLND in cN0 papillary thyroid carcinoma is associated with lower postoperative Tg levels and reduces the need for reoperation in the central compartment.

▶ The debate about the role of prophylactic central neck dissection (CND) in patients undergoing total thyroidectomy for papillary thyroid cancer goes on. In this article, the discussion that ensued after it was presented and in the accompanying editorial by McHenry,[1] the pros and cons of central neck dissection are detailed. It is clear that this question will be answered only by a large, multicenter, randomized, prospective study—and hopefully there will be funding for such a study in the United States soon. In the absence of this, there is a suggestion that there is a reduction in central neck recurrence of papillary thyroid cancer (PTC) with the addition of a prophylactic CND. There is no question that the addition of CND should only be done by surgeons who feel comfortable with the operation. However, using surgical inadequacy as an argument against its use is specious and goes against surgical dogma. For virtually any other elective operation in surgery, if the surgeon cannot do the operation with accepted rates of morbidity, then we would all recommend that the surgeon refer the patient to someone who can do the operation properly. Why should this be different for patients undergoing thyroidectomy for thyroid cancer? Finally, not mentioned by the authors, discussants, or by Dr McHenry in his editorial is the potential benefit of a negative CND—avoidance of radioactive iodine (RAI). There have been significant data published in recent years that there are short-term and potential long-term side effects of RAI, and both patients and doctors are increasingly leery about routine adjuvant RAI treatment. Patients with PTC—especially those with papillary microcarcinomas—with negative central nodes can be more confidently advised that they can forgo postoperative RAI.

T. J. Fahey, MD

Reference

1. McHenry CR. Prophylactic central compartment neck dissection for papillary thyroid cancer: the search for justification continues. *Surgery.* 2011;150:1058-1060.

Recurrent Laryngeal Nerve Monitoring Versus Identification Alone on Post-Thyroidectomy True Vocal Fold Palsy: A Meta-Analysis

Higgins TS, Gupta R, Ketcham AS, et al (Eastern Virginia Med School, Norfolk; Osborne Head and Neck Inst, Los Angeles, CA; et al)

Laryngoscope 121:1009-1017, 2011

Objectives/Hypothesis.—To compare by meta-analysis the effect of recurrent laryngeal nerve (RLN) monitoring versus RLN identification alone on true vocal fold palsy rates after thyroidectomy.

Study Design.—Systematic review and meta-analysis.

Methods.—A search of MEDLINE (1966–July 2008), EMBASE (1980–July 2008), Cochrane Central Register of Clinical Trials (CENTRAL), Cochrane Database of Systematic Reviews, clinicaltrials.gov, and The National Guideline Clearinghouse databases was performed. References from retrieved articles, presentation data, and correspondence with experts was also included. All authors used a detailed list of inclusion/exclusion criteria to determine articles eligible for final inclusion. Two authors independently extracted data including study criteria, methods of vocal fold function assessment, laryngeal nerve monitor type, and surgical procedure. Odds ratios (OR) were pooled using a random-effects model. Associations with patient and operative characteristics were tested in subgroups.

Results.—One randomized clinical trial, seven comparative trials, and 34 case series evaluating 64,699 nerves-at-risk were included. The overall incidence of true vocal fold palsy (TVFP) was 3.52% for intraoperative nerve monitoring (IONM) versus 3.12% for nerve identification alone (ID) (OR 0.93; 95% confidence interval [CI], 0.76-1.12]. No statistically significant difference in transient TVFP (2.74% IONM vs. 2.49% ID [OR 1.07, 95% CI, 0.95-1.20]), persistent TVFP (0.75% IONM vs. 0.58% ID [OR 0.99, 95% CI, 0.79-1.23]), or unintentional RLN injury (0.12% IONM vs. 0.33% ID [OR 0.50, 95% CI, 0.15-1.75]) was found.

Conclusions.—This meta-analysis demonstrates no statistically significant difference in the rate of true vocal fold palsy after using intraoperative

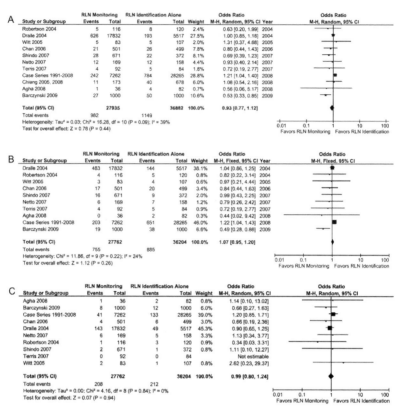

FIGURE 3.—Forest plots showing the distribution of (A) overall true vocal fold palsy (TVFP). (B) Transient TVFP. (C) Persistent TVFP. RLN = recurrent laryngeal nerve; CI = confidence interval. (Reprinted from Higgins TS, Gupta R, Ketcham AS, et al. Recurrent laryngeal nerve monitoring versus identification alone on post-thyroidectomy true vocal fold palsy: a meta-analysis. *Laryngoscope*. 2011;121:1009-1017, John Wiley and Sons (www.interscience.wiley.com).

neuromonitoring versus recurrent laryngeal nerve identification alone during thyroidectomy (Fig 3).

▶ Like the debate about prophylactic central neck dissection, the debate regarding whether to use routine recurrent laryngeal nerve (RLN) monitoring is sometimes contentious and also equally unlikely to be resolved without a large, randomized, multicenter trial. As with prophylactic central neck dissection, such a trial may never happen. Here the authors attempt to provide some insight using a meta-analysis of available data already published. The results demonstrate that there is no discernible difference in RLN injury rate whether intraoperative nerve monitoring is performed or the nerve is identified only visually. Fig 3 contains the critical data from the article. The Forest plots detail the studies that were used to derive the data, the confidence intervals for RLN injury rates in each of the studies, and the combined data conclusion. The authors further conclude that intraoperative nerve monitoring should not be considered standard of care. This conclusion may have important implications for surgeons who have had an RLN injury and are the focus of a malpractice case. There is also a suggestion that a randomized trial may be difficult to conduct in the standard sense because surgeons who are used to using nerve monitoring may not feel comfortable operating without it. Thus, any randomized trial would have to pit 1 surgeon or center against another. Finally, there is simply no replacement for visual identification of the nerve, even if the surgeon uses routine RLN monitoring.

T. J. Fahey, MD

The value of detectable thyroglobulin in patients with differentiated thyroid cancer after initial ^{131}I therapy

van Dijk D, Plukker JTM, van der Horst-Schrivers ANA, et al (Univ of Groningen, The Netherlands)
Clin Endocrinol 74:104-110, 2011

Objective.—To assess the prognostic value of detectable thyroglobulin (Tg) after initial surgery and radioactive iodine (^{131}I) therapy by comparing patients with a negative post-therapeutic whole body scan (WBS) with either detectable or undetectable Tg.

Background.—Differentiated thyroid cancer has a good prognosis. However, recurrences can occur up to 30 years after initial treatment. Because life-long follow-up is necessary, it is important to explore possible risk factors associated with recurrence and mortality.

Design, Patients and Measurements.—We studied 539 patients who were treated between 1980 and 2007. After the last therapeutic dosage of 5550 MBq ^{131}I, 72 patients had negative post-therapeutic WBS and positive Tg levels (Tg+ group) and 399 patients had negative post-therapeutic WBS and negative Tg (Tg− group). The 68 remaining patients had proven residual macroscopic disease. We investigated recurrences and overall mortality in the Tg+ and Tg− group compared with the Dutch population.

Results.—In the Tg+ group, detectable recurrences occurred significantly earlier and more frequently than in the Tg− group (19% vs 13%, $P = 0 \cdot 024$). Survival between these groups was comparable, but shorter than the general Dutch population [Standardised Mortality Rate (SMR) $1 \cdot 38$ (95% CI $1 \cdot 12;1 \cdot 63$) ($P = 0 \cdot 003$)]. Disease-free survival in the Tg groups was comparable and not significantly different from the Dutch population [SMR $= 1 \cdot 09$ (95% CI $0 \cdot 81;1 \cdot 34$) ($P = 0 \cdot 569$)].

Conclusion.—Patients with detectable Tg during the last ^{131}I treatment and a negative post-therapeutic WBS have significant earlier and more recurrences than patients without detectable Tg. Survival in both groups is comparable. After initial therapy, the combination of a negative high dose post-therapeutic WBS with detectable Tg is a valuable predictor for earlier and more recurrences, but is not associated with survival.

▶ The use of thyroglobulin assay (Tg) in the follow up of patients with differentiated thyroid cancer is accepted as standard of care. The authors here have shown what could be considered common sense—that if a patient has an elevated Tg level after initial treatment is completed, then their risk of recurrence is significantly higher than patients who do not have detectable Tg after treatment (19% vs 13%). One attribute of the study is a very long follow-up. A possible detractor—acknowledged by the authors—was the change in the Tg assay that was used over the course of the study period. Also of note, the protocol for treatment of patients with radioactive iodine seemed quite aggressive, with some patients getting repeated doses to try to eliminate residual Tg levels.

The authors did note that the overall mortality between Tg+ and Tg− patients was equivalent, but decreased compared with the general Dutch population. Although it is not easy to dissect this out in the article, this decrease appeared to be entirely accounted for by patients who developed macroscopic recurrent disease—disease that could be identified radiographically or clinically—and this became evident in only 20% of the patients who had persistent Tg elevation. This may be one of the most important observations in the study; patients who either have persistent elevation in Tg or who develop biochemical evidence for recurrence usually do not go on to develop identifiable disease and have a normal lifespan—at least within the limits of this study. The implication is that patients who have a biochemical recurrence should be reassured that they are not likely to die of their disease in the absence of macroscopic disease.

T. J. Fahey, MD

Current Thyroglobulin Autoantibody (TgAb) Assays Often Fail to Detect Interfering TgAb that Can Result in the Reporting of Falsely Low/Undetectable Serum Tg IMA Values for Patients with Differentiated Thyroid Cancer

Spencer C, Petrovic I, Fatemi S (Univ of Southern California, Los Angeles; Kaiser Permanente, Panorama City, CA)
J Clin Endocrinol Metab 96:1283-1291, 2011

Context.—Specimens have thyroglobulin antibody (TgAb) measured prior to thyroglobulin (Tg) testing because the qualitative TgAb status (positive or negative) determines risk for Tg assay interference, and the quantitative TgAb concentration serves as a surrogate tumor marker for differentiated thyroid cancer.

Objective.—This study assessed the reliability of four TgAb methods to detect interfering TgAb [as judged from abnormally low Tg immunometric assay (IMA) toTgRIA ratios] and determine whether between method conversion factors might prevent a change in method from disrupting TgAb monitoring.

Methods.—Sera from selected and unselected TgAb-negative and TgAb-positive differentiated thyroid cancer patients had serum Tg measured by both IMA and RIA and TgAb measured by a reference method and three additional methods.

Results.—The Tg IMA and Tg RIA values were concordant when TgAb was absent. Tg IMA to Tg RIA ratios below 75% were considered to indicate TgAb interference. Manufacturer-recommended cutoffs were set in the detectable range, and when used to determine the presence of TgAb misclassified many specimens displaying Tg interference as TgAb negative. False-negative misclassifications were virtually eliminated for two of four methods by using the analytical sensitivity (AS) as the detection limit for TgAb. Relationships between values for different specimens were too variable to establish between-method conversion factors.

Conclusions.—Many specimens with interfering TgAb were misclassified as TgAb negative using manufacturer-recommended cutoffs. It is recommended that assay AS limits be used to detect TgAb to minimize false-negative misclassifications. However, for two of four assays, AS limits failed to detect interfering TgAb in 20—30% of cases. TgAb methods were too qualitatively and quantitatively variable to establish conversion factors that would allow a change in method without disrupting serial TgAb monitoring.

▶ The fact that thyroglobulin antibodies (TgAb) can affect the use of thyroglobulin (Tg) assays for follow-up of patients with differentiated thyroid cancers is well known. In this study, Carole Spencer, a leader in the field of TgAb, delineates nicely the pitfalls of TgAB assays. It is clear that some assays are more sensitive than others and thus presumably more accurate. Although the names of the different assays are not revealed in the article, the competitive immunoassays appear to generally be more sensitive for measuring TgAb and thus ultimately more accurate. One of the important take-home messages is that Tg assays are not all equivalent, and there is no means for accounting for the differences between assays. Thus, once an assay or laboratory test is chosen for follow-up, the most reliable way to follow up with the patient is to stick with that assay. Finally, even though Dr Spencer reports that interfering antibodies may be present in 20% to 30% of cases, the actual effect of this finding is not clear because there are in fact very few cases of thyroglobulin-negative recurrent thyroid cancers.

T. J. Fahey, MD

Does an undetectable rhTSH-stimulated Tg level 12 months after initial treatment of thyroid cancer indicate remission?
Klubo-Gwiezdzinska J, Burman KD, Van Nostrand D, et al (Washington Hosp Ctr, DC)
Clin Endocrinol 74:111-117, 2011

Objectives.—Routine monitoring after the initial treatment of differentiated thyroid cancer (DTC) includes periodic cervical ultrasonography (US) and measurement of serum thyroglobulin (Tg) during thyrotrophin (TSH) suppression and after recombinant human TSH (rhTSH) stimulation. The aim of our study was to evaluate the utility of repeated rhTSH-stimulated Tg measurements in patients with DTC who have had no evidence of disease at their initial rhTSH stimulation test performed 1 year after the treatment.

Material and Methods.—A retrospective chart review of 278 patients with DTC who had repeated rhTSH stimulation testing after an initial undetectable rhTSH-stimulated serum Tg level.

Results.—The number of rhTSH stimulation tests performed on individual patients during the follow-up period (3—12 years, mean 6·3) varied from two to seven. Biochemical and/or cytological evidence of potential persistent/recurrent disease based on detectable second or third rhTSH-stimulated Tg values and US findings was observed in 11 (4%) patients. Subsequent follow-up data revealed that in five cases, the results of the second stimulation were false positive, in one case — false negative. Combined with the negative neck US, the negative predictive value for disease-free survival was 98% after the first undetectable rhTSH-stimulated Tg and 100% after the second one.

Conclusions.—In patients with DTC, the intensity of follow-up should be adjusted to new risk estimates evolving with time. The first rhTSH-stimulated Tg is an excellent predictor for remission, independent of clinical stage at presentation. Second negative rhTSH-Tg stimulation is additionally reassuring and can guide less aggressive follow-up by the measurement of nonstimulated Tg and neck US every few years.

▶ Recommendations for follow-up of patients with differentiated thyroid cancer are generally lacking. In this article from the Washington Hospital Center, the authors review their experience using thyrogen-stimulated thyroglobulin (Tg). In a large retrospective study carried out over 13 years, the authors document that a single thyrogen-stimulated Tg level done 1 year after radioiodine is highly predictive of cure. Less than 4% of patients who had a negative 1-year thyrogen-stimulated Tg went on to have an elevation of Tg on a second thyrogen-stimulated test 1—3 years after the first one. The authors conclude that follow-up can be modified after the second test by reducing the interval for follow-up. Given the cost associated with thyrogen, it would have been interesting to see a cost analysis for the use of thyrogen—incorporating the pathologic characteristics of the initial primary tumor into the equation. Is it possible that a single thyrogen stimulation test is all that is needed? Other studies have suggested that this is the case. Nevertheless, the data are very useful for focusing long-term follow-up for patients with negative scans and thyrogen stimulation tests.

T. J. Fahey, MD

In Differentiated Thyroid Cancer, an Incomplete Structural Response to Therapy Is Associated with Significantly Worse Clinical Outcomes Than Only an Incomplete Thyroglobulin Response

Vaisman F, Tala H, Grewal R, et al (Universidade Federal do Rio de Janeiro and Instituto Nacional do Cancer, Brazil; Clínica Alemana/Universidad del Desarrollo, Santiago, Chile; Memorial Sloan-Kettering Cancer Ctr, NY)
Thyroid 21:1317-1322, 2011

Background.—We previously demonstrated the clinical utility of using response to therapy variables obtained during the first 2 years of follow-up to actively modify initial risk estimates which were obtained using standard clinic-pathologic staging systems. While our proposed dynamic risk stratification system accurately reclassified patients who demonstrated an excellent response to therapy as low-risk patients, it grouped patients with either biochemical or structural evidence of disease into a single incomplete response to therapy cohort. This cohort included a wide variety of patients ranging from very minor thyroglobulin (Tg) elevations in the absence of structurally identifiable disease to widespread, progressive structural disease. Here we determined whether subdivision of the incomplete response to therapy category more precisely predicted clinical outcomes. We hypothesized that patients with an incomplete response to therapy based on persistently abnormal Tg values alone would have better clinical outcomes than patients having structurally identifiable disease.

Methods.—Following total thyroidectomy and radioactive iodine (RAI) ablation, 192 adult thyroid cancer patients were retrospectively identified as having either a biochemical incomplete response (abnormal Tg without structural evidence of disease) or structural incomplete response (structurally identifiable disease with or without abnormal Tg) as the best response to initial therapy within the first 24 months after RAI ablation. Clinical outcomes evaluated included structural disease progression, biochemical disease progression, and overall survival.

Results.—Sixty-three patients (33%) had a biochemical incomplete response while 129 (67%) had a structural incomplete response. Eleven to 156 months after evaluation of their responses (mean = 70 months), patients with structural incomplete response were significantly more likely to have structural evidence of disease at final follow-up (37% vs. 17%, $p = 0.0004$), structural progression (52% vs. 5%, $p < 0.001$), biochemical progression (45% vs. 11%, $p < 0.001$), and death from disease (38% vs. 0%, $p < 0.0001$) than patients demonstrating a biochemical incomplete response. Overall survival was significantly better in patients with either a biochemical incomplete response or a loco-regional structural incomplete response than patients demonstrating a structural incomplete response with distant metastasis (Kaplan-Meier analysis, $p < 0.0001$).

TABLE 2.—Description of the Cohort

	Biochemical Incomplete Response (n = 63)	Structural Incomplete Response (n = 129)	p-Value
Age (years)			
Mean ± SD	43 ± 14	50 ± 16	0.002
Median	39	52	
Range	21−79	18−82	
Gender			
Female	49 (77.8%)	69 (53.5%)	0.001
Male	14 (22.2%)	60 (46.5%)	
Histology			
Papillary	54 (85.7%)	94 (72.9%)	0.22
Poorly differentiated	5 (7.9%)	20 (15.5%)	
Follicular	2 (3.2%)	9 (7%)	
HCC	2 (3.2%)	6 (4.6%)	
Preparation for ablation			
rhTSH	28 (44.4%)	53 (41.1%)	0.59
THW	35 (55.6%)	76 (58.9%)	
PET/CT			
Positive	0	58 (45%)	<0.0001
Negative	31 (49.2%)	44 (34.1%)	
Nonavailable	32 (50.8%)	27 (20.9%)	
RAI avid disease			
Yes	49 (77.8%)	77 (59.7%)	0.015
No	14 (22.2%)	52 (40.3%)	
AJCC/UICC stage			
I	37 (58.7%)	27 (20.9%)	<0.0001
II	4 (6.3%)	15 (11.6%)	
III	14 (22.2%)	6 (4.7%)	
IVa	6 (9.5%)	24 (18.6%)	
IVb	0	2 (1.6%)	
IVc	2 (3.2%)	55 (42.6%)	
ATA initial risk			
Low	10 (15.9%)	3 (2.3%)	< 0.0001
Intermediate	40 (63.5%)	40 (31%)	
High	13 (20.6%)	86 (66.7%)	
Follow-up duration (months)			
Mean ± SD	98.4 ± 30	90.1 ± 34.8	0.115
Median	98	42	
Range	40−160	9−180	
RAI ablation activity (mCi)	100 (29−150)	150 (28−590)	<0.0001
Time (months) to additional therapy (after initial surgery and RRA)	13 (5−160)	12 (4−180)	<0.0001
Additional therapy during follow-up			
Surgery	4 (6.3%)	74 (57.3%)	<0.0001
RAI	53 (84.1%)	106 (82.3%)	
EBRT	0	45 (34.9%)	
Systemic therapy	1 (1.6%)	17 (13.2%)	
Lowest suppressed Tg in the first 2 years			
Mean	3.6	726.8	<0.0001
Median	3.6 (<0.3−36)	20.3 (<0.3−43500)	
Structural Progression			
Yes	3 (4.8%)	67 (51.9%)	<0.0001
No	60 (95.2%)	62 (48.1%)	
Biochemical Progression			
Yes	7 (11.1%)	58 (45%)	<0.0001
No	56 (88.9%)	71 (55%)	

SD, standard deviation; HCC, Hurthle cell carcinoma; rhTSH, recombinant human thyroid-stimulating hormone; THW, thyroid hormone withdrawal; PET, positron emission tomography; CT, computerized tomography; RAI, radioactive iodine; AJCC, American Joint Committee on Cancer; UICC, Union Internationale Contre le Cancer; ATA, American Thyroid Association; RRA, RAI remnant ablation; EBRT, external beam radiation therapy.

Conclusions.—A structural incomplete response to initial therapy is associated with significantly worse clinical outcome than a biochemical incomplete response to therapy (Table 2).

▶ This article from Mike Tuttle's group at Memorial Sloan-Kettering Cancer Center documents that disease that can be seen on imaging after initial treatment for differentiated thyroid cancer is more significant than disease that can be detected only by biochemical tests. Although this seems self-evident, the characterization and quantification of this difference is important because small molecular tyrosine kinase inhibitors are introduced into the management of patients with differentiated thyroid cancer. What is not addressed in the article itself but is evident from Table 2 is that the patients in the structural incomplete response group are a substantially higher risk group of patients to begin with. More than 60% of the patients who did not respond presented with stage IV disease versus only 12% who did respond. So it would appear that these patients are destined for poor outcome based on their initial presentation. Given that there is a 38% risk of dying of thyroid cancer in this group of patients (over a mean of just 70 months), it would appear that early identification of these patients may be beneficial so that they can be directed toward novel therapies.

T. J. Fahey, MD

The Outcomes of First Reoperation for Locoregionally Recurrent/Persistent Papillary Thyroid Carcinoma in Patients Who Initially Underwent Total Thyroidectomy and Remnant Ablation

Yim JH, Kim WB, Kim EY, et al (Univ of Ulsan College of Medicine, Seoul, Korea)
J Clin Endocrinol Metab 96:2049-2056, 2011

Context.—The primary treatment of locoregionally recurrent/persistent papillary thyroid cancer (PTC) is surgical removal by reoperation. However, there had been only limited number of reports on the outcome of reoperation.

Objective.—This study was to evaluate the efficacy of the first reoperation for locoregionally recurrent/persistent papillary thyroid carcinoma and the usefulness of stimulated thyroglobulin for evaluating efficacy of reoperation.

Design and Settings.—This was a retrospective observational cohort study in a tertiary referral hospital.

Patients.—A total of 83 patients, who underwent initial total thyroidectomy and nodal dissection with radioactive iodine remnant ablation, received reoperation for locoregionally recurrent/persistent PTC and were included in this study. Stimulated thyroglobulin levels were assessed before and after reoperation.

Main Outcome Measures.—We assessed biochemical remission (stimulated thyroglobulin <1 ng/ml) after reoperation and evaluated second clinical recurrence-free survival rate according to stimulated thyroglobulin value.

TABLE 1.—Comparisons of Clinical Characteristics of Patients According to Status of Biochemical Remission After First Reoperation

	No Biochemical Remission (n = 41)[a]	Biochemical Remission (n = 42)[b]	P
Initial characteristics			
Male (%)	14 (34)	10 (24)	0.34
Initial operation extent			0.17
Total thyroidectomy (%)	0 (0)	1 (2)	
Plus central neck dissection (%)	28 (68)	34 (81)	
Plus MRND (%)	13 (32)	7 (17)	
Size or tumor (cm in diameter)	2.8 ± 1.3	2.3 ± 1.1	0.07
Number of pathologically proven malignant lymph node	6 (0–26)	4 (0–26)	0.09
T stage			1.00
pT1 (%)	3 (7)	4 (10)	
pT2 (%)	4 (10)	4 (10)	
pT3 (%)	31 (76)	32 (76)	
pT4 (%)	3 (7)	2 (5)	
N stage			0.38
pN0 (%)	3 (7)	5 (12)	
pN1a (%)	26 (63)	30 (71)	
pN1b (%)	12 (29)	7 (17)	
AJCC TNM staging			1.00
I/II (%)	25 (61)	26 (62)	
III/IV (%)	16 (39)	16 (38)	
Characteristics at reoperation			
Age at reoperation	43 ± 12	47 ± 12	0.12
Prereop stim Tg (ng/ml)	31.1 (2.0–592.0)	5.6 (0.1–106.0)	<0.01
Number of removed lymph node at reoperation	31 (1–90)	34 (11–100)	0.16
Number of pathologically proven malignant lymph node at reoperation	4 (1–31)	3 (1–9)	0.05
Reoperation extent			0.09
Unilateral MRND (%)	27 (66)	36 (86)	
Bilateral MRND (%)	10 (24)	6 (14)	
Simple lymph node excision (%)	4 (10)	0	
Adjuvant RAI treatment after reoperation (%)	12 (29)	6 (14)	0.12

MRND, Modified radical neck dissection; AJCC, American Joint Committee on Cancer (6th ed., 2002); TNM, tumor node metastasis; RAI, radioactive iodine.
[a]Stim Tg less than 1 ng/ml after reoperation.
[b]Stim Tg 1 ng/ml or greater after reoperation.

Results.—There was a significant positive correlation between the numbers of resected malignant lymph nodes and the reduction in stimulated thyroglobulin level after reoperation. Biochemical remission was achieved in 51% of patients who underwent first reoperation. Patients with stimulated thyroglobulin level greater than 5 ng/ml after first reoperation had a greater chance of a second clinical recurrence (the estimated 5 yr clinical recurrence free survival rate, 94 ± 3 *vs.* 74 ± 9%, log rank statistics 15.8, df = 1, P < 0.001).

Conclusion.—Surgery is an effective option for managing locally recurrent/persistent PTC. Stimulated thyroglobulin is a useful marker for evaluating efficacy of reoperation and predicting second recurrence in locoregionally recurrent/persistent PTC.

▶ The value of stimulated thyroglobulin (Tg) for excluding the presence of persistent disease has been well characterized, as noted previously in this chapter. Here the authors examined patients who had undergone a first reoperation for persistent or recurrent disease after total thyroidectomy + radioactive iodine ablation and analyzed the stimulated Tg level as a predictor of future recurrence. The second operations were generally either unilateral or bilateral modified radical neck dissections. The authors note in the conclusion that surgery was an effective treatment option, but it should be noted that only 51% of the patients in the study enjoyed a biochemical remission, and Table 1 shows that mean stimulated Tg in those patients who had a biochemical remission was 5.6 versus 31 in those who did not enter a biochemical remission. The authors go on to demonstrate that a postoperative stimulated Tg > 5 was associated with a significantly higher chance of a second clinical recurrence. While they note in the abstract that the difference at 5 years is 94% recurrence with a stimulated Tg < 5 versus 74% with a stimulated Tg > 5, Fig 4 from the original article demonstrates that the 10-year clinical recurrence with a stimulated Tg > 5 appears to be about 60%. This study shows that the stimulated Tg is highly predictive of both persistent disease and potential for another recurrence but also reinforces the observation made by others that biochemical cure in patients with recurrent disease should not be an expected outcome. This is an important point to discuss with patients prior to embarking on reoperative surgery for papillary thyroid carcinoma.

T. J. Fahey, MD

Central Compartment Reoperation for Recurrent/Persistent Differentiated Thyroid Cancer: Patterns of Recurrence, Morbidity, and Prediction of Postoperative Hypocalcemia

Roh J-L, Kim J-M, Park CI (Univ of Ulsan College of Medicine, Seoul, Republic of Korea; Chungnam Natl Univ College of Medicine, Daejeon, Republic of Korea)

Ann Surg Oncol 18:1312-1318, 2011

Background.—Incidence rates of hypoparathyroidism and vocal cord paralysis are high following central compartment reoperation, but few prospective studies have assessed morbidities and factors predictive of hypocalcemia after reoperation. We investigated recurrence patterns, morbidity, and factors predictive of postoperative hypocalcemia in patients undergoing central compartment reoperation for recurrent/persistent differentiated thyroid cancer (DTC).

Methods.—We prospectively evaluated 45 consecutive patients with recurrent/persistent DTC. Thyroid remnants or recurrent cancers were removed in 16 patients, the unilateral or bilateral central compartment was cleared in all patients, and the lateral compartment on the diseased side was comprehensively removed from 24 patients. Recurrence patterns were assessed histopathologically, morbidities were monitored, and serum concentrations of calcium and intact parathyroid hormone (iPTH) were measured in all patients.

Results.—Eleven patients (24.4%) had tumor invasion into the recurrent laryngeal nerve and/or the tracheoesophagus. Central nodal involvement occurred frequently (86.7%), and the ipsilateral jugular nodes of the lateral compartment were frequently involved. Temporary and permanent vocal cord paralysis developed in 10 (22.2%) and 8 (17.8%) patients, respectively, due primarily to intentional nerve resection following tumor invasion. Of 41 patients without preoperative hypoparathyroidism, 21 (46.3%) had temporary and 2 (4.9%) had permanent hypocalcemia. Multivariate analysis showed that bilateral central compartment dissection and low iPTH levels (<12.0 pg/ml) were independent predictors of postoperative hypocalcemia.

Conclusions.—Most patients with recurrent/persistent DTC harbor lesions in the central compartment. Central compartment reoperation may lead to high rates of morbidity, including hypoparathyroidism, which can be predicted by surgical extent and low serum iPTH levels.

▶ The morbidity of reoperative central neck dissection has recently been the subject of some debate. Some authors have suggested that reoperative central neck dissection is associated with low or no excess morbidity. This report from 2 busy centers in Korea suggests that reoperative central neck dissection is associated with significant short- and long-term morbidity. Although the tumors may have been more infiltrative than those documented in other recent reports—as evidenced by the fact that 11 patients had tumors invading the recurrent laryngeal nerve, trachea, or esophagus—it is likely that these were not all poorly differentiated carcinomas because the mean time to relapse was 6 years. Although this manuscript will not settle any debates regarding the question of whether morbidity is increased with reoperative central neck exploration, it demonstrates that these operations cannot be taken lightly and that morbidity can be substantial.

T. J. Fahey, MD

Long-Term Outcome of Comprehensive Central Compartment Dissection in Patients with Recurrent/Persistent Papillary Thyroid Carcinoma
Clayman GL, Agarwal G, Edeiken BS, et al (The Univ of Texas M.D. Anderson Cancer Ctr, Houston)
Thyroid 21:1309-1316, 2011

Background.—Persistent or recurrent papillary thyroid carcinoma (PTC) occurs in some patients after initial thyroid surgery and often, radioactive iodine treatment. Here, we identify the efficacy, safety, and long-term outcome of our current surgical management paradigm for persistent/recurrent PTC in the central compartment in an interdisciplinary thyroid cancer clinical and research program at a tertiary thyroid cancer referral center.

Methods.—We retrospectively analyzed our standardized approach of comprehensive bilateral level VI/VII lymph node dissection (SND [VI, VII]) for cytologically confirmed PTC in the central compartment.

Results.—From 1994 to 2004, 210 patients, median age 42 (range 12–82) underwent SND (VI, VII). Most patients (106, 51%) had already undergone ≥2 surgical procedures for persistent or recurrent disease, and 31 (15%) had distant metastases at presentation. Postoperatively, 104 (71%) of the 146 patients who were thyroglobulin (Tg) positive had no evidence of disease. Anti-Tg antibodies were present in 38 patients (18%), 17 of whom (53%) did not have anti-Tg antibodies postoperatively. Fourteen patients (7%) were hypoparathyroid at presentation, and 2 more (1%) became permanently hypoparathyroid after surgery. Four patients (2%) experienced recurrent laryngeal nerve paralysis (RLNP) of a previously functioning nerve. Unanticipated RLNP was observed in only one nerve at risk. External beam radiation was given to 33 patients (17%). An additional 17 patients (8%) developed distant metastases during follow-up. At the last follow-up, 130 (66%) of the 196 patients had no detectable Tg; of these, 99 (76%) had no further evidence of disease. A median of 7.25 years after surgery, 167 (90%) of the 185 patients were without evidence of central disease, and 18 (10%) had developed central compartment recurrences within a median interval of 24.3 months. Of those with recurrence, 16 out of 18 patients (89%) underwent a subsequent surgical procedure, thus resulting in an overall 98% central compartment control rate. Kaplan–Meier disease-specific survival at 10 years was 98.9% for patients <45 years old and 77.9% for those ≥45 years old (log-rank $p < 0.00001$). The only predictor of central compartment recurrence was malignancy in a thyroid remnant noted within the central compartment surgical specimen.

Conclusions.—Bilateral comprehensive level VI/VII dissections are safe and effective for long-term control of recurrent/persistent PTC in the central lymphatic compartment.

▶ This large series of reoperative central neck dissections from the group at MD Anderson suggests that reoperative central neck surgery can be done safely and with a high degree of success. The long-term follow-up (a median of more than 7 years) demonstrates that the most significant risk factor for dying of thyroid cancer was age > 45 years (Fig 1 in the original article). Older men (> 45 years) tended to have a worse survival than their female counterparts, although this did not reach statistical significance. This is an interesting observation that appears to parallel the risk that older age and, to a lesser extent, male gender confer on patients presenting with primary papillary thyroid carcinoma (PTC).

While the article is an excellent analysis of a long-term database, the authors do suggest that prophylactic central neck dissection may have little effect in reducing the incidence of persistent or recurrent PTC in the central neck. Because the study is in no way designed to assess this question, this is a surprising suggestion from the authors. They do note that surgical treatment of central neck recurrences remains the gold standard and should be the treatment of choice for patients with central neck recurrences. Given the excellent results seen here, this is a justifiable conclusion, although it is worth remembering again that these operations are not for the occasional central neck surgeon.

T. J. Fahey, MD

Adjuvant Radioactive Therapy after Reoperation for Locoregionally Recurrent Papillary Thyroid Cancer in Patients Who Initially Underwent Total Thyroidectomy and High-Dose Remnant Ablation

Yim JH, Kim WB, Kim EY, et al (Univ of Ulsan College of Medicine, Seoul, Korea)
J Clin Endocrinol Metab 96:3695-3700, 2011

Context.—Some patients have elevated stimulated thyroglobulin (sTg) concentrations after reoperation for locoregionally recurrent/persistent papillary thyroid cancer (PTC). Little is known, however, about the efficacy of adjuvant radioactive iodine (RAI) therapy in these patients.

Objective.—The objective of the study was to evaluate the efficacy of adjuvant RAI therapy in patients with elevated sTg after reoperation for locally recurrent/persistent PTC.

Design and Settings.—This was a retrospective observational cohort study in a tertiary referral hospital.

Patients.—We evaluated 45 consecutive patients with sTg greater than 2 ng/ml after reoperation for locoregionally recurrent PTC, all of whom had previously undergone initial total thyroidectomy followed by high-dose RAI remnant ablation. Of these 45 patients, 23 received adjuvant RAI therapy (adjuvant group) and 22 did not (control group).

Main Outcome Measures.—Main outcome measures included changes in sTg concentration after reoperation and disease-free survival.

Results.—Over time, there were no significant differences inmean sTg concentration in the adjuvant ($P = 0.35$) and control ($P = 0.74$) groups. Only 15% of patients in the adjuvant group and 33% in the control group showed a greater than 50% decrease in sTg level from baseline. There were no between-group differences in changes ($P = 0.83$) or percent decrease ($P = 0.97$) in sTg concentration and no difference in clinical recurrence-free survival ($P = 0.20$).

Conclusion.—In patients who still have elevated sTg after reoperation for locally recurrent/persistent PTC, adjuvant RAI therapy compared with no additional RAI therapy resulted in no significant differences in the subsequent sTg changes or the recurrence-free survival.

▶ The decision as to whether to give a patient a follow-up dose of radioactive iodine (RAI) after a reoperation for recurrent papillary thyroid cancer (PTC) is one that had not previously been formally addressed. The immediate natural response would be to give an additional dose of RAI. However, in theory, this is unlikely to be effective because cells that grew after RAI are likely to stem from cells that were resistant to the initial treatment with RAI. The data presented in Fig 2 in the original article summarize the findings. Clearly there is no difference in the serum thyroglobulin levels in patients who received RAI versus those who did not. It is worth noting that the authors excluded patients who had only 30 mCi of RAI after the first operation, and thus it is possible that patients who had a low dose of RAI after initial surgical treatment of PTC may have some benefit from additional RAI after a reoperation. It is likely that even patients who had a low initial dose of RAI would not derive any additional benefit from a subsequent larger dose; however, this remains to be studied.

While the study is relatively small and retrospective, it lends support to the belief that additional RAI in the postoperative setting does not provide any benefit. A prospective study that examines this question is necessary to definitively prove this, although it is unlikely that such a study will be done. Thus it is reasonable to conclude that the only patients who should receive RAI after reoperative surgery for PTC recurrence are those who did not receive it after their initial surgery.

T. J. Fahey, MD

Invasive Fibrous Thyroiditis (Riedel Thyroiditis): The Mayo Clinic Experience, 1976–2008
Fatourechi MM, Hay ID, McIver B, et al (Mayo Clinic, Rochester, MN)
Thyroid 21:765-772, 2011

Background.—Invasive fibrous thyroiditis (IFT) is the rarest form of thyroiditis, and reports are often limited to case reports and small case series. In this study, we aimed to summarize our institutional experience with IFT since 1976.

Methods.—We retrospectively reviewed the cases of all patients with IFT evaluated at Mayo Clinic, Rochester, Minnesota, from 1976 through 2008, with special emphasis on clinical presentation, associated risk factors, associated comorbid conditions, complications, and treatment.

Results.—Twenty-one patients met our inclusion criteria of (i) IFT confirmed by pathologic review at our institution and (ii) evidence of extension of fibrosis outside the thyroid capsule. Most patients (17, 81%) were women (mean age, 42 years). Presenting symptoms included pain (24%), dysphagia (33%), vocal cord paralysis (29%), and tracheal narrowing (48%). Three patients had associated hypoparathyroidism. Sixteen (76%) had a history of tobacco use, and 10 (48%) were current smokers. Fibrosing mediastinitis was present in four, orbital fibrosis in one, retroperitoneal fibrosis in three, and pancreatic fibrosis in one (38% had extracervical fibrotic processes). Eighteen patients had partial thyroidectomy, 7 (39%) of whom had surgical complications involving vocal cords and parathyroid. Two required tracheostomy. Thirteen had corticosteroid therapy; six received tamoxifen. There was no cause-specific mortality, and the fibrotic process stabilized or partially resolved in all patients.

Conclusions.—IFT often is associated with a systemic extracervical fibrotic process and tobacco use. Attempted thyroid resection often results

TABLE 2.—Treatment and Outcomes in Patients with Invasive Fibrous Thyroiditis

Patient	Age at Diagnosis, Year/Sex	Intervention	Outcome	Follow-up, Years[a]
1	43/F	Prednisone, 18 months	Shrinkage of goiter; alive, doing well at last follow-up	10.5
2	31/M	Subtotal thyroidectomy; two courses of prednisone	Initial good response with later relapse; transient vocal cord paralysis improved	13.5
3	47/M	Subtotal thyroidectomy	No change in goiter size; follow-up not available	0.2
4	53/F	Subtotal thyroidectomy	Partial resolution of ophthalmopathy; symptoms resolved	1.0
5	54/F	Subtotal thyroidectomy; corticosteroids	Postoperative dysphonia; increased erythrocyte sedimentation rate resolved; stable	14.6
6	58/F	Subtotal thyroidectomy; tracheostomy; 221 weeks of prednisone	Continued right vocal cord paralysis; resolution of symptoms at last followup; died age 70 years of nonthyroid metastatic adenocarcinoma	11.1
7	35/M	Lobectomy; isthmectomy; long-term prednisone and tamoxifen	Dysphagia and neck pain continued several years, then improved; alive at last follow-up, age 60 years	30.5
8	39/F	Isthmectomy; tracheostomy; long-term prednisone; methimazole for Graves' hyperthyroidism with ophthalmopathy	Vocal cord paralysis resolved; tracheostomy closed; hypoparathyroidism; hypothyroidism on T4 therapy; alive age 61 years	20.5
9	35/F	Right lobectomy; isthmectomy; 55 weeks of prednisone	Resolution of symptoms, decrease in mass size; alive age 47 years; no progression	10.7
10	65/F	No specific therapy other than thyroxine replacement for hypothyroidism and large goiter	Keratoconjunctivitis sicca, process stable	22.7
11	49/F	Corticosteroid therapy	Good short-term clinical response	0.6
12	35/F	Subtotal thyroidectomy; declined prednisone therapy	Resolution of dysphonia; long-term follow-up not available	0.6
13	61/F	Thyroidectomy; partial isthmectomy; tamoxifen 4 months	Dysphagia, dyspnea resolved	1.5
14	38/F	Three courses of prednisone; chlorambucil; isthmectomy	After 8 years fibrosis stabilized; alive and stable age 47 years	8.3
15	38/M	Three courses of prednisone; intravenous dexamethasone; tamoxifen	Thyroid mass decreased	1.6
16	35/F	Subtotal thyroidectomy; prednisone therapy	Stable after subtotal thyroidectomy and corticosteroid therapy	0.6
17	23/F	Right partial lobectomy; isthmectomy	Ankylosing spondylitis and hydrocephalus developed; thyroid mass stable; alive age 70 years	47.2
18	44/F	Left lobectomy and isthmectomy; two courses of prednisone	Symptoms including dysphonia improved; on long-term tamoxifen	1.6
19	39/F	Isthmectomy; long-term tamoxifen; prednisone, two courses, last course for 1 year	Improved dysphagia, dyspnea; stable	2
20	38/F	Left lobectomy; tracheostomy; two courses prednisone; short course methotrexate; tamoxifen 1 year	Tracheostomy dependent; neck mass decreased	5.5

(Continued)

TABLE 2.—(*Continued*)

Patient	Age at Diagnosis, Year/Sex	Intervention	Outcome	Follow-up, Years[a]
21	26/F	Tracheostomy; prednisone 3 months plus tamoxifen; 4 years later, radioactive iodine therapy for new Graves' hyperthyroidism (11)	Unilateral invasive fibrous thyroiditis; needed radioactive iodine therapy; invasive fibrous thyroiditis stable	4.2

F, female; M, male.
[a]Measured from the time of diagnosis.

in postoperative complications. Long-term follow-up showed no deaths from IFT and showed stability of the thyroiditis (Table 2).

▶ Invasive fibrous thyroiditis is a rare disorder that is considered an autoimmune thyroiditis. Patients present with signs of local compressive symptoms and pain and typically a diffuse firm fixed thyroid mass. Table 2 from this article delineates the outcomes of all 21 patients in the series. There are several important points:

- Surgical treatment should probably be restricted to establishing a diagnosis (ie, biopsy) and/or airway decompression, generally by isthmus resection. While additional surgery is noted to have a high likelihood of leading to additional complications, it is evident in Table 2 that a few patients who were able to undergo partial or subtotal thyroidectomy did have a good initial response. It is likely that those patients who underwent resection had less aggressive disease than other patients who did not undergo resection.

- Despite the infiltrating nature of the disease, patients generally tend to have stabilization of the disease with medical treatment.

- Although tamoxifen has been advocated for the treatment of invasive fibrous thyroiditis, its efficacy as a single agent cannot be assessed in this study and probably should be used in combination with corticosteroids in treating these rare patients.

T. J. Fahey, MD

Normocalcemic parathormone elevation after successful parathyroidectomy: Long-term analysis of parathormone variations over 10 years

Goldfarb M, Gondek S, Irvin GL III, et al (Univ of Miami Leonard M. Miller School of Medicine, FL; Harvard Med School, Boston, MA)
Surgery 150:1076-1084, 2011

Background.—The long-term significance of normocalcemic parathormone elevation (NPE) after successful parathyroidectomy for sporadic primary hyperparathyroidism remains unclear.

Method.—Of 239 consecutive patients who underwent targeted para-thyroidectomy with intraoperative parathormone monitoring, 96 were fol-lowed for ≥10 years. NPE was defined as a normal serum calcium level and parathormone (PTH) above the normal reference range ≥6 months after successful parathyroidectomy. Recurrence was defined as elevated serum calcium and PTH levels ≥6 months after parathyroidectomy. Risk factors for NPE, patterns of postoperative PTH variation, and 10-year outcomes were analyzed.

Results.—Of 96 patients followed ≥10 years, 42 had postoperative NPE. Only male gender ($P = .008$) was a risk factor for NPE, and NPE did not predict recurrence. Three patterns of postoperative NPE were iden-tified in patients with ≥3 PTH measurements over this 10-year period. Group 1 ($n = 11$): 1 to 2 consecutive PTH elevations; none recurred, and most were explained by physiologic variation. Group 2 ($n = 23$): multiple PTH fluctuations; 3 recurred, and almost all had physiologic vari-ations. Group 3 ($n = 4$): PTH always elevated; 2 recurred.

Conclusion.—Postoperative NPE may be a dynamic, reversible, and tran-sient clinical entity that does not predict recurrence. Nevertheless, patients with postoperative NPE should be monitored and an attempt made to correct any obvious potential causes of PTH elevation.

▶ The problem of an elevated parathyroid hormone level after apparently successful parathyroidectomy can be a vexing one. Previous studies have noted that this can happen in up to 30% to 40% of patients who undergo parathyroid-ectomy. Here, the Miami group looks at long-term follow-up of a group of patients who underwent focused parathyroidectomy guided by intraoperative parathyroid hormone (IOPTH) monitoring and had rebound elevations in the parathyroid hormone levels. The authors identify 3 patterns of rebound elevation and conclude that postoperative normocalcemic elevation in parathyroid hormone is not predictive of recurrence. However, it would seem that the results for these 3 groups should not be lumped together. Although it seems clear that having 1 or 2 elevated postoperative levels is not predictive of recurrence, having a persistent elevation of parathormone (PTH) postoperatively certainly seems worrisome given that 50% of this small group did recur. Furthermore, 3 of 23 patients (13%) in Group 2—the group that fluctuated over the years—recurred, a number higher than what would be expected for patients with surgically cor-rected primary hyperparathyroidism.

Most of the patients in this study appear to have had significant hyperparathy-roidism because the preoperative calcium and PTH levels were quite high: 11.7 and 150 to 190 in the controls and patients, respectively (Table 1). It does appear that the patients in the persistent PTH elevation group (NPE) were less likely to have had a drop of the IOPTH into the normal range. This is not discussed either in the article or in the accompanying discussion at the meeting, but there are now ample data that IOPTH drops into the normal range, but above a level of 30 or 40 pg/mL, it is associated with a higher recurrence rate. It would be interesting to see whether the patients who recurred were those who may not have an adequate drop in the IOPTH.

TABLE 1.—Univariate Analysis for Predictors of Postoperative Normocalcemic
PTH Elevation

	Normal Calcium and PTH Throughout (%)	Normocalcemic PTH Elevation NPE (%)	*P* Value (chi-square [C] or Fisher Exact [F])
Pre-op variables			
Gender			
Male	4 (28.5)	10 (71.4)	.041 (F)
Female	48 (60.0)	32 (40.0)	
Race			
White	27 (52.9)	24 (47.1)	.936 (C)
Black	15 (55.6)	12 (44.4)	
Hispanic	7 (58.3)	5 (41.7)	
Age (years)	58.3 ± 2.9	59.7 ± 4.3	.581
Calcium (mg/dL)	11.7 ± .2	11.7 ± .3	.861
PTH (pg/mL)	145.8 ± 15.0	187.9 ± 41.8	.048
Symptoms			
Bone pain	17 (63.0)	10 (37.0)	.407 (C)
Stones	12 (63.2)	7 (36.8)	.498 (C)
Mental	1 (50.0)	1 (50.0)	1.00 (F)
Fatigue	3 (60.0)	2 (40.0)	1.00 (F)
Asymptomatic	11 (47.8)	12 (52.2)	.350 (C)
Crisis	0 (0)	1 (100)	.437 (F)
Calcium >11.2	33 (57.9)	24 (42.1)	.696 (C)
Age <40	12 (57.1)	9 (42.9)	.926 (C)
High urinary Ca	3 (37.5)	5 (62.5)	.292 (F)
Cr ≥1.5	1 (33.3)	2 (66.7)	.585 (F)
Intraop variables			
Correct preop localization*	43 (52.4)	39 (47.6)	.215 (F)
BNE	7 (50)	7 (50)	.773 (F)
MGD	0 (0)	3 (100)	.086 (F)
% IPM drop	77.6 ± 2.7	77.0 ± 3.1	.774
>50% PTH drop to normal range at 10 min	36 (63.2)	21 (36.8)	.058 (F)
>50% PTH drop from preincision at 10 min	47 (57.3)	35 (42.7)	.362 (F)
Postop variables			
Immediate calcium level (within 7 days)	9.15 ± .18	9.08 ± .20	.546
Elevated PTH in first 6 months	6 (30.0)	14 (70.0)	.050 (C)

BNE, Bilateral neck exploration; *IPM*, intraoperative parathormone monitoring; *MGD*, multiglandular disease; *NPE*, normocalcemic parathormone elevation; *PTH*, parathormone.
*According to sestamibi scan.

In sum, this article highlights an important area of controversy in parathyroid surgery and one that clearly requires further study. Whether groups that do routine 4-gland exploration and excise any abnormal appearing gland (eg, Cleveland, Tampa) see similar percentages of patients with NPE may help to better understand this phenomenon.

T. J. Fahey, MD

Parathyroid Carcinoma: A 43-Year Outcome and Survival Analysis

Harari A, Waring A, Fernandez-Ranvier G, et al (Univ of California, Los Angeles; Univ of California, San Francisco; Loma Linda Univ, CA)
J Clin Endocrinol Metab 96:3679-3686, 2011

Context.—Parathyroid carcinoma is a rare but ominous cause of primary hyperparathyroidism.

Objectives and Main Outcome Measures.—The objective of the study was to review the outcomes of parathyroid cancer patients and to evaluate the factors associated with mortality.

Design, Setting, and Patients.—This was a retrospective review performed on 37 patients with parathyroid cancer treated at a single university tertiary care center between 1966 and 2009.

Results.—The average age at cancer diagnosis was 53 yr (range 23–75 yr), and 23 patients (62%) were men. Eighteen patients (49%) recurred after their initial cancer operation. The average number of neck dissections done for cancer was three (range 1–11). After initial diagnosis, 22 patients (60%) eventually developed complications, including unilateral (n = 11) or bilateral (n = 3) vocal cord paralysis (38%). Eight patients (22%) had, at some point, an associated benign parathyroid adenoma. Median overall survival was 14.3 yr (range 10.5–25.7 yr) from the date of diagnosis. Factors associated with increased mortality included lymph node or distant metastases, number of recurrences, higher calcium level at recurrence, and a high number of calcium-lowering medications. Factors not associated with mortality included age, race, tumor size, time to first recurrence, and extent of initial operation. Initial operations done at our center had improved survival ($P = 0.037$) and decreased complication rates ($P < 0.001$) *vs.* those done elsewhere.

Conclusion.—Parathyroid cancer patients typically have a long survival, which often includes multiple reoperations for recurrence and thus a high rate of surgical complications. Patients in whom there is a high index of suspicion for parathyroid cancer should be referred to a dedicated endocrine surgery center for their initial operation (Table 3).

▶ Parathyroid carcinoma is rare. This review from the University of California, San Francisco, of 43 years of experience with just 37 patients demonstrates just how uncommon this disease is. The report demonstrates that this is not just a disease of advanced age, as the mean age at diagnosis was just 53 years. In addition, not all patients with parathyroid carcinoma have to have markedly elevated calcium levels, although most do.

Table 3 from the article provides the most important information regarding patients with parathyroid carcinoma. It is clear that lymph node and distant metastases are the major factors associated with mortality from parathyroid carcinoma. Although the authors note that there is no statistical difference between lymph node metastases and distant metastases and their impact on survival, Fig 2 in the original article suggests that patients with distant metastases do succumb more quickly than those with lymph node metastases. The figure also demonstrates

TABLE 3.—Survival Analysis and Factors Associated with Mortality

Factor	Hazard Ratio	Confidence Interval
Lymph node metastasis[a]	4.27[b]	1.19−15.30
Distant metastases[a]	3.50[b]	1.60−7.64
Initial operation done at UCSF (endocrine surgery center)	0.17[b]	0.04−0.78
Higher calcium level at recurrence	1.35[b]	1.09−1.68
Calcium level at diagnosis	1.09	0.93−1.27
Calcium level before diagnosis	1.08	0.93−1.25
High number of calcium lowering medications	1.49[b]	1.18−1.87
Gender (male reference group)	0.77	0.25−2.40
Age (yr)	1.04	0.99−1.09
Race (white reference group)	0.40	0.14−1.19
Number of recurrences	1.18[b]	1.02−1.36
Number of neck dissections	1.14	0.98−1.32
Time to first recurrence	0.83	0.62−1.12
Extent of operation (parathyroidectomy alone *vs.* parathyroidectomy with partial or total thyroidectomy)	1.12	0.44−2.86
XRT	0.41	0.12−1.38
Years that patients were initially treated for cancer: first 20 yr (reference group) *vs.* second 20 yr	0.75	0.26−2.17

Cox proportional hazards analysis was used. UCSF, University of California, San Francisco.
[a]*vs.* no metastases.
[b]$P < 0.05$.

that patients tend to live a relatively long time after diagnosis, although, as noted in the text, patients frequently require multiple reoperations and suffer from complications of multiple reoperative neck procedures: recurrent laryngeal nerve injuries and hypoparathyroidism.

T. J. Fahey, MD

Is genetic screening indicated in apparently sporadic pheochromocytomas and paragangliomas?

Iacobone M, Schiavi F, Bottussi M, et al (Univ of Padua, Italy; Veneto Inst of Oncology - IRCSS, Padua, Italy)
Surgery 150:1194-1201, 2011

Background.—Pheochromocytoma (Pheo) is usually considered a sporadic disease. Recently, an increasing rate of genetically based tumors has been reported. However, the need for systematic screening of unsuspected germline mutations in apparently sporadic forms is still debated. This study aimed to assess the effective rate of germline mutations causing Pheo and Paraganglioma (PGL), and the role of systematic genetic screening.

Methods.—Demographics, clinical, and genetic evaluation were performed in a series of 71 patients with Pheo and/or PGL.

Results.—Twelve patients had evident inherited/familial disease at presentation: NF1 $(n = 4)$; MEN2 $(n = 4)$, and familial Pheo/PGL $(n = 4)$. Among 59 patients with apparently sporadic disease, unsuspected germline mutations occurred in 8 cases: TMEM127 ($n = 4$), SDHB ($n = 2$), VHL ($n = 1$), SDHC ($n = 1$). No differences were found between hereditary and sporadic disease concerning age, sex, and tumor size; bilateral Pheo and/or PGL and recurrences occurred most often in hereditary disease.

Conclusion.—Hereditary Pheo and/or PGL are frequent (28.2%). Inheritance is evident at presentation only in 16.9% of cases; 13.6% of apparently sporadic variants are genetically determined. Despite increased costs, systematic genetic screening might be useful because it might lead to a stricter follow-up, early diagnosis of recurrences in index cases and presymptomatic detection of disease in relatives (Fig 2).

▶ The role for genetic testing in patients presenting with pheochromocytoma or paraganglioma is still debated. This single-center series looks at 71 patients presenting with either pheochromocytoma or paraganglioma and determined the rate of known germline mutations. They note an overall rate of 28% of patients who had hereditary disease. However, only 13% of those patients presenting with apparently sporadic disease were found to have germline mutations. The question is whether mutation analysis in these patients is worthwhile.

The authors do not provide an answer to this question, as there are no data presented about the cost of the genetic testing. However, they do note that selective screening on the basis of demographics, including age, sex, and tumor size, was

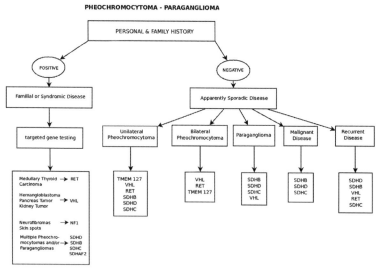

FIGURE 2.—Flow chart suggested for genetic analysis in patients affected by Pheo or PGL. The genes reported in the boxes are those more likely to be found mutated according to the clinical picture. Prioritization may be also guided by the biochemical phenotype: *VHL*-related tumors are characterized by exclusive noradrenergic hypersecretion; *SDH*-related tumors by exclusive noradrenergic or dopaminergic hypersecretion; and *RET, NF1*, and *TMEM127*-related tumors by both noradrenergic and adrenergic hypersecretion.[10] *Editor's Note*: Please refer to original journal article for full references. (Reprinted from Surgery, Iacobone M, Schiavi F, Bottussi M, et al. Is genetic screening indicated in apparently sporadic pheochromocytomas and paragangliomas? *Surgery.* 2011;150:1194-1201. Copyright 2011, with permission from Elsevier, Inc.)

not helpful in predicting who might have genetic disease. So why test everyone who present with a pheochromocytoma or paraganglioma? There are 2 important reasons: First, the presence of a germline mutation was highly correlated with the development of recurrent disease, and this information would be useful to know for planning follow-up for patients with pheochromocytoma or paraganglioma. Second, the information is useful in advising family members to get screened regularly for the development of either pheochromocytoma or paraganglioma. Fig 2 from the article summarizes current thinking regarding who to test and for what mutations. As the authors note, as other mutations responsible for hereditary pheochromocytoma or paraganglioma are identified, this list will need to be updated.

T. J. Fahey, MD

Urine Steroid Metabolomics as a Biomarker Tool for Detecting Malignancy in Adrenal Tumors

Arlt W, Biehl M, Taylor AE, et al (Univ of Birmingham, UK; Univ of Groningen, The Netherlands; et al)
J Clin Endocrinol Metab 96:3775-3784, 2011

Context.—Adrenal tumors have a prevalence of around 2% in the general population. Adrenocortical carcinoma (ACC) is rare but accounts for 2—11% of incidentally discovered adrenal masses. Differentiating ACC from adrenocortical adenoma (ACA) represents a diagnostic challenge in patients with adrenal incidentalomas, with tumor size, imaging, and even histology all providing unsatisfactory predictive values.

Objective.—Here we developed a novel steroid metabolomic approach, mass spectrometry-based steroid profiling followed by machine learning analysis, and examined its diagnostic value for the detection of adrenal malignancy.

Design.—Quantification of 32 distinct adrenal derived steroids was carried out by gas chromatography/mass spectrometry in 24-h urine samples from 102 ACA patients (age range 19—84 yr) and 45 ACC patients (20—80 yr). Underlying diagnosis was ascertained by histology and metastasis in ACC and by clinical follow-up [median duration 52 (range 26—201) months] without evidence of metastasis in ACA. Steroid excretion data were subjected to generalized matrix learning vector quantization (GMLVQ) to identify the most discriminative steroids.

Results.—Steroid profiling revealed a pattern of predominantly immature, early-stage steroidogenesis in ACC. GMLVQ analysis identified a subset of nine steroids that performed best in differentiating ACA from ACC. Receiver-operating characteristics analysis of GMLVQ results demonstrated sensitivity = specificity = 90% (area under the curve = 0.97) employing all 32 steroids and sensitivity = specificity = 88% (area under the curve = 0.96) when using only the nine most differentiating markers.

Conclusions.—Urine steroid metabolomics is a novel, highly sensitive, and specific biomarker tool for discriminating benign from malignant adrenal tumors, with obvious promise for the diagnostic work-up of patients with adrenal incidentalomas.

▶ Preoperative identification of malignancy in adrenal masses is useful for surgical planning. Additionally, if a mass is known to be benign, it is possible that surgery may be avoided. The authors here have identified a noninvasive urine-based test as a potentially very useful tool in helping to make this determination.

The data confirm what has been suspected happens in adrenal cortical carcinoma cells: inability to complete the enzymatic steps necessary to produce the final active steroid products, presumably due to loss of the final enzymes as a consequence of dedifferentiation of the cells. Although the authors have used a comprehensive analysis of either 32 or 9 adrenal steroids, the data in Figure 2 in the original article seem to indicate that there are several measured precursor metabolites that show no evidence of overlap between benign adrenal cortical adenomas and carcinomas. Specifically, the lowest levels of androgen, mineralocorticoid and glucocorticoid precursors in carcinomas are all higher than the corresponding highest levels in adenomas.

The authors conclude that a prospective study is warranted, which is appropriate. What will also have to be determined in such a study is just how commonly such a test needs to be obtained to figure out whether to operate on a patient with an adrenal mass. It may be that such a test is required uncommonly—73% of the 45 patients had routine biochemical evidence of excess hormone production.

T. J. Fahey, MD

Everolimus plus octreotide long-acting repeatable for the treatment of advanced neuroendocrine tumours associated with carcinoid syndrome (RADIANT-2): a randomised, placebo-controlled, phase 3 study
Pavel ME, for the RADIANT-2 Study Group (Charité-Universitätsmedizin Berlin/Campus Virchow Klinikum, Germany; et al)
Lancet 378:2005-2012, 2011

Background.—Everolimus, an oral inhibitor of the mammalian target of rapamycin (mTOR), has shown antitumour activity in patients with advanced pancreatic neuroendocrine tumours. We aimed to assess the combination of everolimus plus octreotide long-acting repeatable (LAR) in patients with low-grade or intermediate-grade neuroendocrine tumours (carcinoid).

Methods.—We did a randomised, double-blind, placebo-controlled, phase 3 study comparing 10 mg per day oral everolimus with placebo, both in conjunction with 30 mg intramuscular octreotide LAR every 28 days. Randomisation was by interactive voice response systems. Participants were aged 18 years or older, with low-grade or intermediate-grade advanced (unresectable locally advanced or distant metastatic) neuroendocrine tumours, and disease progression established by radiological assessment within the past 12 months. Our primary endpoint was progression-free survival. Adjusted for two interim analyses, the prespecified boundary at final analysis was p≤0·0246. This study is registered at ClinicalTrials.gov, number NCT00412061.

Findings.—429 individuals were randomly assigned to study groups; 357 participants discontinued study treatment and one was lost to follow-up. Median progression-free survival by central review was 16·4 (95% CI 13·7—21·2) months in the everolimus plus octreotide LAR group and 11·3 (8·4—14·6) months in the placebo plus octreotide LAR group (hazard ratio 0·77, 95% CI 0·59—1·00; one-sided log-rank test p=0·026). Drug-related adverse events (everolimus plus octreotide LAR vs placebo plus octreotide LAR) were mostly grade 1 or 2, and adverse events of all grades included stomatitis (62% *vs* 14%), rash (37% *vs* 12%), fatigue (31% *vs* 23%), and diarrhoea (27% *vs* 16%).

Interpretation.—Everolimus plus octreotide LAR, compared with placebo plus octreotide LAR, improved progressionfree survival in patients with advanced neuroendocrine tumours associated with carcinoid syndrome (Fig 2).

▶ Treatment of patients with metastatic carcinoid has largely been confined to the use of long-acting octreotide to inhibit excess hormone production and to slow growth. The authors report here a large randomized prospective study that documents the addition of everolimus to the treatment regimen results in

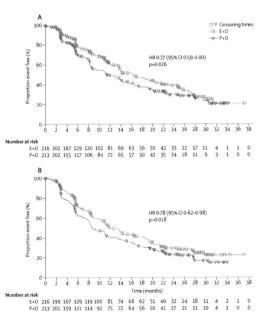

FIGURE 2.—Kaplan-Meier plots of progression-free events. Assessed by central radiology review (A) and local investigator review (B). E+O=everolimus plus octreotide LAR. P+O=placebo plus octreotide LAR. HR=hazard ratio. (Reprinted from The Lancet, Pavel ME, for the RADIANT-2 Study Group, Everolimus plus octreotide long-acting repeatable for the treatment of advanced neuroendocrine tumours associated with carcinoid syndrome (RADIANT-2): a randomised, placebo-controlled, phase 3 study. *Lancet.* 2011;378:2005-2012. © 2011, with permission from Elsevier.)

improved progression-free survival. While the results are encouraging, they will probably not bring much excitement to physicians treating these patients or much comfort to the patients themselves. Fig 2 from the article shows the Kaplan-Meier curves of the 2 groups for progression-free events. While there is some separation of the 2 curves from 8 to 20 months, the curves are unfortunately quite similar. When breaking down the benefit by site of origin of the tumor, small intestinal carcinoids, which were more than half of the tumors, showed a median progression-free survival of 18.6 months in the group treated with everolimus versus 14 months in the group treated with only long-acting octreotide. The data were much more promising for colon primaries (30 vs 13 months). Overall, while the data are encouraging, it is clear that everolimus will not be a panacea for patients with metastatic carcinoid and much work still needs to be done to better understand these tumors.

T. J. Fahey, MD

Closure of cutaneous incision after thyroid surgery: a comparison between metal clips and cutaneous octyl-2-cyanoacrylate adhesive. A prospective randomized clinical trial
Pronio A, Di Filippo A, Narilli P, et al (Sapienza Univ of Rome, Italy)
Eur J Plast Surg 34:103-110, 2011

Octyl-2-cyanoacrylate (Dermabond, Ethicon Inc.) has been introduced in clinical practice as an ideal system of closure of wounds, but no studies have confirmed the advantages of wound closure performed with Dermabond compared to skin staples (Proximate, Ethicon Inc.) in thyroid surgery. The objective of this study is to evaluate the short- and long-term results of wound closure in thyroid surgery performed with Dermabond (DERM) versus Proximate (PROX). Seventy patients after thyroidectomy were randomly assigned into the two groups (DERM vs PROX). The postoperative and the long-term outcomes were clinically evaluated by physicians, and the Stony Brook scar evaluation scale has also been used. The patients' satisfaction with the early postoperative management and with the cosmetic outcomes has been assessed by a numerical scale ranging from 0 to 10. Results were compared using appropriate statistical tests. Thirty-two patients used DERM, while 38 patients used PROX. Immediate results showed difficult application in two cases DERM (6.2%) and hyperemia in one case DERM (3.1%). Early results showed edema in eight cases DERM (25%) vs two cases PROX (5.2%; $p<0.05$); patients' satisfaction: optimum judgement in 100% DERM vs 15.7% PROX ($p<0.001$); patients' self aesthetic evaluation: PROX higher percentage of excellent results vs DERM ($p<0.005$). After one month, results showed edema in nine cases DERM (28.8%) vs two cases PROX (5.2%; $p<0.01$), while after 6 months, DERM had lesser symptoms than PROX ($p<0.01$). Octyl-2-cyanoacrylate has proven to be effective and reliable in the skin closure of cervical incision similar to suture with staples and yields similar final cosmetic outcomes. Because Dermabond offers the advantage of better management in the early postoperative phase, the patients' satisfaction is clearly better.

▶ In this study, the authors evaluated 70 patients who underwent thyroidectomy using an average incision length of 5 cm. The authors randomly assigned patients after the closure of the platysma muscle to either use Dermabond or to use skin staples to close the skin incision. They evaluated the patient's wounds carefully; in addition to evaluating the wound from the surgeon's perspective, the patients were asked to fill out a survey with self-evaluation for both cosmesis and pain.

Interestingly, there was no substantial difference between the 2 methods of closure with the exception that pain was greater in those treated with staples during the early postoperative period. Edema was more common in the Dermabond group compared with the stapled group. The final incision outcome months after the procedure was similar between the 2 groups.

The authors suggest that either closure method is equivalent but felt that Dermabond may offer some advantages in terms of improved patient self-assessment of their incision and their ability to shower and get the neck wet almost immediately after the operation. Of note, the authors closed the platysma muscle layer making certain that the skin edges were relaxed and able to come together easily without tension. For Dermabond to be efficacious, it will require that skin edges are easily opposed. One criticism of the study is the small number of patients who were entered into the trial, which might have led to a type II error in their conclusions.

J. M. Daly, MD

8 Nutrition

A contemporary analysis of parenteral nutrition—associated liver disease in surgical infants

Javid PJ, Malone FR, Dick AAS, et al (Univ of Washington, Seattle)
J Pediatr Surg 46:1913-1917, 2011

Background/Purpose.—Despite advances in pediatric nutritional support and a renewed focus on management of intestinal failure, there are limited recent data regarding the risk of parenteral nutrition (PN)—associated liver disease in surgical infants. This study investigated the incidence of cholestasis from PN and risk factors for its development in this population.

Methods.—A retrospective review was performed of all neonates in our institution who underwent abdominal surgery and required postoperative PN from 2001 to 2006. Cholestasis was defined as 2 conjugated bilirubin levels greater than 2 mg/dL over 14 days. Nonparametric univariate analyses and multivariate logistic regression were used to model the likelihood of developing cholestasis. Median values with range are presented.

Results.—One hundred seventy-six infants met inclusion criteria, and patients received PN for 28 days (range, 2-256 days). The incidence of cholestasis was 24%. Cholestatic infants were born at an earlier gestational age (34 vs 36 weeks; $P < .01$), required a 3-fold longer PN duration (76 vs 21 days; $P < .001$), had longer inpatient stays (86 vs 29 days; $P < .001$), and were more likely to be discharged on PN. The median time to cholestasis was 23 days. Cholestasis was an early development; 77% of cholestatic infants developed cholestasis by 5 weeks of PN exposure. On multivariate regression, only prematurity was significantly associated with development of cholestasis $(P < .05)$.

Conclusion.—In this analysis, the development of PN-associated liver disease occurred early in the course of exposure to PN. These data help to define the time course and prognosis for PN-associated cholestasis in surgical infants.

▶ The development of parenteral nutrition—associated liver disease is a significant problem in neonates. Older studies have characterized prematurity (gestational age) and associated conditions as important factors in the development of cholestasis. This report is a more contemporary evaluation of parenteral nutrition—associated liver disease in a single institution. It is a retrospective review subject to all the bias associated with this type of analysis. Nevertheless, the authors noted that duration of parenteral nutrition and prematurity were significant factors associated with cholestasis. Interestingly, cholestasis was an early event occurring at a median time of 28 days.

As the authors point out in their discussion, there are a number of ways to help lessen this problem using enteral nutrition as well as omega-3 fatty acids, but unfortunately, the liver dysfunction still occurs in more than 20% of patients. It will be important to use data such as presented in this article to identify those patients at greater risk for cholestasis and implement aggressive preventive therapy.

J. M. Daly, MD

Characterization of Posthospital Bloodstream Infections in Children Requiring Home Parenteral Nutrition

Mohammed A, Grant FK, Zhao VM, et al (Emory Univ School of Medicine, Atlanta, GA; Cincinnati Childeren's Hosp Med Ctr, OH)
JPEN J Parenter Enteral Nutr 35:581-587, 2011

Background.—Home parenteral nutrition (HPN) is lifesaving for children with intestinal failure. Catheter-associated bloodstream infections (CA-BSI) are common in hospitalized patients receiving parenteral nutrition (PN), but data evaluating CA-BSI in children receiving HPN are limited.

Objective.—To determine the incidence and characteristics of CA-BSI in children receiving HPN.

Methods.—Medical records of 44 children receiving HPN during a 3-year period were reviewed. End points were CA-BSI during the initial 6 months after discharge. CA-BSI was defined as isolation of pathogens from blood requiring antimicrobial therapy.

Results.—The primary indication for HPN was short bowel syndrome (46%), and 59 BSI were documented during the initial 6 months of HPN in 29 (66%) children. Of CA-BSI, polymicrobial infections accounted for 52%; gram-positive, 29%; gram-negative, 17%; and fungal, 2%. CA-BSI incidence per 1000 catheter-days was highest during the first month posthospital discharge (72 episodes; 95% confidence interval [CI], 45.4−109.6). CA-BSI incidence density ratio for children receiving HPN for >90 days compared with those receiving HPN for <30 days was 2.2 ($P < .05$). Logistic regression revealed that Medicaid insurance and age <1 year were associated with increased risk for CA-BSI (odds ratio [OR], 4.4 [95% CI, 1.13−16.99] and 6.6 [1.50−28.49], respectively; $P < .05$).

Conclusions.—The incidence of CA-BSI in children receiving HPN is highest during the first month posthospital discharge. Strategies to address care in the immediate posthospital discharge period may reduce the burden of infectious complications of HPN.

▶ Total parenteral nutrition is an important component in the management of children with short bowel syndrome. The major difficulty with long-term parenteral nutrition is that of catheter-based infections. When patients are discharged home, it is important to understand at what times and with what frequency catheter-based infections may occur.

In this retrospective study, 44 children were followed for at least 6 months to determine whether a bloodstream infection occurred. Nearly half of these children had short gut syndrome. Forty-four percent of the children developed bloodstream infection that was associated with the catheter during this time. Most developed the infection during the first 30 days after discharge from the hospital. The catheter-based infections were polymicrobial in the majority, and Gram-positive bacteria were the next most common isolates. Children under age 1 year and those on Medicaid were most likely to develop catheter-based infection.

Studies such as these are very important to help document when catheter-based infections may occur. For example, the results of this study suggest that better education of caregivers for children at home receiving parenteral nutrition and particularly for caregivers of those receiving Medicaid and for children less than 1 year of age is critically important to prevent catheter-based infection and readmission to the hospital.

J. M. Daly, MD

Cisapride Improves Enteral Tolerance in Pediatric Short-Bowel Syndrome With Dysmotility

Raphael BP, Nurko S, Jiang H, et al (Harvard Med School, Boston, MA)
J Pediatr Gastroenterol Nutr 52:590-594, 2011

Background and Objectives.—Gastrointestinal dysmotility is common in pediatric short-bowel syndrome, leading to prolonged parenteral nutrition dependence. There is limited literature regarding the safety and efficacy of cisapride for this indication. The aim of the study was to describe the safety and efficacy of cisapride for enteral intolerance in pediatric short-bowel syndrome.

Methods.—Open-labeled pilot study in a limited access program for cisapride. Indications were short-bowel syndrome with underlying dysmotility and difficulty advancing enteral feeds despite standard therapies and without evidence of anatomic obstruction. Patients received cisapride 0.1 to 0.2 mg/kg per dose for 3 to 4 doses per day. We collected electrocardiogram, nutrition, and anthropometric data prospectively at study visits.

Results.—Ten patients with mean (SD) age of 30.3 (30.5) months were enrolled in our multidisciplinary pediatric intestinal rehabilitation program. Median (interquartile range [IQR]) duration of follow-up was 8.7 (3.1—14.3) months. Median (IQR) residual bowel length was 102 (85—130) cm. Median (IQR) citrulline level was 14.5 (10.5—31.3) µmol/L. Diagnoses included isolated gastroschisis (n = 3), gastroschisis with intestinal atresia (n = 4), necrotizing enterocolitis (n = 2), and long-segment Hirschsprung disease (n = 1). Six subjects had at least 1 prior bowel-lengthening procedure. Median (IQR) change in percentage enteral energy intake was 19.9% (15.4%—29.8%) during follow-up ($P = 0.01$). Seven patients improved in enteral tolerance during treatment and 2 were weaned completely from parenteral nutrition. Complications during therapy were prolonged corrected QT interval (n = 2), gastrointestinal bleeding (n = 2), D-lactic acidosis (n = 1), and death due to presumed sepsis (n = 1). Longitudinal analysis (general estimating equation model) showed a strong positive association between cisapride duration and improved enteral tolerance. Mean percentage of enteral intake increased by 2.9% for every month of cisapride treatment ($P < 0.0001$).

Conclusions.—Cisapride is a potentially useful therapy in patients with pediatric short-bowel syndrome with gastrointestinal dysmotility. We observed modest improvement in feeding tolerance where prior treatments failed; however, patients treated with cisapride require careful cardiac monitoring because corrected QT prolongation occurred in 20% of our cohort.

▶ Children who require home total parenteral nutrition need to be treated carefully and need to be aggressively weaned toward receiving most of their dietary needs from enteral nutrition. Often this is difficult either because of short gut syndrome or dysmotility. It has been suggested that promotility agents can in fact improve the use of enteral nutrition in children with short gut and other dysmotility syndromes. Other investigators have used glutamine, growth hormone, and products that increase short chain fatty acids to improve the absorption and use of enteral nutrients.

In this study, the authors treated 10 children who required total parenteral nutrition for long periods. They placed them on divided doses of cisapride administered 3 or 4 times daily. They monitored the children carefully for any cardiac electrical abnormalities such as prolongation of the QT interval. The authors noted improvement in 7 children with 2 being weaned completely from parenteral nutrition to enteral nutrition. There were complications associated with the long-term use of parenteral nutrition and cisapride. One child died from sepsis, and 2 had gastrointestinal bleeding episodes. Nevertheless, the authors noted improvement (approximately 3% per month) in the intake of enteral nutrition while these children were receiving cisapride.

The long-term management of children who require home total parenteral nutrition is extremely difficult. It is important to continue to attempt weaning from total parenteral nutrition to enteral nutrition to avoid problems related to catheter-based sepsis.

J. M. Daly, MD

Commercial Enteral Formulas and Nutrition Support Teams Improve the Outcome of Home Enteral Tube Feeding
Klek S, Szybinski P, Sierzega M, et al (Nutrimed Med Corporation, Krakow, Poland; Jagiellonian Univ Med College, Krakow, Poland)
JPEN J Parenter Enteral Nutr 35:380-385, 2011

Background.—The benefits of home enteral tube feeding (HETF) provided by nutrition support teams (NSTs) have been questioned recently, given the growing costs to the healthcare system. This study examined the effect of a specialized home enteral nutrition program on clinical outcome variables in HETF patients.

Methods.—The observational study included 203 patients (103 women, 100 men; mean age 52.5 years) receiving HETF with homemade diets for at least 12 months before starting a specialized home nutrition program for another 12 months consisting of provision of commercial enteral formulas and the guidance of an NST. Both study periods were compared regarding the number of hospital admissions, length of hospital and intensive care unit (ICU) stay, and costs of hospitalization.

Results.—A specialized HETF program significantly reduced the number of hospital admissions and the duration of hospital and ICU stays. The need for hospitalization and ICU admission was significantly reduced, with odds ratios of 0.083 (95% confidence interval, 0.051—0.133, $P < .001$) and 0.259 (95% confidence interval, 0.124—0.539, $P < .001$), respectively. Specialized HETF was associated with a significant decrease in the prevalence of pneumonia (24.1% vs 14.2%), respiratory failure (7.3% vs 1.9%), urinary tract infection (11.3% vs 4.9%), and anemia (3.9% vs 0%) requiring hospitalization. The average yearly cost of hospital treatment decreased from $764.65 per patient to $142.66 per year per patient.

Conclusions.—The specialized HETF care program reduces morbidity and costs related to long-term enteral feeding at home.

▶ In this observational study, the authors sought to understand the costs involved and hospital readmission rates in patients managed with home enteral tube feeding either done within their families or tube feedings carried out under the observation and guidance of a nutrition support team. They noted a significant decrease in hospital admission rates over a 12-month period using the nutrition support team to manage home enteral tube feedings compared with the previous 12-month observational period. A significant decrease in pneumonia, respiratory infections, anemia, and other tube feeding complications were also noted. When calculating costs related to hospital treatment, there was an approximately $600 per patient per year decrease in hospitalization costs in those patients managed with the nutrition support team.

Importantly, the authors should have calculated all costs associated with nutritional support team management, including the costs associated with visits to the patient. The cost of tube feeding would have been similar, as these were blended home diets. However, the morbidity associated with complications of tube feeding and the need for hospital readmissions is a significant quality of care issue and an important finding.

At this time, it is important for us to be able to better manage patients in the home setting. This requires greater use of the specialized personnel such as ostomy nurses, wound nurses, and health care personnel providing antibiotic administration and nutrition support therapy. This study documents the benefit of nutrition support teams in providing care to patients in the home setting.

J. M. Daly, MD

Delayed enteral feeding impairs intestinal carbohydrate absorption in critically ill patients

Nguyen NQ, Besanko LK, Burgstad C, et al (Royal Adelaide Hosp, Australia)
Crit Care Med 40:50-54, 2012

Objectives.—Delay in initiating enteral nutrition has been reported to disrupt intestinal mucosal integrity in animals and to prolong the duration of mechanical ventilation in humans. However, its impact on intestinal absorptive function in critically ill Patients is unknown. The aim of this study was to examine the impact of delayed enteral nutrition on small intestinal absorption of 3-O-methyl-glucose.

Design.—Prospective, randomized study.

Setting.—Tertiary critical care unit.

Patients.—Studies were performed in 28 critically ill Patients.

Interventions.—Patients were randomized to either enteral nutrition within 24 hrs of admission (14 "early feeding": 8 males, 6 females, age 54.9 ± 3.3 yrs) or no enteral nutrition during the first 4 days of admission (14 "delayed feeding": 10 males, 4 females, age 56.1 ± 4.2 yrs).

Measurements and Main Results.—Gastric emptying (scintigraphy, 100 mL of Ensure (Abbott Australia, Kurnell, Australia) with 20 MBq ^{99m}Tc-sulphur colloid), intestinal absorption of glucose (3 g of 3-O-methyl-glucose), and clinical outcomes were assessed 4 days after intensive care unit admission. Although there was no difference in gastric emptying, plasma 3-O-methyl-glucose concentrations were less in the Patients with delayed feeding compared to those who were fed earlier (peak: 0.24 ± 0.04 mmol/L vs. 0.37 ± 0.04 mmol/L, $p < .02$) and integrated (area under the curve at 240 mins: 38.5 ± 7.0 mmol/min/L vs. 63.4 ± 8.3 mmol/min/L, $p < .04$). There was an inverse correlation between integrated plasma concentrations of 3-O-methyl-glucose (area under the curve at 240 mins) and the duration of ventilation ($r = -.51$; $p = .006$). In the delayed feeding group, both the duration of mechanical ventilation (13.7 ± 1.9 days vs. 9.2 ± 0.9 days; $p = .049$) and length of stay in the intensive care unit (15.9 ± 1.9 days vs. 11.3 ± 0.8 days; $p = .048$) were greater.

Conclusions.—In critical illness, delaying enteral feeding is associated with a reduction in small intestinal glucose absorption, consistent with the reduction in mucosal integrity after nutrient deprivation evident in animal models. The duration of both mechanical ventilation and length of stay in the intensive care unit are prolonged. These observations support recommendations for "early" enteral nutrition in critically ill Patients.

▶ The administration of early enteral feeding in critically ill patients in the intensive care unit (ICU) continues to be controversial. As the authors note, most patients do not receive enteral feeding during the first 3 to 5 days in the ICU, and most receive less than 70% of their needed calories and protein while in the ICU. This situation occurs despite some prospective trials that have documented improved outcomes when ICU patients receive early enteral nutrition. This study sought to determine whether early enteral nutrition maintained intestinal function better by randomizing 28 patients to either early or delayed enteral feeding. They noted improved enteral absorptive function in the group receiving early enteral nutrition, but importantly, they also noted decreased time on mechanical ventilation and less time on average in the ICU.

It is often difficult to administer early enteral nutrition in critically ill ICU patients. Proper placement of the tube, monitoring of gastrointestinal function, along with cardiovascular function, fluid administration, glucose monitoring, and hemodynamic stability, require close attention to detail and enteral feeding is often put off until the patient is better controlled. This study suggests that early feeding is important and should be used more frequently and aggressively in critical ill ICU patients.

J. M. Daly, MD

Early use of supplemental parenteral nutrition in critically ill patients: Results of an international multicenter observational study
Kutsogiannis J, Alberda C, Gramlich L, et al (Univ of Alberta, Edmonton, Canada; et al)
Crit Care Med 39:2691-2699, 2011

Objective.—To evaluate the effect of using supplemental parenteral nutrition compared to early enteral nutrition alone on nutritional and clinical outcomes.

Design.—A multicenter, observational study.

Setting.—Two hundred twenty-six intensive care units from 29 Countries.

Patients.—Mechanically ventilated critically ill adult patients that remained in the intensive care unit for >72 hrs and received early enteral nutrition within 48 hrs from admission.

Interventions.—Data were collected on patient characteristics and daily nutrition practices for up to 12 days. Patient outcomes were recorded after 60 days.

Measurements and Main Results.—We compared the outcomes of patients who received early enteral nutrition alone, early enteral nutrition + early parenteral nutrition, and early enteral nutrition + late parenteral nutrition (after 48 hrs of admission). Cox regression analyses were conducted to determine the effect of feeding strategy, adjusted for other confounding variables, on time to being discharged alive from hospital. A total of 2,920 patients were included in this study; 2562 (87.7%) in the early enteral nutrition group, 188 (6.4%) in the early parenteral nutrition group, and 170 (5.8%) in the late parenteral nutrition group. Adequacy of calories and protein was highest in the early parenteral nutrition group (81.2% and 80.1%, respectively) and lowest in the early enteral nutrition group (63.4% and 59.3%) ($p < .0001$). The 60-day mortality rate was 27.8% in the early enteral nutrition group, 34.6% in the early parenteral nutrition group, and 35.3% in the late parenteral nutrition group ($p = .02$). The rate of patients discharged alive from hospital was slower in the group that received early parenteral nutrition (unadjusted hazard ratio 0.75,

95% confidence interval 0.59–0.96) and late parenteral nutrition (hazard ratio 0.64, 95% confidence interval 0.51–0.81) ($p = .0003$) compared to early enteral nutrition. These findings persisted after adjusting for known confounders.

Conclusions.—The supplemental use of parenteral nutrition may improve provision of calories and protein but is not associated with any clinical benefit.

▶ This interesting observational study evaluated more than 5700 patients from 29 countries in hundreds of intensive care units. The study retrospectively reviewed hospital discharge information on patients who were mechanically ventilated and who had received early (within 48 hours upon admission to the intensive care unit [ICU]) enteral nutritional support. Patients were then divided into 3 groups: those who received early enteral nutrition alone, those who received early enteral nutrition and early parenteral nutrition, and those who received early enteral nutrition and late intervention with parenteral nutrition. Several thousand patients accumulated to the early enteral nutrition alone group while only 188 and 177 patients accrued to the latter 2 groups receiving parenteral nutrition. The study found that there was a higher mortality rate in those that received parenteral nutrition along with enteral nutrition either early or late. In addition, there were more days in the ICU and infectious complications were higher in those fed parenterally.

The study is important because it was carried out across 29 countries in hundreds of ICUs. However, it is subject to all the biases of a retrospective review and observational report in that each institution and each physician within that institution was free to institute nutritional support of any type during the patient's hospitalization and mechanical ventilation in the intensive care unit. The decisions to institute earlier enteral nutrition might have been due to patients who were unable to be enterally nourished. Those who received later intervention with parenteral nutrition were those who did not respond to enteral nutritional support because of a variety of factors. Nevertheless, the study does not show benefit to the addition of parenteral nutrition on top of enteral nutritional support. These results are supportive of the American Society of Parenteral and Enteral Nutrition guidelines on the use of nutrition support in the ICU suggesting that patients receive enteral nutrition and perhaps only if failure occurs with this mode of treatment should they receive parenteral nutrition. The importance of this study is that it would allow future randomized, prospective trials to be carried out, which would not be subject to the same observational retrospective bias.

J. M. Daly, MD

Early versus late Parenteral Nutrition in Critically Ill Adults

Casaer MP, Mesotten D, Hermans G, et al (Univ Hosps of the Catholic Univ of Leuven, Belgium; et al)
N Engl J Med 365:506-517, 2011

Background.—Controversy exists about the timing of the initiation of parenteral nutrition in critically ill adults in whom caloric targets cannot be met by enteral nutrition alone.

Methods.—In this randomized, multicenter trial, we compared early initiation of parenteral nutrition (European guidelines) with late initiation (American and Canadian guidelines) in adults in the intensive care unit (ICU) to supplement insufficient enteral nutrition. In 2312 patients, parenteral nutrition was initiated within 48 hours after ICU admission (early-initiation group), whereas in 2328 patients, parenteral nutrition was not initiated before day 8 (late-initiation group). A protocol for the early initiation of enteral nutrition was applied to both groups, and insulin was infused to achieve normoglycemia.

Results.—Patients in the late-initiation group had a relative increase of 6.3% in the likelihood of being discharged alive earlier from the ICU (hazard ratio, 1.06; 95% confidence interval [CI], 1.00 to 1.13; P = 0.04) and from the hospital (hazard ratio, 1.06; 95% CI, 1.00 to 1.13; P = 0.04), without evidence of decreased functional status at hospital discharge. Rates of death in the ICU and in the hospital and rates of survival at 90 days were similar in the two groups. Patients in the late-initiation group, as compared with the early-initiation group, had fewer ICU infections (22.8% vs. 26.2%, P = 0.008) and a lower incidence of cholestasis (P < 0.001). The late-initiation group had a relative reduction of 9.7% in the proportion of patients requiring more than 2 days of mechanical ventilation (P = 0.006), a median reduction of 3 days in the duration of renal-replacement therapy (P = 0.008), and a mean reduction in health care costs of €1,110 (about $1,600) (P = 0.04).

Conclusions.—Late initiation of parenteral nutrition was associated with faster recovery and fewer complications, as compared with early initiation. (Funded by the Methusalem program of the Flemish government and others; EPaNIC ClinicalTrials.gov number, NCT00512122.)

▶ This large, multicenter study sought to understand whether early initiation of parenteral nutrition (PN) as a supplement to enteral nutrition would be beneficial in critically ill intensive care unit (ICU) patients. More than 4600 patients were randomized in multiple centers and in multiple types of ICUs to receive either early addition of PN to enteral nutrition (early-intervention PN) or to receive late intervention (day 8) with PN as a supplement to their enteral feedings (late-intervention PN). All patients were treated with insulin administration for tight blood glucose control, and average blood sugars were in the 100 to 108 mg/dL levels.

As expected, those receiving early PN as a supplement had much higher early (days 1–7) calorie and protein intake compared with results in the late-intervention group. Insulin requirements were greater in the former group as well. Results also showed a shorter length of ICU stay in patients receiving late intervention as well as fewer overall respiratory and wound infections compared with results in the early-intervention group. Interestingly, patients receiving early-intervention PN had less of a systemic inflammatory response as determined by circulating levels of C reactive protein. Functional status and time to discharge from the hospital were similar in both groups.

Current dogma suggests that patients should receive targeted goals of calories and protein while in the ICU. This has resulted in a standard of care in which enteral tubes are inserted and enteral tube feedings started. While this is being done, PN is used as a supplement. This well-done, prospective, randomized trial in a large number of patients suggests that enteral nutrition alone should be used in the ICU with late initiation of PN as a supplement to enteral nutrition alone if targeted goals are not met by day 8 of ICU care. In this trial, patients who were able to achieve 80% of their target calorie goals did not receive PN. This level of caloric intake could be used as a benchmark in the treatment of patients in the ICU setting. As noted, standard parenteral formulas were used in this study and immunonutrition was not used. Nevertheless, this study is important in setting a new standard for our nutritional care of critically ill patients in the ICU.

J. M. Daly, MD

Effect of Early Compared With Delayed Enteral Nutrition on Endocrine Function in Patients With Traumatic Brain Injury: An Open-Labeled Randomized Trial

Chourdakis M, Kraus MM, Tzellos T, et al (Aristotle Univ of Thessaloniki, Greece)
JPEN J Parenter Enteral Nutr 36:108-116, 2012

Background.—Traumatic brain injury (TBI) results in a hypermetabolic and hypercatabolic status in which adequate nutrition support is essential to improve clinical outcome. The endocrine system of a patient with TBI is also affected and may play a critical role in either the metabolic or the immunologic response to the trauma. In the present study, the effect of standard, delayed enteral feeding (DEF), compared with early (within 24–48 hours) enteral feeding (EEF), on the endocrine function of patients with TBI was investigated.

Methods.—This comparative, prospective, open-labeled, randomized study included TBI patients admitted to the intensive care unit (ICU). Injury severity was assessed by the Glasgow Coma Scale and predicted mortality by the Acute Physiology and Chronic Health Evaluation II. Twenty-five patients received DEF and 34 patients received EEF. The effect of the onset of nutrition on pituitary, thyroidal, gonadal, and adrenal function was investigated on days 6 and 12 after admission to the hospital.

Results.—Levels of thyroid-stimulating hormone, free triiodothyronine, free thyroxine, and testosterone (in males) of DEF patients declined in comparison to levels of the day of admission to the ICU. The decrease of hormonal values was less pronounced in the EEF group. Cortisol concentrations rose in the DEF group; a lesser hormonal change was found in the EEF group. Deaths during the study for the DEF group and EEF group were 2 and 3, respectively.

Conclusions.—EEF may exert beneficial effects on the hormonal profile of TBI patients, possibly contributing to a better clinical outcome in this patient group.

▶ This prospective, randomized trial evaluated the hormonal effects of early versus delayed enteral nutrition in patients suffering traumatic brain injury. Fifty-nine patients were randomly assigned to receive either early enteral nutrition (within 48 hours of admission to the intensive care unit [ICU]) or delayed enteral nutrition (once gastroparesis was resolved but within 5 days of admission to the ICU). Interestingly, patients who received delayed enteral nutrition had a marked reduction in almost all hormonal values that were measured including free triiodothyronine, free thyroxine, thyroid-stimulating hormone, and testosterone. Patients who received early enteral nutritional support within 48 hours of admission to the ICU had less reduction of these hormone levels. While cortisol levels increased in the delayed enteral feeding group, there was less elevation in the early enteral feeding group. There were too few deaths in this series of 59 patients to assess any effect on mortality, and there was no reported effect on infections or other types of complications in the ICU.

Other studies have evaluated the use of nutritional support in patients suffering traumatic brain injury and have found no effect on overall outcome. This is understandable in that the major prognostic variable is the degree of injury and not necessarily the use of nutritional support or many other interventions. It would be interesting to understand the immunologic effects of enteral nutritional support in this group of patients given the changes that were observed in systemic hormonal levels.

J. M. Daly, MD

Effect of titrated parenteral nutrition on body composition after allogeneic hematopoietic stem cell transplantation in children: A double-blind, randomized, multicenter trial

Sharma TS, Bechard LJ, Feldman HA, et al (Children's Hosp, Boston, MA; et al)
Am J Clin Nutr 95:342-351, 2012

Background.—Children undergoing hematopoietic stem cell transplantation (HSCT) often require parenteral nutrition (PN) to optimize caloric intake. Standard approaches to nutritional supplementation provide 130–150% of estimated energy expenditure, but resting energy expenditure (REE) may be lower than expected after HSCT. Provision of PN exceeding energy needs may lead to overfeeding and associated complications.

Objective.—We conducted a blinded, randomized, controlled, multicenter trial in children undergoing HSCT to determine the effect on body composition of 2 different approaches of nutrition support: standard amounts of energy from PN (130–150% of REE) compared with PN titrated to match measured REE.

Design.—Twenty-six children undergoing HSCT were randomly assigned to standard or titrated PN. Energy intake was monitored until day 30 after HSCT. Body-composition and anthropometric measures were obtained through day 100. The primary outcome variable was percentage body fat (%BF) measured by dual energy X-ray absorptiometry.

Results.—The estimated change in %BF from baseline to day 30 was 1.2 ± 0.5% in the standard group and 0.1 ± 0.5% in the experimental group, but the overall time course of %BF did not differ significantly by treatment ($P = 0.39$ for time × treatment interaction). A profound loss of lean body mass (LBM) occurred in both groups during the intervention period and persisted through day 100.

Conclusions.—Parenteral energy intake titrated to energy expenditure does not result in a lower accumulation of BF than does standard energy intake. Neither titrated nor standard PN regimens during HSCT preserve LBM. Alternative approaches to preserve LBM are needed. This trial is registered at clinicaltrials.gov as 00115258.

▶ Children who undergo bone marrow transplantation are at a substantial risk of developing malnutrition. The use of parenteral nutrition is necessary because often they cannot take adequate amounts of enteral nutrition. However, despite the general use of parenteral nutrition, these children lose lean body mass while increasing body fat and may develop cholestasis. This randomized, prospective, blinded trial sought to determine if provision of parenteral nutrition calories based on measured energy expenditures might preserve lean body mass and avoid complications of nutritional therapy.

The study found fewer increases in body fat percentage in those children who had energy supplied according to their individual energy expenditure; however, all lost lean body mass and complications appeared similar. Thus, as the authors suggested, other strategies, such as use of different nutritional formulae, deliberate exercise regimens, or other means, should be tried in an effort to reduce the losses of lean body mass in these children.

J. M. Daly, MD

Effects of Long-term Parenteral Nutrition on Serum Lipids, Plant Sterols, Cholesterol Metabolism, and Liver Histology in Pediatric Intestinal Failure
Kurvinen A, Nissinen MJ, Gylling H, et al (Univ of Helsinki, Finland)
J Pediatr Gastroenterol Nutr 53:440-446, 2011

Background and Objective.—Plant sterols (PS) in parenteral nutrition (PN) may contribute to intestinal failure—associated liver disease. We investigated interrelations between serum PS, liver function and histology, cholesterol metabolism, and characteristics of PN.

Patients and Methods.—Eleven patients with intestinal failure (mean age 6.3 years) receiving long-term PN were studied prospectively (mean

254 days) and underwent repeated measurements of serum lipids, noncholesterol sterols, including PS, and liver enzymes. PS contents of PN were analyzed. Liver biopsy was obtained in 8 patients. Twenty healthy children (mean age 5.7 years) served as controls.

Results.—Median percentage of parenteral energy of total daily energy (PN%) was 48%, including 0.9 $g \cdot kg^{-1} \cdot day^{-1}$ of lipids. Respective amounts of PN sitosterol, campesterol, avenasterol, and stigmasterol were 683, 71, 57, and 45 $\mu g \cdot kg^{-1} \cdot day^{-1}$. Median serum concentrations of sitosterol (48 vs 7.5 $\mu mol/L$, $P < 0.001$), avenasterol (2.9 vs 1.9, $P < 0.01$), stigmasterol (1.9 vs 1.2, $P < 0.005$), but not that of campesterol (9.8 vs 12, $P = 0.22$), were increased among patients in relation to controls, and correlated with PN% ($r = 0.81-0.88$, $P < 0.005$), but not with PN fat. Serum cholesterol precursors were higher in patients than in controls. Serum liver enzymes remained close to normal range. Glutamyl transferase correlated with serum PS ($r = 0.61-0.62$, $P < 0.05$). Liver fibrosis in 5 patients reflected increased serum PS ($r = 0.55-0.60$, $P = 0.16-0.12$).

Conclusions.—Serum PS moderately increase during olive oil–based PN, and correlate positively with PN% and glutamyl transferase. Despite well-preserved liver function, histology often revealed significant liver damage.

▶ Intestinal failure in children and its management with long-term parenteral nutrition are fraught with many complications. The most serious of these are infection and associated liver failure. This study evaluated the relationship of plant sterols thought to be present in parenteral nutrition formulas and the development of liver dysfunction. As noted previously by others, mean serum total cholesterol, low-density lipoprotein and high-density lipoprotein cholesterol serum levels were lower in nutritionally supported children than the 20 controls. Circulating plant sterol levels were higher. Interestingly, liver biopsies showed inflammatory reaction ranging to fibrotic changes despite relatively normal serum liver enzyme levels. These results demonstrate the need to ameliorate the liver dysfunction that occurs with parenteral nutrition support for children with intestinal failure and the need to better monitor the occurrence of liver histologic changes to intervene earlier, preventing liver failure.

J. M. Daly, MD

Evaluation of effects of nutrition intervention on healing of pressure ulcers and nutritional states (randomized controlled trial)

Ohura T, Nakajo T, Okada S, et al (Pressure Ulcers and Wound Healing Res Ctr (Kojin-Kai), Sapporo, Japan; Aoba Hosp, Tokyo, Japan; Kitamihara Clinic, Hakodate, Japan; et al)
Wound Repair Regen 19:330-336, 2011

The objective of this study was to evaluate the effects of nutrition intervention on nutritional states and healing of pressure ulcers by standardizing or unified factors including nursing, care and treatment in a multicenter open randomized trial. Tube-fed patients with Stage III—IV pressure ulcers were selected. The control group (30 patients) received the same nutrition management as before participating in this trial, whereas the intervention group (30 patients) was given calories in the range of Basal Energy Expenditure (BEE)×1.1×1.3 to 1.5. The intervention period was 12 weeks. The efficacy and safety were evaluated based on the nutritional states and the sizes of ulcers (length×width), and on the incidence of adverse events related to the study, respectively. The calories administered to the control and intervention groups were 29.1 ± 4.9 and 37.9 ± 6.5 kcal/kg/day, respectively. Significant interactions between the presence or absence of the intervention and the intervention period were noted for nutritional states ($p < 0.001$ for body weight, $p < 0.05$ for prealbumin). Similarly, the size of ulcers differed significantly between subjects in the intervention group and in the control group ($p < 0.001$). The results suggest that nutrition intervention could directly enhance the healing process in pressure ulcer patients.

▶ This prospective, randomized Japanese study evaluated the healing response of patients with stage III-IV pressure ulcers to enhanced nutritional support. For example, during the study period, those receiving nutritional intervention received an average of 38 cal/kg/d compared with 29 kcal/kg/d in those that received standard treatment. Protein intake was also significantly higher in the nutritional intervention group. There was a marked improvement in nutritional indices such as serum proteins and body anthropometrics. In addition, there was a significant reduction in the mean pressure ulcer size in the intervention group compared with the controls who received standard of nursing care. Finally, the duration of feeding was important and correlated with response to therapy as the healing process was prolonged. Studies such as these emphasize the importance of multidisciplinary care for patients with these complex wound problems. Nursing, rehabilitation therapy, and nutritional care are critical to success.

J. M. Daly, MD

Growth Hormone to Improve Short Bowel Syndrome Intestinal Autonomy: A Pediatric Randomized Open-Label Clinical Trial
Peretti N, Loras-Duclaux I, Kassai B, et al (Université Lyon 1, France; Nutrition Pédiatrique, Lyon, France; et al)
JPEN J Parenter Enteral Nutr 35:723-731, 2011

Background.—The ability of growth hormone (GH) to promote the weaning-off of parenteral nutrition (PN) in short bowel syndrome (SBS) is unclear. No randomized controlled study is available in children. This study was undertaken to determine if GH could enhance the weaning off of PN in PN-dependent children with SBS.

Methods.—A prospective randomized open-label multicenter study was performed in 14 patients (mean age, 9 ± 1.4 years) with SBS (average small bowel length, 33 cm) and long-term PN dependency (8 years) on an unrestricted diet. A standardized PN decrease with and without GH (0.14 mg/kg/d) was conducted. The patients were randomized to either a GH group (4 months of GH) or a control (CTR) group (4 months without GH, followed by 4 months with GH). Blood tests and a nutrition assessment of enteral and parenteral intakes were performed. Groups were compared with the Wilcoxon test.

Results.—Treatment with GH did not improve the weaning off of PN (decrease in PN caloric intake of 32.5% ± 9.6% in the GH group vs 35.2% ± 8.7% in the CTR group, nonsignificant). In the CTR group, GH treatment induced an additional but not statistically significant decrease of 8.8% ± 12.4% in daily calories. Parenteral needs returned to near basal rates 6 months after GH discontinuation (GH: 77.6% ± 10.6% vs CTR: 73.2% ± 7.4%). Weight decreased slightly in both groups. No biological parameters varied significantly.

Conclusions.—GH did not improve the weaning off of PN in PN-dependent children with SBS.

▶ Previous reports have suggested that the use of growth hormone in individuals with short bowel syndrome could help in the weaning of these individuals from total parenteral nutrition. Some studies have used glutamine and bulking fiber agents as well. However, many studies have not been randomized, prospective trials but studies of groups who have been on long-term total parenteral nutrition.

In this report, investigators sought to determine whether the administration of growth hormone would help in the weaning of these children from total parenteral nutrition. Fourteen children with short bowel syndrome were randomly assigned to 2 groups. In one group, the children received growth hormone daily in the evening by injection for 4 months; weaning of parenteral nutrition was conducted similarly between groups. The control group received no growth hormone during this 4-month period. The control group was then administered growth hormone for 4 months, and weaning was again attempted. Following cessation of growth hormone, both groups were followed for a 6-month period.

As stated, administration of growth hormone did not improve the weaning off of total parenteral nutrition in these children. During the weaning period, weight decreased slightly in both groups. In all groups, requirements for intravenous calories and protein returned to basal levels toward the end of the 6-month period following cessation of growth hormone.

Thus, this prospective, randomized trial has found that growth hormone administration in children with short bowel syndrome does not improve the weaning off of parenteral nutrition. The long-term use of parenteral nutrition in children with short bowel syndrome results in many complications, including sepsis and intestinal failure—associated liver failure. Therefore, it is important to use multiple medical approaches in an effort to wean these children from the necessity of total parenteral nutrition.

J. M. Daly, MD

Increased protein-energy intake promotes anabolism in critically ill infants with viral bronchiolitis: a double-blind randomised controlled trial

de Betue CT, van Waardenburg DA, Deutz NE, et al (Maastricht Univ Med Ctr, The Netherlands; et al)

Arch Dis Child 96:817-822, 2011

Objective.—The preservation of nutritional status and growth is an important aim in critically ill infants, but difficult to achieve due to the metabolic stress response and inadequate nutritional intake, leading to negative protein balance. This study investigated whether increasing protein and energy intakes can promote anabolism. The primary outcome was whole body protein balance, and the secondary outcome was first pass splanchnic phenylalanine extraction (SPE_{Phe}).

Design.—This was a double-blind randomised controlled trial. Infants (n=18) admitted to the paediatric intensive care unit with respiratory failure due to viral bronchiolitis were randomised to continuous enteral feeding with protein and energy enriched formula (PE-formula) (n=8; 3.1 ± 0.3 g protein/kg/24 h, 119 ± 25 kcal/kg/24 h) or standard formula (S-formula) (n=10; 1.7 ± 0.2 g protein/kg/24 h, 84 ± 15 kcal/kg/24 h; equivalent to recommended intakes for healthy infants <6 months). A combined intravenous-enteral phenylalanine stable isotope protocol was used on day 5 after admission to determine whole body protein metabolism and SPE_{Phe}.

Results.—Protein balance was significantly higher with PE-formula than with S-formula (PE-formula: 0.73 ± 0.5 vs S-formula: 0.02 ± 0.6 g/kg/24 h) resulting from significantly increased protein synthesis (PE-formula: 9.6 ± 4.4, S-formula: 5.2 ± 2.3 g/kg/24 h), despite significantly increased protein breakdown (PE-formula: 8.9 ± 4.3, S-formula: 5.2 ± 2.6 g/kg/24 h). SPE_{Phe} was not statistically different between the two groups (PE-formula: $39.8 \pm 18.3\%$, S-formula: $52.4 \pm 13.6\%$).

Conclusions.—Increasing protein and energy intakes promotes protein anabolism in critically ill infants in the first days after admission. Since this is an important target of nutritional support, increased protein and energy intakes should be preferred above standard intakes in these infants.

Dutch Trial Register number: NTR 515.

▶ In critically ill infants, protein anabolism, growth, and achievement of positive nutritional status are important goals. Infants have fewer reserves during critical illnesses such as infectious viral bronchiolitis; thus, it has been suggested that aggressive nutritional support is indicated. Often, the volume of nutritional support is limited because of the infant's size, approximating 120 mL/kg.

This randomized, prospective trial examined the effects of increasing protein and energy intake on promoting nutritional status and protein metabolism. Eighteen critically ill infants with viral bronchiolitis were entered into this multi-center trial. They received either standard enteral formulation or a formula with increased protein and energy content. On day 5, protein turnover was measured using an intravenous-enteral phenylalanine stable isotope protocol. Results of the study showed that increasing protein and energy in the diet improved protein synthesis. Thus, results of this study showed that infants who are critically ill should certainly receive supplemented protein and energy intake during the period of their critical illness.

J. M. Daly, MD

Optimal Protein and Energy nutrition decreases Mortality in Mechanically Ventilated, Critically Ill Patients: A Prospective Observational Cohort Study
Weijs PJM, Stapel SN, de Groot SDW, et al (VU Univ Med Ctr, Amsterdam, Netherlands)
JPEN J Parenter Enteral Nutr 36:60-68, 2012

Background.—Optimal nutrition for patients in the intensive care unit has been proposed to be the provision of energy as determined by indirect calorimetry and the provision of protein of at least 1.2 g/kg.

Methods.—Prospective observational cohort study in a mixed medical-surgical intensive care unit in an academic hospital. In total, 886 consecutive mechanically ventilated patients were included. Nutrition was guided by indirect calorimetry and protein provision of at least 1.2 g/kg. Cumulative intakes were calculated for the period of mechanical ventilation. Cox regression was used to analyze the effect of protein + energy target achieved or energy target achieved versus neither target achieved on 28-day mortality, with adjustments for sex, age, body mass index, Acute Physiology and Chronic Health Evaluation II, diagnosis, and hyperglycemic index.

Results.—Patients' mean age was 63 ± 16 years; body mass index, 26 ± 6; and Acute Physiology and Chronic Health Evaluation II, 23 ± 8. For neither target, energy target, and protein + energy target, energy intake was 75% ± 15%, 96% ± 5%, and 99% ± 5% of target, and protein intake was 72% ± 20%, 89% ± 10%, and 112% ± 12% of target, respectively. Hazard ratios (95% confidence interval) for energy target and protein + energy target were 0.83 (0.67−1.01) and 0.47 (0.31−0.73) for 28-day mortality.

Conclusions.—Optimal nutritional therapy in mechanically ventilated, critically ill patients, defined as protein and energy targets reached, is associated with a decrease in 28-day mortality by 50%, whereas only reaching energy targets is not associated with a reduction in mortality.

▶ Controversy exists as to the optimal level of nutrition to provide to patients in the intensive care unit. This observational study evaluated the levels of energy and protein intake in intensive care unit patients requiring mechanical ventilation. This study is subject to all the biases inherent in such observations.

Investigators assigned patients based on their observations; some received energy intake less than optimal (defined as 10% greater than that measured by indirect calorimetry) and some received energy and protein intake that was optimal, reaching their targets. Patients received an average of 75%, 96%, and 99% of target energy requirements and 72%, 89%, and 112% of protein requirements. In the group achieving target energy and protein requirements, morbidity and mortality of these mechanically ventilated intensive care unit patients was lowest.

Results of this study suggest that obtaining optimal protein intake along with optimal energy intake reaching target result in the best outcome for these critically ill patients. Of note, 73% of these patients received enteral feeding alone. One percent received parenteral feeding alone, and the remainder received a combination. Thus, the results of this study suggest that protein and energy intake is more important than that of energy intake alone in these critically ill patients.

J. M. Daly, MD

Parenteral fish-oil—based lipid emulsion improves fatty acid profiles and lipids in parenteral nutrition—dependent children
Le HD, de Meijer VE, Robinson EM, et al (Children's Hosp Boston, MA; et al)
Am J Clin Nutr 94:749-758, 2011

Background.—Total parenteral nutrition (PN), including fat administered as a soybean oil—based lipid emulsion (SOLE), is a life-saving therapy but may be complicated by PN-induced cholestasis and dyslipidemia. A fish-oil—based lipid emulsion (FOLE) as a component of PN can reverse PN-cholestasis and has been shown to improve lipid profiles.

Objective.—The objective was to describe changes in the fatty acid and lipid profiles of children with PN-cholestasis who were treated with a FOLE.

Design.—Lipid and fatty acid profiles of 79 pediatric patients who developed PN-cholestasis while receiving standard PN with a SOLE were examined before and after the switch to a FOLE. All patients received PN with the FOLE at a dose of $1 \text{ g·kg}^{-1} \text{·d}^{-1}$ for ≥ 1 mo.

Results.—The median (interquartile range) age at the start of the FOLE treatment was 91 (56—188) d. After a median (interquartile range) of 18.3 (9.4—41.4) wk of receiving the FOLE, the subjects' median total and direct bilirubin improved from 7.9 and 5.4 mg/dL to 0.5 and 0.2 mg/dL, respectively ($P < 0.0001$). Serum triglyceride, total cholesterol, LDL, and VLDL concentrations significantly decreased by 51.7%, 17.4%, 23.7%, and 47.9%, respectively.

Conclusions.—The switch from a SOLE to a FOLE in PN-dependent children with cholestasis and dyslipidemia was associated with a dramatic improvement in serum triglyceride and VLDL concentrations, a significant increase in serum omega-3 (n−3) fatty acids (EPA and DHA), and a decrease in serum omega-6 fatty acids (arachidonic acid). A FOLE may be the preferred lipid emulsion in patients with PN-cholestasis, dyslipidemia, or both. This trial is registered at clinicaltrials.gov as NCT00910104.

▶ The development of cholestasis in children who require long-term parenteral nutrition is a major problem, resulting in severe morbidity. Alternative therapies include weaning the child from parenteral nutrition to increase enteral intake and potentially altering the composition and amounts of lipid intake during continual parenteral nutrition. This longitudinal study retrospectively reviewed prospectively gathered data on 79 children, nearly 50% of whom had short gut syndrome from necrotizing enterocolitis. The children who were noted to develop cholestasis were switched from a soybean-derived lipid emulsion to a fish oil—based lipid emulsion (FOLE) and followed for lipid and liver profile analysis over time. As noted, serum triglyceride, very low density lipoprotein, direct and total bilirubin levels diminished markedly over time after starting the FOLE. Appropriate elevations in serum omega-3 fatty acid levels were also noted.

Although not a prospective study, the results were impressive in this report. As the authors noted, since marked improvements in cholestasis were seen, it will be important to determine whether the long-term use of FOLE can prevent cholestasis from occurring and if there is a need to alternate FOLE and SOLE over the long term to prevent essential fatty acid deficiency, although none was found in this study.

J. M. Daly, MD

Parenteral Nutrition Supplementation in Biliary Atresia Patients Listed for Liver Transplantation

Sullivan JS, Sundaram SS, Pan Z, et al (Children's Hosp Colorado and Univ of Colorado School of Medicine, Aurora)
Liver Transpl 18:121-129, 2012

The objective of this study was to determine the impact of parenteral nutrition (PN) on the outcomes of biliary atresia (BA) patients listed for liver transplantation (LT). We retrospectively reviewed the charts of all BA patients at our institution who underwent hepatoportoenterostomy and were listed for LT before the age of 36 months between 1990 and 2010. The initiation of PN was based on clinical indications. Twenty-five PN subjects and 22 non-PN subjects (74% female) were studied. The median PN initiation age was 7.7 months, the mean duration was 86 days, and the mean amount of energy supplied by PN was 77 kcal/kg/day. Before PN, the triceps skinfold thickness (TSF) and the mid-arm circumference (MAC) z scores were decreasing. After PN, TSF ($P < 0.001$) and MAC ($P < 0.001$) improved significantly. The PN group had lower MAC and TSF scores than the non-PN group at the time of LT listing. Between listing and LT, MAC and TSF improved in the PN group and worsened in the non-PN groups; as a result, the 2 groups had the same z scores at LT. The PN group had a higher incidence of gastrointestinal bleeding and ascites before LT, but there were no differences in the rates of pre-LT bacteremia, days in the intensive care unit after LT, or patient or graft survival. In conclusion, PN improves the nutritional status of malnourished BA patients awaiting LT, and this is associated with post-LT outcomes comparable to those of patients not requiring PN.

▶ The use of parenteral nutrition in patients awaiting liver transplantation may be life saving, but few studies have examined its role in children with biliary atresia. Compared with adults, these children are at the greatest risk for malnutrition as they await a liver donor. This retrospective report examined the role of parenteral nutrition in children with biliary atresia awaiting transplantation. The indications for parenteral nutritional support were clearly present as the children had lower body fat and muscle mass. Administration of total parenteral nutrition (TPN) was safe as similar rates of infection occurred as in the group who did not receive TPN. Importantly, use of TPN resulted in marked improvement of nutritional indices, bringing the treated group to the same level as those who did not require nutritional intervention. Thus, use of TPN in these children should be advocated when they are malnourished to maintain their nutritional status and maximize their opportunities for safe recovery after liver transplant.

J. M. Daly, MD

Provision of Balanced Nutrition Protects Against Hypoglycemia in the Critically Ill Surgical Patient

Kauffmann RM, Hayes RM, Jenkins JM, et al (Vanderbilt Univ Med Ctr, Nashville, TN)

JPEN J Parenter Enter Nutr 35:686-694, 2011

Background.—Intensive insulin therapy lowers blood glucose and improves outcomes but increases the risk of hypoglycemia. Typically, insulin protocols require a dextrose solution to prevent hypoglycemia. The authors hypothesized that the provision of balanced nutrition (enteral nutrition [EN] or parenteral nutrition [PN]) would be more protective against hypoglycemia ($\geq$50 mg/dL) than carbohydrate alone.

Methods.—A retrospective analysis was performed of patients treated with intensive insulin therapy and surviving $\geq$24 hours. The computer-based insulin protocol requires infusion of D10W at 30 mL/h if EN or PN is not provided. Nutrition provision was assessed in 2-hour increments, comparing periods of blood glucose control with and without balanced nutrition. The risk of hypoglycemia for each blood glucose measurement was estimated by multivariable regression.

Results.—In total, 66,592 glucose measurements were collected on 1392 patients. Hypoglycemic events occurred in 5.8/1000 glucose tests after 2 hours without balanced nutrition compared to 2.2/1000 tests when balanced nutrition was given in the preceding 2 hours. In multivariable regression models, balanced nutrition was the strongest protective factor against hypoglycemia. Patients who did not receive balanced nutrition in the preceding 2 hours had a 3 times increase in the odds of a hypoglycemic event at their next glucose check (odds ratio = 3.6, $P < .001$). Providing carbohydrate alone was not protective.

Conclusions.—Balanced nutrition is associated with reduced risk of hypoglycemia. These results suggest that balanced nutrition should be given when insulin therapy is initiated. Future studies should evaluate the efficacy of EN vs PN in preventing hypoglycemia.

▶ There continues to be some controversy regarding the efficacy of intensive insulin therapy in critically ill patients. An early prospective randomized study suggested benefit, although later studies were less positive. In this report, the authors retrospectively reviewed records of critically ill patients in the intensive care unit who underwent care using an intensive insulin therapy protocol. The protocol called for D10W to be infused if other nutrition was stopped for a period of 30 minutes.

Interestingly, in those receiving balanced nutrition within the preceding 2 hours, episodes of hypoglycemia were far less frequent, suggesting that its provision was protective. However, one must bear in mind that this was a retrospective study that might show association but does not show causation. Episodes of hypoglycemia are more frequent in those who are septic, already diabetic, and receiving vasopressors, and so on. Thus, the true mechanisms behind the potential protective effect of balanced nutrition remain unclear.

J. M. Daly, MD

Randomised placebo-controlled trial of teduglutide in reducing parenteral nutrition and/or intravenous fluid requirements in patients with short bowel syndrome

Jeppesen PB, Gilroy R, Pertkiewicz M, et al (Rigshospitalet, Copenhagen, Denmark; Kansas Univ Med Ctr; Med Univ of Warsaw, Poland; et al)
Gut 60:902-914, 2011

Background and Aims.—Teduglutide, a GLP-2 analogue, may restore intestinal structural and functional integrity by promoting repair and growth of the mucosa and reducing gastric emptying and secretion, thereby increasing fluid and nutrient absorption in patients with short bowel syndrome (SBS). This 24-week placebo-controlled study evaluated the ability of teduglutide to reduce parenteral support in patients with SBS with intestinal failure.

Methods.—In 83 patients randomised to receive subcutaneous teduglutide 0.10 mg/kg/day (n=32), 0.05 mg/kg/day (n=35) or placebo (n=16) once daily, parenteral fluids were reduced at 4-week intervals if intestinal fluid absorption (48 h urine volumes) increased ≥10%. Responders were subjects who demonstrated reductions of ≥20% in parenteral volumes from baseline at weeks 20 and 24. The primary efficacy end point, a graded response score (GRS), took into account higher levels and earlier onset of response, leading to longer duration of response. The intensity of the response was defined as a reduction from baseline in parenteral volume (from 20% to 100%), and the duration of the response was considered the response at weeks 16, 20 and 24. The results were tested according to a step-down procedure starting with the 0.10 mg/kg/day dose.

Results.—Using the GRS criteria, teduglutide in a dose of 0.10 mg/kg/day did not have a statistically significant effect compared with placebo (8/32 vs 1/16, p=0.16), while teduglutide in a dose of 0.05 mg/kg/day had a significant effect (16/35, p=0.007). Since parenteral volume reductions were equal (353±475 and 354±334 ml/day), the trend towards higher baseline parenteral volume (1816±1008 vs 1374±639 ml/day, p=0.11) in the 0.10 mg/kg/day group compared with the 0.05 mg/kg/day group may have accounted for this discrepancy. Three teduglutide-treated patients were completely weaned off parenteral support. Serious adverse events were distributed similarly between active treatment groups and placebo. Villus height, plasma citrulline concentration and lean body mass were significantly increased with teduglutide compared with placebo.

Conclusions.—Teduglutide was safe, well tolerated, intestinotrophic and suggested pro-absorptive effects facilitating reductions in parenteral support in patients with SBS with intestinal failure. ClinicalTrials.gov number: NCT00172185.

▶ This prospective, randomized trial is the largest to date in patients with short bowel syndrome. It is well known that patients with short bowel syndrome requiring long-term parenteral nutrition suffer from episodes of catheter-related sepsis and intestinal failure—associated liver failure. These are the 2 main complications along with fluid and electrolyte abnormalities that can occur with deficiencies in certain nutrients. Thus, it is incumbent upon physicians treating patients with short bowel syndrome to attempt to wean patients from parenteral nutrition and satisfy their nutritional requirements using enteral nutrition. A variety of methods have been described, including administration of growth hormone, use of glutamine, and use of short-chain and omega-3 fatty acids in the diet.

This study used teduglutide to improve intestinal function and absorption and allow for weaning from parenteral nutrition. Interestingly, subjects receiving teduglutide at a dose of 0.10 mg had nonsignificant effects on intestinal function whereas those receiving a lesser dose (0.05 mg) demonstrated a significant improvement in intestinal absorption along with increases in plasma citrulline levels, suggesting structural changes in the small intestine as well. Three patients were able to be weaned off parenteral nutrition during treatment. However, even after 6 months of treatment, the intestinal function seemed to regress back to baseline levels 3 months after cessation of teduglutide.

Results of this study are extremely important for those who care for patients with short gut syndrome. These patients suffer fluid and electrolyte disturbances during oral intake due to loss of fluid, flatulence, dehydration, and abdominal pain. Nevertheless, it should be the ultimate goal to wean patients from parenteral nutrition, reducing the complications associated with intravenous feeding and allowing patients to lead a more normal life. Teduglutide appears to be very useful in optimizing intestinal function and weaning from parenteral nutrition in those patients with short bowel syndrome.

J. M. Daly, MD

Randomized clinical trial of omega-3 fatty acid-supplemented enteral nutrition *versus* standard enteral nutrition in patients undergoing oesophagogastric cancer surgery

Sultan J, Griffin SM, Di Franco F, et al (Royal Victoria Infirmary, Newcastle upon Tyne, UK; et al)
Br J Surg 99:346-355, 2012

Background.—Oesophagogastric cancer surgery is immunosuppressive. This may be modulated by omega-3 fatty acids (O-3FAs). The aim of this study was to assess the effect of perioperative O-3FAs on clinical outcome and immune function after oesophagogastric cancer surgery.

Methods.—Patients undergoing subtotal oesophagectomy and total gastrectomy were recruited and allocated randomly to an O-3FA enteral immunoenhancing diet (IED) or standard enteral nutrition (SEN) for 7 days before and after surgery, or to postoperative supplementation alone (control group). Clinical outcome, fatty acid concentrations, and HLA-DR expression on monocytes and activated T lymphocytes were determined before and after operation.

Results.—Of 221 patients recruited, 26 were excluded. Groups (IED, 66; SEN, 63; control, 66) were matched for age, malnutrition and co-morbidity. There were no differences in morbidity ($P = 0 \cdot 646$), mortality ($P = 1 \cdot 000$) or hospital stay ($P = 0 \cdot 701$) between the groups. O-3FA concentrations were higher in the IED group after supplementation ($P < 0 \cdot 001$). The ratio of omega-6 fatty acid to O-3FA was $1 \cdot 9{:}1$, $4 \cdot 1{:}1$ and $4 \cdot 8{:}1$ on the day before surgery in the IED, SEN and control groups ($P < 0 \cdot 001$). There were no differences between the groups in HLA-DR expression in either monocytes ($P = 0 \cdot 538$) or activated T lymphocytes ($P = 0 \cdot 204$).

Conclusion.—Despite a significant increase in plasma concentrations of O-3FA, immunonutrition with O-3FA did not affect overall HLA-DR expression on leucocytes or clinical outcome following oesophagogastric cancer surgery. Registration number: ISRCTN43730758 (http://www.controlledtrials.com).

▶ This prospective, randomized, and blinded (except for the control group) study carried out in patients who underwent esophagogastrectomy was well done. The authors stratified patients for the presence or absence of malnutrition, with 1 group receiving an omega-3 fatty acid—enriched formula by mouth, 1 group receiving a standard nutritional formula, and a control group that received no particular dietary intervention. No statistical differences in postoperative morbidity or mortality were noted, yet there were differences in blood levels of omega-3 fatty acids in line with the patients' supplementation.

Some previous studies have shown differences in postoperative outcomes in patients receiving immunonutrition with omega-3 fatty acids, arginine, RNA, and perhaps glutamine supplementation, but it was unclear which of the supplemental ingredients were helpful in terms of postoperative outcomes. However, not all such studies showed differences, perhaps because of the degree of malnutrition noted in these patients with upper gastrointestinal cancers. It is critically important that negative studies such as this one be published to balance others that often have positive results with interventions.

J. M. Daly, MD

Substitution of Standard Soybean Oil with Olive Oil-Based Lipid Emulsion in Parenteral Nutrition: Comparison of Vascular, Metabolic, and Inflammatory Effects

Siqueira J, Smiley D, Newton C, et al (Emory Univ, Atlanta, GA; et al)
J Clin Endocrinol Metab 96:3207-3216, 2011

Context.—Soybean oil-based lipid emulsions are the only Food and Drug Administration-approved lipid formulation for clinical use in parenteral nutrition (PN). Recently concerns with its use have been raised due to the proinflammatory effects that may lead to increased complications because they are rich in ω-6 polyunsaturated fatty acids.

Methods.—This was a prospective, randomized, controlled, crossover study comparing the vascular, metabolic, immune, and inflammatory effects of 24-h infusion of PN containing soybean oil-based lipid emulsion (Intralipid), olive oil-based (ClinOleic), lipid free, and normal saline in 12 healthy subjects.

Results.—Soybean oil-PN increased systolic blood pressure compared with olive oil-PN ($P < 0.05$). Soybean oil PN reduced brachial artery flow-mediated dilatation from baseline (-23% at 4 h and -25% at 24 h, both $P < 0.01$); in contrast, olive oil PN, lipid free PN, and saline did not change either systolic blood pressure or flow-mediated dilatation. Compared with saline, soybean oil PN, olive oil PN, and lipid free PN similarly increased glucose and insulin concentrations during infusion ($P < 0.05$). There were no significant changes in plasma free fatty acids, lipid profile, inflammatory and oxidative stress markers, immune function parameters, or sympathetic activity between soybean oil- and olive oil-based lipid emulsions.

Conclusion.—The 24-h infusion of PN containing soybean oil-based lipid emulsion increased blood pressure and impaired endothelial function compared with PN containing olive oil-based lipid emulsion and lipid-free PN in healthy subjects. These vascular changes may have significant implications in worsening outcome in subjects receiving nutrition support. Randomized controlled trials with relevant clinical outcome measures are needed in patients receiving PN with olive oil-based and soybean oil-based lipid emulsions.

▶ Although olive oil—based lipid emulsions are not currently in use in the United States, there is a significant interest in their use to reduce the inflammatory response to lipid emulsions and to underlying disease processes such as the systemic inflammatory response syndrome. This short-term study evaluated the physiologic responses to soybean oil—based lipid and olive oil—based lipid emulsion infusions over 24 hours. Interestingly, the soybean oil emulsion increased significantly mean systemic blood pressure and reduced mean brachial artery flow dilation compared with the other 3 infusions. These short-term physiologic responses are interesting in that no effect was noted in serum levels of fatty acid or c-reactive protein levels, suggesting another mechanism than that which was postulated. It remains to be seen whether these physiologic responses to soybean oil—based lipid emulsions persist over a longer term.

J. M. Daly, MD

The effect of L-alanyl-L-glutamine dipeptide supplemented total parenteral nutrition on infectious morbidity and insulin sensitivity in critically ill patients
Grau T, for the Metabolism, Nutrition Working Group, SEMICYUC, Spain (Hospital Universitario Doce de Octubre, Madrid, Spain; et al)
Crit Care Med 39:1263-1268, 2011

Objective.—The aim of this study was to assess the clinical efficacy of alanine-glutamine dipeptide-supplemented total parenteral nutrition defined by the occurrence of nosocomial infections. Secondary parameters included Sequential Organ Failure Assessment score, hyperglycemia and insulin needs, intensive care unit and hospital length of stay, and 6-month mortality.

Design.—Multicenter, prospective, double-blind, randomized trial.

Setting.—Twelve intensive care units at Spanish hospitals.

Patients.—One hundred twenty-seven patients with Acute Physiology and Chronic Health Evaluation II score >12 and requiring parenteral nutrition for 5—9 days.

Intervention.—Patients were randomized to receive an isonitrogenous and isocaloric total parenteral nutrition or alanine-glutamine dipeptide-supplemented total parenteral nutrition. Nutritional needs were calculated: 0.25 g N/kg^{-1}/d^{-1} and 25 kcal/kg^{-1}/d^{-1}. The study group received 0.5 g/kg^{-1}/d^{-1} of glutamine dipeptide and the control total parenteral nutrition group a similar amount of amino acids. Hyperglycemia was controlled applying an intensive insulin protocol with a target glycemia of 140 mg/dL.

Measurements and Main Results.—The two groups did not differ at inclusion for the type and severity of injury or the presence of sepsis or septic shock. Caloric intake was similar in both groups. Preprotocol analysis showed that treated patients with alanine-glutamine dipeptide-supplemented total parenteral nutrition had lesser nosocomial pneumonia, 8.04 vs. 29.25 episodes-‰ days of mechanical ventilation (p = .02), and urinary tract infections, 2.5 vs. 16.7 episodes-‰ days of urinary catheter (p = .04). Intensive care unit, hospital, and 6-month survival were not different. Mean plasmatic glycemia was 149 ± 46 mg/dL in the alanine-glutamine dipeptide-supplemented total parenteral nutrition group and 155 ± 51 mg/dL in the control total parenteral nutrition group (p < .04), and mean hourly insulin dose was 4.3 ± 3.3 IU in the alanine-glutamine dipeptide-supplemented total parenteral nutrition group and 4.7 ± 3.7 IU in control total parenteral nutrition group (p < .001). Multivariate analysis showed a 54% reduction of the amount of insulin for the same levels of glycemia in the alanine-glutamine dipeptide-supplemented total parenteral nutrition group.

Conclusions.—Total parenteral nutrition supplemented with alanine-glutamine in intensive care unit patients is associated with a reduced rate of infectious complications and better glycemic control.

▶ This interesting study was conducted at multiple centers in a randomized, prospective, double-blinded fashion. It sought to determine the effects of total parenteral nutrition (TPN) supplemented with alanine-glutamine dipeptide compared with standard TPN in critically ill patients. The hypothesis was that the supplemented formula would improve nitrogen balance, increase the patient's immune function both directly and through the positive effects on the patient's intestinal function, and might reduce both intensive care unit complications and length of stay. The patients were appropriately stratified and randomized, and proper endpoints were measured.

As shown, the supplemented patients had fewer nosocomial pneumonias and urinary tract infections. Other endpoints were similar in outcomes between groups. Interestingly, the amount of insulin used in the supplemented group was significantly less in comparison with the control group to maintain the same level of glycemia. This is a very important study to help define the use of the alanine-glutamine dipeptide in this group of critically ill patients.

J. M. Daly, MD

Vitamin D Status in Relation to Glucose Metabolism and Type 2 Diabetes in Septuagenarians
Dalgård C, Petersen MS, Weihe P, et al (Univ of Southern Denmark, Odense, Denmark; Faroese Hosp System, Tórshavn, Denmark)
Diabetes Care 34:1284-1288, 2011

Objective.—Vitamin D deficiency is thought to be a risk factor for development of type 2 diabetes, and elderly subjects at northern latitudes may therefore be at particular risk.

Research Design and Methods.—Vitamin D status was assessed from serum concentrations of 25-hydroxyvitamin D_3 [25(OH)D_3] in 668 Faroese residents aged 70–74 years (64% of eligible population). We determined type 2 diabetes prevalence from past medical histories, fasting plasma concentrations of glucose, and/or glycosylated hemoglobin (HbA$_{1c}$).

Results.—We observed 70 (11%) new type 2 diabetic subjects, whereas 88 (13%) were previously diagnosed. Having vitamin D status < 50 nmol/L doubled the risk of newly diagnosed type 2 diabetes after adjustment for BMI, sex, exposure to polychlorinated biphenyls, serum triacylglyceride concentration, serum HDL concentration, smoking status, and month of blood sampling. Furthermore, the HbA$_{1c}$ concentration decreased at higher serum 25(OH)D_3 concentrations independent of covariates.

Conclusions.—In elderly subjects, vitamin D sufficiency may provide protection against type 2 diabetes. Because the study is cross-sectional, intervention studies are needed to elucidate whether vitamin D could be used to prevent development of type 2 diabetes.

▶ An association has been drawn previously between serum concentrations of vitamin D and the occurrence of type 2 diabetes. It is unclear as to the mechanisms involved. It is possible that vitamin D has a direct effect on beta cells enhancing insulin production or may have an effect on insulin resistance. Nevertheless, vitamin D deficiency has been suggested to be correlated with the development of type 2 diabetes.

This interesting report investigated circulating vitamin D levels in elderly patients between the ages of 70 and 74 on Faroe Island. A total of 668 patients were studied. As noted, 70 patients were newly diagnosed with type 2 diabetes. When vitamin D levels were less than 50 nmol/L, the risk of newly diagnosed type 2 diabetes doubled even after adjusting for body mass index, gender, and other factors. The study is also interesting in that the cohort examined represented more than 60% of the population of Faroe Island. While this island lies midway between Norway and Iceland in the northern latitude, the population has prolonged exposure to the sun during the summer months but much less during the winter months. Thus, one wonders whether time of the year has an influence on the incidence of type 2 diabetes as reflective of circulating vitamin D level. Results of the study also suggest that elderly patients are at substantial risk for the development of vitamin D deficiency and should have such levels measured routinely. Proof of concept will require intervention in this population by administration of vitamin D to prevent the development of type 2 diabetes.

J. M. Daly, MD

9 Gastrointestinal

A Stepwise Approach and Early Clinical Experience in Peroral Endoscopic Myotomy for the Treatment of Achalasia and Esophageal Motility Disorders

Swanström LL, Rieder E, Dunst CM (The Oregon Clinic, Portland; Legacy Health System, Portland, OR)
J Am Coll Surg 213:751-756, 2011

Background.—Peroral endoscopic myotomy (POEM) has recently been described in humans as a treatment for achalasia. This concept has evolved from developments in natural orifice translumenal endoscopic surgery (NOTES) and has the potential to become an important therapeutic option. We describe our approach as well as our initial clinical experience as part of an ongoing study treating achalasia patients with POEM.

Study Design.—Five patients (mean age 64 ± 11 years) with esophageal motility disorders were enrolled in an IRB-approved study and underwent POEM. This completely endoscopic procedure involved a midesophageal mucosal incision, a submucosal tunnel onto the gastric cardia, and selective division of the circular and sling fibers at the lower esophageal sphincter. The mucosal entry was closed by conventional hemostatic clips. All patients had postoperative esophagograms before discharge and initial clinical follow-up 2 weeks postoperatively.

Results.—All (5 of 5) patients successfully underwent POEM treatment, and the myotomy had a median length of 7 cm (range 6 to 12 cm). After the procedure, smooth passage of the endoscope through the gastroesophageal junction was observed in all patients. Operative time ranged from 120 to 240 minutes. No leaks were detected in the swallow studies and mean length of stay was 1.2 ± 0.4 days. No clinical complications were observed, and at the initial follow-up, all patients reported dysphagia relief without reflux symptoms.

Conclusions.—Our initial experience with the POEM procedure demonstrates its operative safety, and early clinical results have shown good results. Although further evaluation and long-term data are mandatory, POEM could become the treatment of choice for symptomatic achalasia.

▶ Swanström et al provide early results of an innovative endoscopic technique for division of the esophageal circular muscle fibers for the treatment of achalasia and esophageal motility disorders. This endoscopic approach is an outgrowth of the research of natural orifice translumenal endoscopic surgery and provides preliminary evidence that endoscopic procedures may be efficacious and should be in the realm of surgeons. Undoubtedly, this work shows that surgical training programs must include an in-depth experience in endo-scopic procedures, including diagnostic and therapeutic maneuvers. Several gastrointestinal medical organizations (American Gastroenterological Associa-tion, American Association for the Study of Liver Diseases, American Society for Gastrointestinal Endoscopy, and American College of Gastroenterology) issued a position paper that was critical of the endoscopic training requirements of surgeons. While the position paper did not reflect the substance of the American Board of Surgery's position on endoscopic training, it is clear that surgeons must be facile with the endoscope. Indeed, this article shows that surgeons are leaders in the field of endoscopic procedures and, furthermore, we must be adept at delivering this surgical care since many potential compli-cations may require a surgical solution. This work nicely outlines a stepwise approach to this operation, and the authors should be credited for their logical approach and for advancing surgical endoscopy.

K. E. Behrns, MD

Atypical Variants of Classic Achalasia Are Common and Currently Under-Recognized: A Study of Prevalence and Clinical Features

Galey KM, Wilshire CL, Niebisch S, et al (Univ of Rochester Med Ctr, NY)
J Am Coll Surg 213:155-163, 2011

Background.—Advances in esophageal manometry have facilitated iden-tification of variants of achalasia, suggesting they are more common than previously thought. This study assesses the frequency and clinical charac-teristics of patients with motility abnormalities similar to, but not meeting criteria for, classic achalasia.

Study Design.—Records of patients undergoing high-resolution esopha-geal manometry between January 2008 and January 2010 were screened for diagnosis of achalasia, impaired lower esophageal sphincter (LES) relax-ation, or severe peristaltic dysfunction of the esophageal body. Forty-four patients with classic achalasia and 31 with variant characteristics were iden-tified. Clinical and manometric characteristics were recorded and compared.

Results.—Variant achalasia was almost as common as the classic type (31 versus 44 patients). Eighty-two percent (36 of 44) of those with classic and 48% (15 of 31) of those with variant characteristics had dysphagia. Classic achalasia patients' mean age was 62 years (SD 19 years) versus 53 years (SD 14 years) in the variant group. The classic achalasia group had 26 male patients and 18 female patients and the variant group had 9 male patients and 22 female patients. Two thirds (21 of 31) of the variant group had impaired LES relaxation. Three variant patterns emerged: impaired LES relaxation with normal/hypertensive peristalsis (n = 10), impaired/borderline LES relaxation with mixed peristalsis/simultaneous contractions (n = 14), and impaired/normal LES and aperistalsis with occasional short segment peristalsis (n = 7). Mean intrabolus pressure was 16.3 mmHg in variant patients with normal LES relaxation and 23.1 mmHg in those with impaired relaxation.

TABLE 4.—Manometric Classification of Types of Variant Achalasia (n = 31)

Characteristic	I	Type II	III
Lower esophageal sphincter			
n	10	14	7
Mean age, y	52	52	58
4 s IRP, mmHg (<14.7 mmHg)	23.3	19.8	12.2
Resting pressure (<48 mmHg)	58.4	38.3	28.5
IBP, mmHg (<17 mmHg)	21.8	22.1	16.2
Esophageal body (swallow characteristics)			
Spastic	0.4	5.6	1.7
Segmentally spastic	0.4	1.3	0.1
Failed	0.1	0.4	1.4
Hypotensive	0.1	0.1	3.9
Hypertensive	4.0	1.1	0.0
Normal	5.0	1.5	2.9
Increased IBP ≥ 17 mmHg	7.2	6.0	4.0
Multiple peaks	1.0	2.7	0.9
DEA	162	159	46
DCI	4735	4518	498

Swallows represent average number of swallows out of ten with each characteristic.
DCI, distal contractile integral; DEA, distal esophageal amplitude; IBP, intrabolus pressure.

Conclusions.—Variants of achalasia are more common than previously recognized. LES dysfunction defined by high relaxation pressure occurs in two-thirds of variant achalasia patients and might be a hallmark that could direct therapy. The notion that esophageal body dysfunction/aperistalsis in achalasia is all or none should be reconsidered (Table 4).

▶ Galey et al conducted an important study examining esophageal motility using state-of-the-art high-resolution esophageal manometry to characterize motility features of classic and variant achalasia. In a short span of 2 years, the authors identified 44 patients with classic achalasia and 31 patients with variant achalasia. Patients with variant achalasia either had a near-normal or abnormal lower esophageal relaxation either alone or in combination with disordered esophageal motility. The authors identified 3 groups of variant achalasia defined by manometric findings. Although these findings are important and incrementally move the study of variant achalasia forward, the manometric features remain quite heterogeneous. As seen in Table 4, the esophageal body manometric features of variant achalasia are characterized by multiple motor patterns. Obviously, these diverse findings make accurate diagnosis and treatment difficult. Wisely, the authors performed surgery infrequently with good results; however, a note of caution, functional gastrointestinal diseases may be difficult to accurately diagnose, and surgical treatment should be used in select cases.

K. E. Behrns, MD

Pneumatic Dilation versus Laparoscopic Heller's Myotomy for Idiopathic Achalasia

Boeckxstaens GE, for the European Achalasia Trial Investigators (Academic Med Ctr, Amsterdam, The Netherlands; et al)
N Engl J Med 364:1807-1816, 2011

Background.—Many experts consider laparoscopic Heller's myotomy (LHM) to be superior to pneumatic dilation for the treatment of achalasia, and LHM is increasingly considered to be the treatment of choice for this disorder.

Methods.—We randomly assigned patients with newly diagnosed achalasia to pneumatic dilation or LHM with Dor's fundoplication. Symptoms, including weight loss, dysphagia, retrosternal pain, and regurgitation, were assessed with the use of the Eckardt score (which ranges from 0 to 12, with higher scores indicating more pronounced symptoms). The primary outcome was therapeutic success (a drop in the Eckardt score to ≤3) at the yearly follow-up assessment. The secondary outcomes included the need for retreatment, pressure at the lower esophageal sphincter, esophageal emptying on a timed barium esophagogram, quality of life, and the rate of complications.

Results.—A total of 201 patients were randomly assigned to pneumatic dilation (95 patients) or LHM (106). The mean follow-up time was 43 months (95% confidence interval [CI], 40 to 47). In an intention-to-treat analysis, there was no significant difference between the two groups in the primary outcome; the rate of therapeutic success with pneumatic dilation was 90% after 1 year of follow-up and 86% after 2 years, as compared with a rate with LHM of 93% after 1 year and 90% after 2 years (P=0.46). After 2 years of follow-up, there was no significant between-group difference in the pressure at the lower esophageal sphincter (LHM, 10 mm Hg [95% CI, 8.7 to 12]; pneumatic dilation, 12 mm Hg [95% CI, 9.7 to 14]; P=0.27); esophageal emptying, as assessed by the height of barium-contrast column (LHM, 1.9 cm [95% CI, 0 to 6.8]; pneumatic dilation, 3.7 cm [95% CI, 0 to 8.8]; P=0.21); or quality of life. Similar results were obtained in the per-protocol analysis. Perforation of the esophagus occurred in 4% of the patients during pneumatic dilation, whereas mucosal tears occurred in 12% during LHM. Abnormal exposure to esophageal acid was observed in 15% and 23% of the patients in the pneumatic-dilation and LHM groups, respectively (P=0.28).

Conclusions.—After 2 years of follow-up, LHM, as compared with pneumatic dilation, was not associated with superior rates of therapeutic success. (European Achalasia Trial Netherlands Trial Register number, NTR37, and Current Controlled Trials number, ISRCTN56304564.)

▶ Boeckxstaens et al published a randomized, multicenter clinical trial comparing the outcomes of laparoscopic esophageal myotomy with endoscopic balloon dilation. This study was performed across 14 medical centers in 5 European countries. The findings demonstrate that laparoscopic myotomy and pneumatic dilation have similar outcomes with regard to control of symptoms from achalasia. This conclusion differs significantly from standard treatment that generally recognizes laparoscopic myotomy as the preferred treatment. Certainly, the data from the article demonstrate no difference in the primary outcome and few, if any, differences in secondary outcomes. However, the definition of treatment failure in the pneumatic dilation group may not be universally accepted. Patients were allowed to have 3 successive dilatations months apart for control of symptoms. Furthermore, the initial protocol for pneumatic dilation resulted in a 31% perforation rate, and these patients were excluded from the study. Of the remaining 95 patients, 4 had no response to the initial therapy, and 23 patients had recurrent symptoms with only 17 of these patients choosing repeat dilation. The redilation data, included in the supplementary appendix, clearly show a progressive failure rate out to 40 months, with some patients needing dilation between 40 and 60 months. Laparoscopic esophageal myotomy certainly had a failure rate as well, but it appears that generally the operation either worked initially or it did not. Although the authors contend that the study protocol to achieve success is internationally accepted and widely used by treating clinicians, their initial protocol was a failure and resulted in an extraordinarily high perforation rate. These data suggest that a well-accepted dilation protocol does not exist, and that some trial and error was introduced at the start of this study. Furthermore, the perforations led to a modification of the protocol. The definition of success may have resulted in pneumatic dilation equivalency with laparoscopic myotomy, but would our patients call the requirement of multiple treatments a success?

K. E. Behrns, MD

Incidence of Adenocarcinoma among Patients with Barrett's Esophagus
Hvid-Jensen F, Pedersen L, Drewes AM, et al (Aarhus Univ Hosp, Denmark; Aarhus Univ Hosp, Aalborg, Denmark; et al)
N Engl J Med 365:1375-1383, 2011

Background.—Accurate population-based data are needed on the incidence of esophageal adenocarcinoma and high-grade dysplasia among patients with Barrett's esophagus.

Methods.—We conducted a nationwide, population-based, cohort study involving all patients with Barrett's esophagus in Denmark during the period from 1992 through 2009, using data from the Danish Pathology Registry and the Danish Cancer Registry. We determined the incidence rates (numbers of cases per 1000 person-years) of adenocarcinoma and high-grade dysplasia. As a measure of relative risk, standardized incidence ratios were calculated with the use of national cancer rates in Denmark during the study period.

Results.—We identified 11,028 patients with Barrett's esophagus and analyzed their data for a median of 5.2 years. Within the first year after the index endoscopy, 131 new cases of adenocarcinoma were diagnosed. During subsequent years, 66 new adenocarcinomas were detected, yielding an incidence rate for adenocarcinoma of 1.2 cases per 1000 person-years

(95% confidence interval [CI], 0.9 to 1.5). As compared with the risk in the general population, the relative risk of adenocarcinoma among patients with Barrett's esophagus was 11.3 (95% CI, 8.8 to 14.4). The annual risk of esophageal adenocarcinoma was 0.12% (95% CI, 0.09 to 0.15). Detection of low-grade dysplasia on the index endoscopy was associated with an incidence rate for adenocarcinoma of 5.1 cases per 1000 person-years. In contrast, the incidence rate among patients without dysplasia was 1.0 case per 1000 person-years. Risk estimates for patients with high-grade dysplasia were slightly higher.

Conclusions.—Barrett's esophagus is a strong risk factor for esophageal adenocarcinoma, but the absolute annual risk, 0.12%, is much lower than the assumed risk of 0.5%, which is the basis for current surveillance guidelines. Data from the current study call into question the rationale for ongoing surveillance in patients who have Barrett's esophagus without dysplasia. (Funded by the Clinical Institute, University of Aarhus, Aarhus, Denmark.) (Fig 1).

▶ Hvid-Jensen et al performed an important population-based study in Denmark to determine the incidence of development of adenocarcinoma of the esophagus in patients with Barrett esophagus. This is a much-needed study because of the varied reports on the incidence of adenocarcinoma and the screening programs

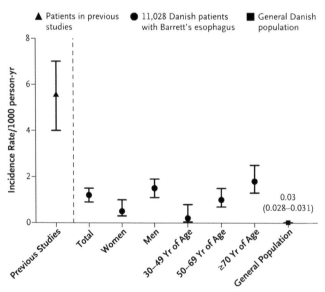

FIGURE 1.—Incidence Rates of Esophageal Adenocarcinoma. Incidence rates of esophageal adenocarcinoma are shown in a cohort of 11,028 Danish patients with Barrett's esophagus, as compared with mean incidence rates in the Danish general population and with mean incidence rates from previous international studies.[9,17,24,25] I bars indicate 95% confidence intervals. *Editor's Note*: Please refer to original journal article for full references. (Reprinted from Hvid-Jensen F, Pedersen L, Drewes AM, et al. Incidence of adenocarcinoma among patients with Barrett's esophagus. *N Engl J Med.* 2011;365:1375-1383. © 2011 Massachusetts Medical Society.)

developed on the existing data. Overall, most studies would suggest that the incidence was approximately 0.5% per year, but this carefully performed work suggests that the incidence is much lower at 0.12% per year—a more than 4-fold difference (Fig 1). In addition, the authors note that the incidence of adenocarcinoma in patients with Barrett esophagus but without dysplasia is negligible, and therefore, screening programs in these patients are likely not worthwhile. Because of the increasing incidence of esophageal adenocarcinoma overall, there is the perception that the outcome of the disease can be impacted markedly by screening programs focused on early identification of adenocarcinoma in the setting of Barrett esophagus. However, a key piece of data in this study shows that only 7.6% of all esophageal adenocarcinomas were associated with known Barrett esophagus. Population-based studies such as this are crucially important and must be conducted assiduously since we base screening decisions on such studies. As surgeons, we need to remember that most cases of esophageal adenocarcinoma do not arise in Barrett esophagus, and thus, we must carefully evaluate patients with symptoms of esophageal disease.

K. E. Behrns, MD

Risk Factors for Progression of Low-Grade Dysplasia in Patients With Barrett's Esophagus

Wani S, Falk GW, Post J, et al (Veterans Affairs Med Ctr and Univ of Kansas School of Medicine, MO; Cleveland Clinic, OH; et al)
Gastroenterology 141:1179-1186, 2011

Background & Aims.—Data vary on the progression of low-grade dysplasia (LGD) in patients with Barrett's esophagus (BE); in patients with LGD, we investigated the incidence of high-grade dysplasia (HGD) and esophageal adenocarcinoma (EAC) and compared progression in patients with different forms of LGD (prevalent vs incident and multifocal vs unifocal). We assessed the effects of consensus diagnosis of LGD on progression rates to HGD and EAC among expert pathologists.

Methods.—In a multicenter outcomes project, 210 patients with BE and LGD (classified as incident, prevalent, or persistent) were included. Patients were followed up for an average of 6.2 years (959.6 patient-years). Persistent LGD was defined as detection of LGD on ≥2 consecutive occasions during the follow-up period and extent as either unifocal (LGD at one level of BE segment) or multifocal (>1 level). Histology specimens were reviewed by 2 blinded pathologists.

Results.—Six patients developed EAC (incidence of 0.44%/year), and 21 developed HGD (incidence of 1.6%/year). The incidence of the combination of HGD and EAC was 1.83%/year. There were no associations between presence of prevalent, incident, or persistent LGD and the extent of LGD with progression rates. Based on consensus diagnosis of 88 reviewed specimens, there was no difference in the progression of LGD to either EAC (the incidence based on analyses by the local pathologist was 0.18%/year, the incidence when there was agreement between the local and one central pathologist was 0.21%/year, and the incidence when all 3 pathologists were in agreement was 0.39%/year) or combined HGD and EAC (0.94%/year, 0.87%/year, and 0.84%/year, respectively).

Conclusions.—Overall, patients with BE and LGD have a low annual incidence of EAC, similar to nondysplastic BE. There are no risk factors for progression and there is significant interobserver variation in diagnosis, even among expert pathologists.

▶ Wani et al performed a multi-institutional investigation of the risk of progression of low-grade dysplasia in patients with Barrett esophagus. Although high-grade dysplasia is a readily identified risk factor for the development of esophageal adenocarcinoma, the finding of low-grade dysplasia has not been definitively identified as a risk factor for progression to either high-grade dysplasia or esophageal adenocarcinoma. Therefore, clinicians frequently face the quandary of what to do with patients who have newly diagnosed low-grade dysplasia. Should the patients have ablative therapy of esophageal mucosa? Is a fundoplication warranted in these patients? In 2264 patients, the incidence of high-grade dysplasia, esophageal adenocarcinoma or combined high-grade dysplasia/esophageal adenocarcinoma after a diagnosis of low-grade dysplasia was 1.6%, 0.44%, and 1.83%, respectively. The shortest time to development of any of these findings was 2.86 years. At 5 years, more than 97% of patients were cancer free. Importantly, this study also investigated the interobserver error between 2 expert gastrointestinal pathologists when examining histopathologic slides for low-grade dysplasia. Surprisingly, these experts agreed on the diagnosis of low-grade dysplasia in only 55.6% of the cases. What do these data tell us? First, as treating clinicians, we should not offer interventional procedures, such as ablative therapy or fundoplication, for low-grade dysplasia. Second, we should realize that the diagnosis of low-grade dysplasia may be incorrect. Finally, surveillance endoscopy should not occur more frequently than every 2 years. Obviously, the diagnosis of low-grade dysplasia does not reliably help clinical decision making, and other biomarkers are needed to better risk stratify these patients.

K. E. Behrns, MD

Association of *Helicobacter pylori* Infection With Reduced Risk for Esophageal Cancer Is Independent of Environmental and Genetic Modifiers
Whiteman DC, for the Australian Cancer Study (Queensland Inst of Med Res, Brisbane, Australia)
Gastroenterology 139:73-83, 2010

Background & Aims.—Infection with *Helicobacter pylori* is associated with reduced risk of esophageal adenocarcinoma (EAC), but it is not clear whether this reduction is modified by genotype, other host characteristics, or environmental factors. Furthermore, little is known about the association between *H pylori* and adenocarcinomas of the esophagogastric junction (EGJAC) or squamous cell carcinomas (ESCC). We sought to measure the association between *H pylori* infection and esophageal cancer and identify potential modifiers.

Methods.—In an Australian, population-based, case-control study, we compared the prevalence of *H pylori* seropositivity and single nucleotide polymorphisms in interleukin (IL)-*1B (−31, −511)* and tumor necrosis factor *(TNF)-α (−308, −238)* among 260 EAC, 298 EGJAC, and 208 ESCC patients and 1346 controls. To estimate relative risks, we calculated odds ratios (OR) and 95% confidence intervals (CI) using multivariable logistic regression in the entire sample and within strata of phenotypic and genotypic risk factors.

Results.—*H pylori* infection was associated with significantly reduced risks of EAC (OR, 0.45; 95% CI: 0.30−0.67) and EGJAC (OR, 0.41; 95% CI: 0.27−0.60) but not ESCC (OR, 1.04; 95% CI: 0.71−1.50). For each cancer subtype, risks were of similar magnitude across strata of reflux frequency and smoking status. We found no evidence that polymorphisms in *IL-1B* or *TNF-α* modified the association between *H pylori* and EAC or EGJAC.

Conclusions.—*H pylori* infection is inversely associated with risks of EAC and EGJAC (but not ESCC); the reduction in risk is similar across subgroups of potential modifiers.

▶ Whiteman et al conducted a retrospective study to determine the association between *Helicobacter pylori* infection and the development of esophageal carcinoma. They studied 3 groups of patients, those with esophageal adenocarcinoma, esophagogastric junction adenocarcinoma, and esophageal squamous cell carcinoma. In addition, they wished to determine the association of infection with the single nucleotide polymorphisms of the proinflammatory cytokines, IL-1B and TNF-α. The data demonstrate that both esophageal adenocarcinoma and esophagogastric junction adenocarcinoma are associated with a lower rate of *H pylori* infection than controls and that patients with squamous cell carcinoma of the esophagus have the same rate of infection as control subjects. No association with the proinflammatory cytokines was evident. Why is this study important? First, it demonstrates that unlike the positive association between *H pylori* infection and gastric adenocarcinoma, a completely different mechanism is in play with esophageal adenocarcinoma. Furthermore, although chronic gastric atrophy and an inflammatory state is implicated in the mechanistic development of gastric cancer, this exact mechanism does not appear to be operative in esophageal adenocarcinoma. Second, this study is an excellent example of the use of epidemiologic data in conjunction with genetic and molecular markers of inflammation and cancer. Even though the cytokine association did not pan out, the experimental design leads toward identifying patients either at risk or protected by single nucleotide polymorphisms. Thus, this study is a step in the direction toward personalized medicine in which patients with risk factors may be more readily identified and treated appropriately. In ensuing years, studies of this type will become more frequent as we further characterize risk factors for specific diseases.

K. E. Behrns, MD

Long-Term Health-Related Quality of Life for Disease-Free Esophageal Cancer Patients

Donohoe CL, McGillycuddy E, Reynolds JV (Trinity College Dublin/St James' Hosp, Ireland)
World J Surg 35:1853-1860, 2011

Background.—Health-related quality of life (HRQL) has been studied extensively during the first year following esophagectomy, but little is known about HRQL in long-term survivors. The aim of this study was to investigate HRQL in patients alive at least 1 year after surgical resection for esophageal cancer using validated European Organisation for Research and Treatment of Cancer (EORTC) quality of life (QOL) questionnaires (QLQ).

Methods.—Eligible patients, without known disease recurrence and at least 1 year after esophagectomy, were identified from a prospectively maintained database. Patients completed general (QLQ-C30) and esophageal cancer-specific (QLQ-OES18, OG25) questionnaires. A numeric score (0−100) was computed in each conceptual area and compared with validated cancer ($n = 1031$) and age-matched ($n = 7802$) healthy populations using two-tailed unpaired t-tests. A cohort of 80 patients had pretreatment scores recorded.

Results.—Altogether, 132 of 156 eligible patients (84%) completed the self-rated questionnaire, 105 (67.3%) were men, and the mean age was 62 years (range 29−84 years). The mean time since esophagectomy was 70.3 months (12−299 months). Global health status was significantly reduced at least 1 year after esophagectomy (mean ± SD score 48.4 ± 18.6) when compared with patients with esophageal cancer prior to treatment (55.6 ± 24.1) and the general population (71.2 ± 22.4) ($p < 0.0001$). In a prospective cohort of eighty patients, symptoms related to swallowing difficulty, reflux, pain, and coughing significantly decreased in the long term ($p < 0.0001$). The degree of subjective swallowing dysfunction was highly correlated with a poor QOL (Spearman's $\rho = 0.508$, $p < 0.01$).

Conclusions.—Global health status remains significantly reduced in long-term survivors after esophagectomy compared with population controls, and swallowing dysfunction is highly associated with this compromised QOL (Fig 2).

▶ Long-term follow-up of functional status after resection of gastrointestinal cancers is uncommon; therefore, management strategies to correct underlying defects are frequently not invoked. Donohoe et al used a validated quality-of-life scoring scale to determine the functional quality of life in patients who were at least 1 year removed from resection of esophageal cancer. The results showed that compared with control groups, patients undergoing esophageal resection had an overall decrease in functional outcome (Fig 2). Furthermore, the decreased overall function was associated with poor functional swallowing. So how can we use these data? Too frequently when we follow up with patients in the clinic, we do not directly address concerns related to functional

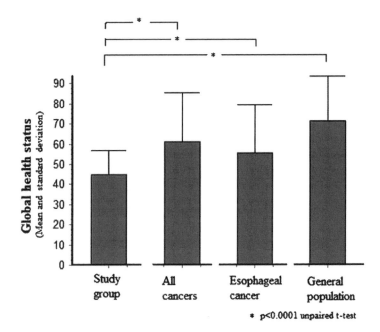

* p<0.0001 unpaired t-test

Global health status	n	Mean	SD	Median	IQR	p-value*
Study group	131	48.35	18.59	50	41.7-50	<0.0001
All cancer types	23553	61.2	24.1	66.7	50-83.3	<0.0001
Esophageal cancer	1031	55.6	24.1	50	41.7-75	<0.0001
General population	7802	71.2	22.4	75	58.3-83.3	<0.0001

*Unpaired t-test with Welch correction applied

FIGURE 2.—Global health status is significantly reduced compared to the reference groups. (With kind permission from Springer Science+Business Media: Donohoe CL, McGillycuddy E, Reynolds JV, Long-term health-related quality of life for disease-free esophageal cancer patients. *World J Surg.* 2011;35:1853-1860, with permission from Société Internationale de Chirurgie.)

outcomes of swallowing, change in bowel habits, etc. This study is an outstanding example of identifying specific, long-term, swallowing problems following esophageal resection. Perhaps, patients who undergo esophageal resection should have prolonged rehabilitation for swallowing difficulties, or patients who do not improve in the short-term (3-6 months) should be referred for rehabilitation. Undoubtedly, we should routinely perform long-term studies to determine how we may assist patients with a full and complete recovery.

K. E. Behrns, MD

Prognostic Significance of Baseline Positron Emission Tomography and Importance of Clinical Complete Response in Patients With Esophageal or Gastroesophageal Junction Cancer Treated With Definitive Chemoradiotherapy

Suzuki A, Xiao L, Hayashi Y, et al (The Univ of Texas MD Anderson Cancer Ctr, Houston)

Cancer 117:4823-4833, 2011

Background.—Metabolic imaging is of interest in esophageal cancer; however, the usefulness of initial standardized uptake value (SUV) in positron emission tomography (PET) is unknown in patients with esophageal or gastroesophageal carcinoma treated with definitive chemoradiotherapy. The authors hypothesized that initial SUV would correlate with patient outcome.

Methods.—The authors retrospectively analyzed esophageal or gastroesophageal carcinoma patients who had baseline PET and endoscopic ultrasonography in addition to other routine staging. All patients received definitive chemoradiotherapy. Multiple statistical methods were used.

Results.—The authors analyzed 209 consecutive esophageal or gastroesophageal carcinoma patients treated with definitive chemoradiation for outcome; of these, 180 had baseline PET for additional analyses. The median overall survival (OS) for all patients was 20.7 months (95% confidence interval, 18.8-26.3). Patients with clinical complete response (CR) lived longer than those with less than clinical CR ($P < .0001$). The median initial SUV was 12.7 (range, 0-51). Higher initial SUV was associated with longer tumors ($P = .0001$), higher T-stage status ($P < .0001$), positive N-stage status ($P = .0001$), higher overall stage ($P < .0001$), lack of clinical CR ($P = .0002$), and squamous cell histology ($P < .0001$). In the univariate analysis, initial SUV was associated with OS (Cox model, $P = .016$; log-rank test, $P = .002$). In the multivariate analysis, initial SUV dichotomized by the median value ($P = .024$) and tumor grade ($P = .016$) proved to be independent OS prognosticators. Median initial SUV for clinical CR patients was 10.2, compared with 15.3 for less than clinical CR patients ($P = .0058$).

Conclusions.—The data indicate that a higher initial SUV is associated with poorer OS in patients with esophageal or gastroesophageal carcinoma receiving definitive chemoradiation. Upon validation, baseline PET may become a useful stratification factor in randomized trials and for individualizing therapy.

▶ This article, along with its parent article[1] by the same group, examined the role of the initial positron emission tomography (PET) in the outcome of patients with esophageal or gastroesophageal cancer. The results of these 2 studies are interesting because the first study showed that patients with a higher standard uptake value (SUV) who underwent trimodal therapy (chemotherapy, radiotherapy, surgery) had a better outcome than patients with a lower SUV prior to treatment. However, this article demonstrates that patients with a higher initial SUV fared worse after undergoing bimodal therapy (chemoradiotherapy) than patients with a lower SUV. The reasons for the discrepancy of findings are not obvious, as the authors point out, and there are many issues with PET and the use of the SUV. However, those issues aside, it appears that surgical resection of these tumors changes the overall response, and this makes one wonder if the removal of the primary tumor environment (even in the absence of identifiable cancer cells) indeed limits the overall systemic tumor burden. Do cancer cells change the local environment such that even after the malignant cells are eradicated there remains a stroma with other surrounding cells that secrete systemic proliferative factors? An intriguing question that seems too far afield—but is it?

K. E. Behrns, MD

Reference

1. Javeri H, Xiao L, Rohren E, et al. Influence of the baseline 18F-fluoro-2-deoxy-D-glucose positron emission tomography results on survival and pathologic response in patients with gastroesophageal cancer undergoing chemoradiation. *Cancer.* 2009;115:624-630.

Surgical Resection for Locoregional Esophageal Cancer Is Underutilized in the United States

Dubecz A, Sepesi B, Salvador R, et al (Univ of Rochester School of Medicine and Dentistry, NY; et al)
J Am Coll Surg 211:754-761, 2010

Background.—Although esophagectomy provides the highest probability of cure in patients with esophageal cancer, many candidates are never referred for surgery. We hypothesized that esophagectomy for esophageal cancer is underused, and we assessed the prevalence of resection in national, state, and local cancer data registries.

Study Design.—Clinical stage, surgical and nonsurgical treatments, age, and race of patients with cancer of the esophagus were identified from the Surveillance, Epidemiology and End Results (SEER) registry (1988 to 2004), the Healthcare Association of NY State registry (HANYS 2007), and a single referral center (2000 to 2007). SEER identified a total of 25,306 patients with esophageal cancer (average age 65.0 years, male-to-female ratio 3:1). HANYS identified 1,012 cases of esophageal cancer (average age 67 years, M:F ratio 3:1); stage was not available from NY State registry data. A single referral center identified 385 patients (48 per year; average age 67 years, M:F 3:1). For SEER data, logistic regression was used to examine determinants of esophageal resection; variables tested included age, race, and gender.

Results.—Surgical exploration was performed in 29% of the total and only 44.2% of potentially resectable patients. Esophageal resection was performed in 44% of estimated cancer patients in NY State. By comparison, 64% of patients at a specialized referral center underwent surgical exploration, 96% of whom had resection. SEER resection rates for esophageal

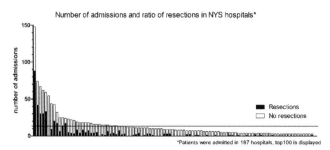

FIGURE 1.—Histogram of esophageal cancer admissions and resections in hospitals in New York State (NYS). Line annotates 13 admissions/year. Patients were admitted in 167 hospitals; top 100 are displayed. (Reprinted from the Journal of the American College of Surgeons, Dubecz A, Sepesi B, Salvador R, et al. Surgical resection for locoregional esophageal cancer is underutilized in the United States. *J Am Coll Surg.* 2010;211:754-761. Copyright 2010, with permission from the American College of Surgeons.)

cancer did not change between 1988 and 2004. Males were more likely to receive operative treatment. Nonwhites were less likely to undergo surgery than whites (odds ratio 0.45, $p < 0.001$).

Conclusions.—Surgical therapy for locoregional esophageal cancer is likely underused. Racial variations in esophagectomy are significant. Referral to specialized centers may result in an increase in patients considered for surgical therapy (Fig 1).

▶ Dubecz et al used the Survelliance, Epidemiology and End Results (SEER) registry, the Healthcare Association of New York State registry (HANY), and their institutional database to assess the use of surgery for esophageal cancer. They hypothesized that surgery was underused for the management of both squamous cell cancer and adenocarcinoma. The SEER and HANY databases provided similar data that suggest that surgical therapy occurs in 44% and 42% of patients, respectively. Furthermore, the survival data demonstrate a distinct benefit for surgical therapy. The univariate analysis showed that patients older than age 65 (and especially older than 80 years), women, and nonwhites were less likely to have surgical therapy. What are the reasons for this underuse of surgery for esophageal cancer? Fig 1 is particularly instructive because it clearly shows that the likelihood of surgery is correlated with the frequency with which a health care center encounters patients with esophageal cancer. Although smaller or rural hospitals may be able to diagnose esophageal cancer, the ability to treat it or to refer a patient for resection may be limited. Although a lack of understanding of the benefit of surgical therapy and persistent nihilism toward the disease may be invoked, dissemination of health care information is broad and ignorance is unlikely to be the major reason for underuse of esophageal resection. Likely, the persistent resistance to regionalization of care is foremost in the minds of referring physicians and medical centers. With intense economic pressure on all hospitals, and especially small hospitals that have limited ability to contract or alter programs, the enthusiasm for sending patients to tertiary centers is likely low. Furthermore, for a variety of reasons, once treated, these patients may not return to their referring physician or center. These referral patterns strongly argue for more transparency and open communication in the care of complex patients. Perhaps sharing medical information through an electronic medical record may transcend these barriers to open communication.

K. E. Behrns, MD

Biologic Prosthesis to Prevent Recurrence after Laparoscopic Paraesophageal Hernia Repair: Long-term Follow-up from a Multicenter, Prospective, Randomized Trial
Oelschlager BK, Pellegrini CA, Hunter JG, et al (Univ of Washington, Seattle; Oregon Health and Sciences Univ, Portland; et al)
J Am Coll Surg 213:461-468, 2011

Background.—In 2006, we reported results of a randomized trial of laparoscopic paraesophageal hernia repair (LPEHR), comparing primary diaphragm repair (PR) with primary repair buttressed with a biologic prosthesis (small intestinal submucosa [SIS]). The primary endpoint, radiologic hiatal hernia (HH) recurrence, was higher with PR (24%) than with SIS buttressed repair (9%) after 6 months. The second phase of this trial was designed to determine the long-term durability of biologic mesh-buttressed repair.

Methods.—We systematically searched for the 108 patients in phase I of this study to assess current clinical symptoms, quality of life (QOL) and determine ongoing durability of the repair by obtaining a follow-up upper gastrointestinal series (UGI) read by 2 radiologists blinded to treatment received. HH recurrence was defined as the greatest measured vertical height of stomach being at least 2 cm above the diaphragm.

Results.—At median follow-up of 58 months (range 42 to 78 mo), 10 patients had died, 26 patients were not found, 72 completed clinical follow-up (PR, n = 39; SIS, n = 33), and 60 repeated a UGI (PR, n = 34; SIS, n = 26). There were 20 patients (59%) with recurrent HH in the PR group and 14 patients (54%) with recurrent HH in the SIS group (p = 0.7). There was no statistically significant difference in relevant symptoms or QOL between patients undergoing PR and SIS buttressed repair. There were no strictures, erosions, dysphagia, or other complications related to the use of SIS mesh.

Conclusions.—LPEHR results in long and durable relief of symptoms and improvement in QOL with PR or SIS. There does not appear to be a higher rate of complications or side effects with biologic mesh, but its benefit in reducing HH recurrence diminishes at long-term follow-up (more than 5 years postoperatively) or earlier.

▶ The laparoscopic approach to paraesophageal hernia repair has benefited a substantial number of patients who otherwise would have undergone major open operations with large incisions through the chest cavity or an abdominal approach. However, the operation is troubled by an Achilles heel, recurrent paraesophageal hernia. Likely, the approach, laparoscopic versus open, would not make a difference in the high rate of hernia recurrence. However, Oelschlager et al have definitively shown that in long-term follow-up of laparoscopic para-esophageal hernia repair, recurrent hernias are surprisingly common (> 50% of patients) regardless of the method of closure—primary repair or biologic mesh-buttressed repair. Obviously, this trial emphasizes the importance of long-term follow-up because the initial published results resoundingly supported the use of a biologic buttress. However, the results also showed that even though many patients had a recurrent paraesophageal hernia, few were symptomatic, and the rare patient required reoperation. This study suggests that despite an excellent experimental design, the primary endpoint may have limited clinical relevance. How should we manage these patients with a recurrent paraesophageal hernia? Likely, no intervention is needed and, indeed, as the authors suggest, perhaps the use of biologic results in a delayed onset of recurrence with minimal symptoms. Nonetheless, is a 2-cm radiologic recurrence the best we can expect after a repair, or should we continue to pursue perfection even in the absence of significant symptoms? This is a difficult and costly question to answer and requires careful consideration in the era of comparative effectiveness research.

K. E. Behrns, MD

Evolving Management Strategies in Esophageal Perforation: Surgeons Using Nonoperative Techniques to Improve Outcomes
Kuppusamy MK, Hubka M, Felisky CD, et al (Virginia Mason Med Ctr, Seattle, WA)
J Am Coll Surg 213:164-172, 2011

Background.—Management of acute esophageal perforation continues to evolve. We hypothesized that treatment of these patients at a tertiary referral center is more important than beginning treatment within 24 hours, and that the evolving application of nonsurgical treatment techniques by surgeons would produce improved outcomes.

Study Design.—Demographics and outcomes of patients treated for esophageal perforation from 1989 to 2009 were recorded in an Institutional Review Board—approved database. Retrospective outcomes assessment was done for 5 separate time spans, including timing and type of treatment, length of stay (LOS), complications, and mortality.

Results.—Eighty-one consecutive patients presented with acute esophageal perforation. Their mean age was 64 years, and 55 patients (68%) had American Society of Anesthesiologists levels 3 to 5; 59% of the study population was referred from other hospitals; 48 patients (59%) were managed operatively, 33 (41%) nonoperatively, and 10 patients with hybrid approaches involving a combination of surgical and interventional techniques; 57 patients (70%) were treated <24 hours and 24 (30%) received treatment >24 hours after perforation. LOS was lower in the early-treatment group; however, there was no difference in complications or mortality. Nonoperative therapy increased from 0% to 75% over time. Nonsurgical therapy was more common in referred cases (48% vs 30%)

and in the >24 hours treatment group (46% vs 38%). Over the period of study, there were decreases in complications (50% to 33%) and LOS (18.5 to 8.5 days). Mortality for the entire series involved 3 patients (4%): 2 operative and 1 nonoperative.

Conclusions.—Results from our series indicate that referral to a tertiary care center is as important as treatment within 24 hours. An experienced surgical management team using a diversified approach, including selective application of nonoperative techniques, can expect to shorten LOS and limit complications and mortality (Fig 2).

▶ Kuppusamy et al report the results of patients treated for esophageal perforations from 1989 to 2009 with an increasing use of nonoperative therapies. The results demonstrate a remarkably low mortality rate of 4% with a decreased rate of complications and a lower length of stay (Fig 2). The authors also emphasize the finding that presentation to a high-volume referral 24 hours or later following a perforation need not be associated with a poor outcome. Furthermore, an experienced team of surgeons, gastroenterologists, and radiologists can effectively manage patients with delayed presentation of an esophageal perforation. However, this finding should not be confused with the notion that all patients with perforations greater than 24 hours will have an outcome equivalent to those patients who present within 24 hours. Likely, there is selection bias in those patients referred after 24 hours and the denominator (total number of

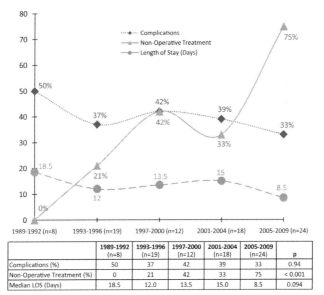

	1989-1992 (n=8)	1993-1996 (n=19)	1997-2000 (n=12)	2001-2004 (n=18)	2005-2009 (n=24)	p
Complications (%)	50	37	42	39	33	0.94
Non-Operative Treatment (%)	0	21	42	33	75	< 0.001
Median LOS (Days)	18.5	12.0	13.5	15.0	8.5	0.094

FIGURE 2.—Graphic description of management and complications over time. Nonoperative treatment has increased significantly, and complications and length of stay (LOS) have decreased, though not to a statistically significant degree. (Reprinted from Journal of American College of Surgeons, Kuppusamy MK, Hubka M, Felisky CD, et al. Evolving management strategies in esophageal perforation: surgeons using nonoperative techniques to improve outcomes. *J Am Coll Surg.* 2011;213:164-172. Copyright 2011, with permission from the American College of Surgeons.)

patients presenting to any institution after 24 hours) is unknown. Another major contribution of this group and the improved outcomes is the use of advances in endoscopic therapy, especially stenting. Placement of covered esophageal stents along with appropriate drainage has markedly altered the care of patients with esophageal perforations. A note of caution, however, is that these stents may migrate (27% in this series) and be associated with an uncontrolled, persistent leak. Therefore, these patients should be followed closely. This study is an excellent example of a team approach that has evolved over the years and resulted in markedly improved patient care.

K. E. Behrns, MD

Laparoscopic Repair of Paraesophageal Hernia: Long-term Follow-up Reveals Good Clinical Outcome Despite High Radiological Recurrence Rate

Dallemagne B, Kohnen L, Perretta S, et al (Univ Hosp of Strasbourg, IRCAD—EITS, France; Les Cliniques Saint-Joseph, Liege, Belgium)
Ann Surg 253:291-296, 2011

Objective.—The purpose of this report is to evaluate and compare the long-term objective and subjective outcome after laparoscopic paraesophageal hernia repair (LPHR).

Background.—Short-term symptomatic results of LPHR are often excellent. However, a high recurrence rate is detected at objective radiographic follow-up.

Methods.—Retrospective review of a prospectively gathered database of consecutive patients undergoing LPHR with and without reinforced crural repair at a single institution. Subjective and objective outcomes were assessed by using a structured symptoms questionnaire, Gastrointestinal Quality-of-Life Index, satisfaction score, and barium esophagogram.

Results.—From September 1991 to September 2005, LPHR was performed in 85 patients (median age, 66 years) with (25 patients) and without (60 patients) reinforced crural repair. Two patients (3%) underwent laparoscopic reoperation, for severe dysphagia and for symptomatic recurrence, respectively. Subjective outcome, available for 64 patients (75%), improved significantly at median follow-up of 118 months with a postoperative median Gastrointestinal Quality-of-Life Index score of 116. Radiographic recurrence (median follow-up, 99 months) occurred in 23 (66%) of the 35 patients, independently of age at operation, type of paresophageal hiatal hernias, and crural reinforcement, and showed no impact on quality of life.

Conclusions.—Although providing excellent symptomatic results, long-term objective evaluation of LPHR reveals a high recurrence rate even with reinforced cruroplasty. A tailored, lengthening gastroplasty and reinforced cruroplasty based on objective intraoperative evaluation, and not only on surgeon's personal judgment, may be the answer to recurrences.

▶ Dallemagne et al stoke the smoldering fire regarding the use of a laparoscopic approach to repair large, paraesophageal hernias. The issue at hand is the radiologic recurrence rate, which is high regardless of an open or laparoscopic approach; however, their data demonstrate that the 66% rate of recurrence is unacceptably high even though the patients had acceptable symptom relief. Early data suggested a high recurrence rate using the laparoscopic approach, and, therefore, the use of mesh to reinforce the crura was introduced. This buttress seemed to be associated with a decreased rate of recurrence; however, the findings in this article indicate that crural reinforcement was not associated with a lower rate of recurrence. These findings leave us scratching our heads about where to go to decrease the recurrence rate; however, even though crural reinforcement did not yield a lower rate of recurrence, Fig 2 in the original article clearly shows a trend for a lower recurrence rate with reinforced crura. Furthermore, only 14 of the 35 patients with long-term objective follow-up had a reinforced crural repair and only 6 of these 14 patients had mesh, whereas the remaining 8 patients had a pledgeted repair. Whether a pledgeted repair is similar to a mesh crural reinforcement will likely engender strong debate. These findings, however, raise the question of early repair of paraesophageal hernias, as elderly patients with markedly attenuated crura obviously do not fare well with the current approach. Should smaller paraesophageal hernias be repaired? Previous data would suggest that these hernias not be repaired, but are we setting patients and surgeons up for failure?

K. E. Behrns, MD

Systematic review and meta-analysis of laparoscopic Nissen fundoplication with or without division of the short gastric vessels

Markar SR, Karthikesalingam AP, Wagner OJ, et al (Univ College London Hosps NHS Foundation Trust, UK; Chelsea and Westminster NHS Foundation Trust, London, UK; Univ of California, San Diego; et al)
Br J Surg 98:1056-1062, 2011

Background.—The aim of this meta-analysis was to provide a pooled analysis of individual trials comparing clinical outcome following laparoscopic Nissen fundoplication with or without division of the short gastric vessels (SGVs).

Methods.—Primary outcome measures were the requirement for reoperation, and the presence of postoperative gastro-oesophageal reflux and postoperative dysphagia. Secondary outcome measures were duration of operation, length of hospital stay, postoperative complications (within 30 days of surgery), postoperative gas bloat syndrome, lower oesophageal sphincter resting pressure and DeMeester score. Pooled odds ratios were calculated for categorical outcomes, and weighted mean differences for secondary continuous outcomes, using random-effects models for meta-analysis.

Results.—Five randomized trials were included in the analysis. There was no statistically significant effect on the requirement for reoperation, or presence of postoperative dysphagia or reflux. SGV division was associated with a longer duration of operation and a reduced postoperative lower oesophageal sphincter pressure. There was no statistically significant difference in length of hospital stay, postoperative complications, postoperative gas bloat syndrome or DeMeester score.

Conclusion.—This meta-analysis has demonstrated that clinical outcome following laparoscopic Nissen fundoplication appears to be similar regardless of whether the short gastric vessels are divided. However, it is not possible to exclude many potentially important clinical differences and further studies are needed.

▶ Surgical treatment of gastroesophageal reflux disease has evolved significantly over the past several decades. During this time, Nissen fundoplication, or total fundoplication, has emerged as the operation of choice for many surgeons. However, some of the technical aspects of the operation remain controversial, especially division of the short gastric vessels. Many surgeons hypothesize division of the short gastric vessels results in a "floppy" fundoplication that permits a 360° volumetric wrap around the esophagus. Furthermore, surgeons opine that nondivided short gastric vessels tether the esophagogastric junction and may be associated with dysphagia. Several randomized trials have addressed outcomes of Nissen fundoplication with or without short gastric division; however, most of these studies are underpowered and do not provide a definitive conclusion. To further address the role of division of the short gastric vessels in Nissen fundoplication, Markar et al performed a meta-analysis of 5 trials. This study demonstrated essentially no difference in clinical outcomes in patients with or without division of the short gastric vessels with Nissen fundoplication. Although these findings may be helpful, as the authors point out, the reasons for these findings are not evident. Perhaps, however, surgeons have continued to evolve technical aspects such as fundic mobilization without division of the short gastric vessels and increased mobilization and, thus, length of the intra-abdominal esophagus. Because Nissen fundoplication is successful in more than 90% of patients, identifying significant technical features that are associated with gross outcome measures will likely be difficult. However, although the operation has an excellent outcome, it is associated with a number of disturbing side effects. Perhaps our investigative focus should be on relief of the side effects of an otherwise highly effective operation.

K. E. Behrns, MD

Bariatric Surgery and Long-term Cardiovascular Events

Sjöström L, Peltonen M, Jacobson P, et al (Univ of Gothenburg, Sweden; Natl Inst for Health and Welfare, Helsinki, Finland; et al)
JAMA 307:56-65, 2012

Context.—Obesity is a risk factor for cardiovascular events. Weight loss might protect against cardiovascular events, but solid evidence is lacking.

Objective.—To study the association between bariatric surgery, weight loss, and cardiovascular events.

Design, Setting, and Participants.—The Swedish Obese Subjects (SOS) study is an ongoing, nonrandomized, prospective, controlled study conducted at 25 public surgical departments and 480 primary health care centers in Sweden of 2010 obese participants who underwent bariatric surgery and 2037 contemporaneously matched obese controls who received usual care. Patients were recruited between September 1, 1987, and January 31, 2001. Date of analysis was December 31, 2009, with median follow-up of 14.7 years (range, 0-20 years). Inclusion criteria were age 37 to 60 years and a body mass index of at least 34 in men and at least 38 in women. Exclusion criteria were identical in surgery and control patients. Surgery patients underwent gastric bypass (13.2%), banding (18.7%), or vertical banded gastroplasty (68.1%), and controls received usual care in the Swedish primary health care system. Physical and biochemical examinations and database cross-checks were undertaken at preplanned intervals.

Main Outcome Measures.—The primary end point of the SOS study (total mortality) was published in 2007. Myocardial infarction and stroke were predefined secondary end points, considered separately and combined.

Results.—Bariatric surgery was associated with a reduced number of cardiovascular deaths (28 events among 2010 patients in the surgery group vs 49 events among 2037 patients in the control group; adjusted hazard ratio [HR], 0.47; 95% CI, 0.29-0.76; $P = .002$). The number of total first time (fatal or nonfatal) cardiovascular events (myocardial infarction or stroke, whichever came first) was lower in the surgery group (199 events among 2010 patients) than in the control group (234 events among 2037 patients; adjusted HR, 0.67; 95% CI, 0.54-0.83; $P < .001$).

Conclusion.—Compared with usual care, bariatric surgery was associated with reduced number of cardiovascular deaths and lower incidence of cardiovascular events in obese adults.

▶ The Swedish Obesity Subjects studies have made several important contributions to the literature of the effects of bariatric surgery on long-term diseases. In 2007, in a *New England Journal of Medicine* article, this group showed that bariatric surgery decreased long-term (nearly 11 years of follow-up) mortality. In addition, in a 2009 study published in *Lancet Oncology*, the group showed that bariatric surgery was associated with a decreased cancer incidence in obese women. In this study, Sjostrom et al found that bariatric surgery was associated with a decreased risk of fatal cardiovascular events and overall cardiovascular events. Although this study was not a randomized trial, it was well controlled, and the 2010 obese patients who underwent surgery were matched across 18 variables to the 2037 nonsurgical patients who were followed for up to 20 years. Notably, the bariatric surgery group included patients that underwent vertical banded gastroplasty (68.1%), gastric banding (18.7%), and gastric bypass (13.2%). Historically, vertical banded gastroplasty was associated with relatively low weight loss and long-term staple line dehiscence; therefore, it was abandoned in favor of gastric bypass. Thus, although the numbers of patients may be low, a subgroup analysis examining cardiovascular events in gastric bypass patients may be educational. It may also provide a clue about the importance of the amount of weight loss needed for a protective cardiovascular effect. Hopefully, the authors will continue this long term study because it permits long-term, longitudinal follow-up, which is exceedingly uncommon.

K. E. Behrns, MD

Fat malabsorption and increased intestinal oxalate absorption are common after roux-en-Y gastric bypass surgery
Kumar R, Lieske JC, Collazo-Clavell ML, et al (Mayo Clinic, Rochester, MN)
Surgery 149:654-661, 2011

Background.—Hyperoxaluria and increased calcium oxalate stone formation occur after Roux-en-Y gastric bypass (RYGB) surgery for morbid obesity. The etiology of this hyperoxaluria is unknown. We hypothesized that after bariatric surgery, intestinal hyperabsorption of oxalate contributes to increases in plasma oxalate and urinary calcium oxalate supersaturation.

Methods.—We prospectively examined oxalate metabolism in 11 morbidly obese subjects before and 6 and 12 months after RYGB ($n = 9$) and biliopancreatic diversion-duodenal switch (BPD-DS) ($n = 2$). We measured 24-hour urinary supersaturations for calcium oxalate, apatite, brushite, uric acid, and sodium urate; fasting plasma oxalate; 72-hour fecal fat; and increases in urine oxalate following an oral oxalate load.

Results.—Six and 12 months after RYGB, plasma oxalate and urine calcium oxalate supersaturation increased significantly compared with similar measurements obtained before surgery (all $P \leq .02$). Fecal fat excretion at 6 and 12 months was increased ($P = .026$ and .055, 0 vs 6 and 12 months). An increase in urine oxalate excretion after an oral dose of oxalate was observed at 6 and 12 months (all $P \leq .02$). Therefore, after bariatric surgery, increases in fecal fat excretion, urinary oxalate excretion after an oral oxalate load, plasma oxalate, and urinary calcium oxalate supersaturation values were observed.

Conclusion.—Enteric hyperoxaluria is often present in patients after the operations of RYGB and BPD-DS that utilize an element of intestinal malabsorption as a mechanism for weight loss.

▶ Kumar et al performed a clinical study of gastrointestinal and renal physiology by studying mechanisms of oxalate absorption in patients who underwent Roux-en-Y gastric bypass for morbid obesity. Patients were studied preoperatively and again 6 and 12 months postoperatively. The findings suggest that postoperative fat malabsorption leads to increased intraluminal binding of calcium to fat. As a consequence of this binding, less calcium is available to bind with oxalate. As a result, free oxalate enters the colon where it is absorbed and excreted into the urine. The increased oxalate in the urine results in a predisposition to oxalate nephrolithiasis. This study is a classic example of basic physiologic studies that were formerly a hallmark of clinical medicine. However, with decreased funding available to study human physiology, it is uncommon to see the type of elegant work presented here. In addition, this work highlights how to effectively enlist our patients in the study of important physiologic questions. We too infrequently ask our patients to participate in clinical studies that will lead to valuable clinical information and drive changes in treatment. Finally, the integrated nature of this study is refreshing because it involves surgeons, nephrologists, biochemists, endocrinologists, radiology, and biostatics.

K. E. Behrns, MD

Predicting Risk for Serious Complications With Bariatric Surgery: Results from the Michigan Bariatric Surgery Collaborative

Finks JF, for the Michigan Bariatric Surgery Collaborative, from the Center for Healthcare Outcomes and Policy (Univ of Michigan, Ann Arbor; et al)
Ann Surg 254:633-640, 2011

Objectives.—To develop a risk prediction model for serious complications after bariatric surgery.

Background.—Despite evidence for improved safety with bariatric surgery, serious complications remain a concern for patients, providers and payers. There is little population-level data on which risk factors can be used to identify patients at high risk for major morbidity.

Methods.—The Michigan Bariatric Surgery Collaborative is a statewide consortium of hospitals and surgeons, which maintains an externally-audited prospective clinical registry. We analyzed data from 25,469 patients undergoing bariatric surgery between June 2006 and December 2010. Significant risk factors on univariable analysis were entered into a multivariable logistic regression model to identify factors associated with serious complications (life threatening and/or associated with lasting disability) within 30 days of surgery. Bootstrap resampling was performed to obtain bias-corrected confidence intervals and c-statistic.

Results.—Overall, 644 patients (2.5%) experienced a serious complication. Significant risk factors ($P < 0.05$) included: prior VTE (odds ratio [OR] 1.90, confidence interval [CI] 1.41—2.54); mobility limitations (OR 1.61, CI 1.23—2.13); coronary artery disease (OR 1.53, CI 1.17—2.02); age over 50 (OR 1.38, CI 1.18—1.61); pulmonary disease (OR 1.37, CI 1.15—1.64); male gender (OR 1.26, CI 1.06—1.50); smoking history (OR 1.20, CI 1.02—1.40); and procedure type (reference lap band): duodenal switch (OR 9.68, CI 6.05—15.49); laparoscopic gastric bypass (OR 3.58, CI 2.79—4.64); open gastric bypass (OR 3.51, CI 2.38—5.22); sleeve gastrectomy (OR 2.46, CI 1.73—3.50). The c-statistic was 0.68 (bias-corrected to 0.66) and the model was well-calibrated across deciles of predicted risk.

Conclusions.—We have developed and validated a population-based risk scoring system for serious complications after bariatric surgery. We expect that this scoring system will improve the process of informed consent, facilitate the selection of procedures for high-risk patients, and allow for better risk stratification across studies of bariatric surgery.

▶ Since the publication of the Institute of Medicine reports "To Err Is Human: Building a Safer Health System" in 1999 and "Crossing the Quality Chasm: Building a New Health System for the 21st Century" in 2001, public interest in the quality of medicine has risen exponentially. The gap between the care delivered and the expected quality of care has given rise to multiple quality programs that are designed to continually improve outcomes. Nowhere is this more measurable than in surgery. The surgical community's response has been expansive and provided new depth to outcome measurements. One of the surgical community's responses has been pay for participation collaboratives such as the Michigan Bariatric Surgery Collaborative. This regional network collectively examines the results of bariatric surgery and implements continual improvements based on the outcomes. In this report, Finks et al identified risk factors for serious complications in patients undergoing bariatric surgery and provided results for the safest bariatric operations. The risk factors for serious complications included venous thromboembolism, lack of mobility, coronary artery disease, age under 50, pulmonary disease, male gender, smoking history, and procedure type. Not surprisingly, in descending order of risk, the operations were duodenal switch procedure, laparoscopic gastric bypass, open gastric bypass, sleeve gastrectomy, and laparoscopic band placement. Importantly, this work led to the generation of a risk calculator that may predict the chance of a serious complication. This collaborative effort to risk stratify an operation(s) based on patient factors represents a major advance in patient assessment. This risk stratification is possible because of the regional collaborative work by many surgeons such that a large number of patients can be examined collectively to enhance results. Clearly, more efforts toward this collaborative end are needed, especially in high-risk operations for benign conditions.

K. E. Behrns, MD

Extent of Gastric Resection Impacts Patient Quality of Life: The Dysfunction After Upper Gastrointestinal Surgery for Cancer (DAUGS32) Scoring System

Nakamura M, Hosoya Y, Yano M, et al (Jichi Med Univ, Shimotsuke, Tochigi, Japan; Osaka Med Ctr for Cancer and Cardiovascular Diseases, Osaka, Japan; et al)
Ann Surg Oncol 18:314-320, 2011

Background.—Quality of life is an important outcome measure in the care of patients with cancer. We developed a new scoring system specifically for the evaluation of patients with upper gastrointestinal cancer and postoperative gastrointestinal dysfunction. This study was undertaken to evaluate the scoring system's validity in comparing outcomes after gastric resection.

Materials and Methods.—Patients with gastric cancer, 3 months to 3 years postoperatively, were surveyed using the survey instrument. Postoperative dysfunction scores and the status of resuming activities of daily living were compared with the surgical procedure performed by analysis of variance and multiple-comparison techniques.

Results.—Of 211 patients surveyed, 165 (119 men, 46 women; mean age, 65.1 ± 10.5 years) responded. Procedures included distal gastrectomy in 100, total gastrectomy in 57, and pylorus-preserving gastrectomy in 8. The overall dysfunction score was 61.8 ± 15.5. The dysfunction score was 58.9 ± 15.0 after distal gastrectomy, 66.8 ± 14.1 after total gastrectomy, and 62.4 ± 21.6 after pylorus-preserving gastrectomy. These values differed significantly among the groups ($P = .007$). Dysfunction scores according to postoperative activity status were 49.1 ± 15.6 in 71 patients who resumed their activities, 56.9 ± 15.7 in 39 patients with reduced activities, 57.3 ± 8.8 in 15 patients with minimal activities, and 63.3 ± 11.8 ($P < .05$) in 16 patients who did not resume activities because of poor physical condition.

Conclusions.—This scoring system for postoperative gastrointestinal dysfunction provides an objective measure of dysfunction related to specific surgical procedures and correlates with activities of daily living in the postoperative period.

▶ Nakamura et al developed a scoring system to assess the quality of life after gastric and esophageal resection for malignancy. The scoring system demonstrated that the quality of life was correlated with the extent of gastric resection. Total gastrectomy was associated with a higher score and, thus, a greater degree of dysfunction than distal gastrectomy. Furthermore, the scoring system was closely associated with the ability to carry out activities of daily living. These findings are helpful in that patients can be thoroughly educated prior to gastric resection. However, the challenge will be to determine whether intervention can improve the quality of life and if this instrument will correlate with improved enteric function. This study is notable because there are virtually no published studies from North America that examine the quality of life after gastroesophageal resection. Although gastric resection is more common in Japan than in North America, patient-centered care in the United States and elsewhere should focus on the quality of life after surgical procedures. Collectively, the aim of the surgical community should be to assess quality of life after all operations and improve the quality of life of our patients.

K. E. Behrns, MD

Tumor Overgrowth After Expandable Metallic Stent Placement: Experience in 583 Patients With Malignant Gastroduodenal Obstruction
Jang JK, Song H-Y, Kim JH, et al (Univ of Ulsan College of Medicine, Seoul, Republic of Korea)
AJR Am J Roentgenol 196:W831-W836, 2011

Objective.—The objective of our study was to assess the incidence, predictive factors, and treatment of tumor overgrowth after placement

of expandable metallic dual stents in patients with malignant gastroduodenal obstruction.

Materials and Methods.—Expandable metallic dual stents were inserted
under fluoroscopic guidance in 583 patients with symptomatic malignant
gastroduodenal obstruction. We retrospectively reviewed prospectively
collected patient records to determine the incidence and treatment of
tumor overgrowth after stent placement and used multivariate analysis
to determine factors predicting tumor overgrowth.

Results.—Tumor overgrowth occurred after stent placement in 22 of 583
patients (3.8%) (range, 41−634 days; mean, 179.0 days). Duodenal lesions
(odds ratio [OR], 4.505; $p = 0.002$), longer survival time (OR, 1.003;
$p = 0.001$), and length of obstruction (OR, 0.783; $p = 0.035$) were independent predictors of tumor overgrowth. Twenty of the 22 patients were
successfully treated by placement of a second dual stent, whereas the
other two patients refused placement of a second stent or other further
treatment. Overall, 19 of 20 patients (95%) showed improvement in symptoms after second stent placement. Duodenal perforation occurred in one of
the 20 patients 125 days after placement of a second stent and was treated
surgically.

Conclusion.—Tumor overgrowth seems to be an uncommon complication of expandable metallic dual stent placement in patients with malignant
gastroduodenal obstruction. Tumor overgrowth is associated with duodenal
lesions, longer survival time, and shorter stricture length. Tumor overgrowth can be successfully managed by coaxial insertion of a second dual-
expandable metallic stent into the obstructed first stent.

▶ Malignant gastric outlet obstruction in patients with locoregional advanced
disease or metastatic disease from gastric, duodenal, or pancreatic cancers presents a management dilemma since these patients often have severely compromised health. Traditionally, surgical approaches to bypass the obstruction have
been used, but too frequently these operations are complicated by long hospital
stays and delayed gastric emptying. In the past several years, endoscopically or
fluoroscopically placed metal stents have been used to treat these obstructions.
However, stenting approaches have not been widely adopted for fear of perforation, stent migration, and tumor overgrowth resulting in recurrent obstruction.
Jang et al, however, have used this procedure frequently and report on 583
patients who were followed at 1-month intervals to assess stent patency.
Surprisingly, in this large series only 3.8% of patients developed recurrence
symptoms caused by tumor overgrowth. Twenty of the 22 recurrences were
treated with placement of a second coaxial stent with only 1 perforation in the
entire series. This perforation occurred after placement of a second stent.
These findings are noteworthy for several reasons. First, the series shows that
stenting can be sucessfully used in a large patient population. Importantly, the
recurrence rate is low, and the risk of perforation is exceedingly small. Finally,
these ill patients can resume a diet in a short period of time and do not need to
spend an inordinate amount of time hospitalized following an operation. The
data in this series should be confirmed in other centers, but certainly the authors

demonstrate the feasibility of this approach and the potential to decrease operative intervention in patients with advanced malignant gastric outlet obstruction.

K. E. Behrns, MD

FOLFIRINOX versus Gemcitabine for Metastatic Pancreatic Cancer

Conroy T, for the Groupe Tumeurs Digestives of Unicancer and the PRODIGE
Intergroup (Nancy Univ and Centre Alexis Vautrin, France; et al)
N Engl J Med 364:1817-1825, 2011

Background.—Data are lacking on the efficacy and safety of a combination chemotherapy regimen consisting of oxaliplatin, irinotecan, fluorouracil, and leucovorin (FOLFIRINOX) as compared with gemcitabine as
first-line therapy in patients with metastatic pancreatic cancer.

Methods.—We randomly assigned 342 patients with an Eastern Cooperative Oncology Group performance status score of 0 or 1 (on a scale of
0 to 5, with higher scores indicating a greater severity of illness) to receive
FOLFIRINOX (oxaliplatin, 85 mg per square meter of body-surface area;
irinotecan, 180 mg per square meter; leucovorin, 400 mg per square meter;
and fluorouracil, 400 mg per square meter given as a bolus followed by
2400 mg per square meter given as a 46-hour continuous infusion, every
2 weeks) or gemcitabine at a dose of 1000 mg per square meter weekly
for 7 of 8 weeks and then weekly for 3 of 4 weeks. Six months of chemotherapy were recommended in both groups in patients who had a response.
The primary end point was overall survival.

Results.—The median overall survival was 11.1 months in the FOLFIR-
INOX group as compared with 6.8 months in the gemcitabine group
(hazard ratio for death, 0.57; 95% confidence interval [CI], 0.45 to 0.73;
P<0.001). Median progression-free survival was 6.4 months in the FOLFIR-
INOX group and 3.3 months in the gemcitabine group (hazard ratio for
disease progression, 0.47; 95% CI, 0.37 to 0.59; P<0.001). The objective
response rate was 31.6% in the FOLFIRINOX group versus 9.4% in the
gemcitabine group (P<0.001). More adverse events were noted in the
FOLFIRINOX group; 5.4% of patients in this group had febrile neutropenia. At 6 months, 31% of the patients in the FOLFIRINOX group had
a definitive degradation of the quality of life versus 66% in the gemcitabine
group (hazard ratio, 0.47; 95% CI, 0.30 to 0.70; P<0.001).

Conclusions.—As compared with gemcitabine, FOLFIRINOX was
associated with a survival advantage and had increased toxicity. FOLFIR-
INOX is an option for the treatment of patients with metastatic pancreatic
cancer and good performance status. (Funded by the French government
and others; ClinicalTrials.gov number, NCT00112658.) (Fig 1A).

▶ Pancreatic adenocarcinoma continues to carry a dismal prognosis with a
5-year survival rate of 6%. Although aggressive, yet increasingly safe, operative
approaches for pancreatic cancer have occurred in the last few decades, improved
survival remains elusive. Obviously, surgery, alone or in combination with recent

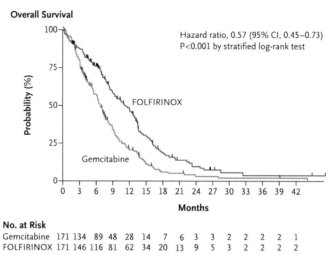

Overall Survival

Hazard ratio, 0.57 (95% CI, 0.45–0.73)
P<0.001 by stratified log-rank test

No. at Risk
Gemcitabine 171 134 89 48 28 14   7   6   3   3   2   2   2   2   1
FOLFIRINOX   171 146 116 81 62 34 20 13   9   5   3   2   2   2   2

FIGURE 1.—Kaplan–Meier Estimates of Overall Survival and Progression-free Survival, According to Treatment Group. Panel A shows overall survival; the median was 11.1 months in the group receiving FOLFIRINOX (oxaliplatin, irinotecan, fluorouracil, and leucovorin). (Reprinted from Conroy T, for the Groupe Tumeurs Digestives of Unicancer and the PRODIGE Intergroup. FOLFIRINOX versus gemcitabine for metastatic pancreatic cancer. N Engl J Med. 2011;364:1817-1825. © 2011 Massachusetts Medical Society.)

chemotherapeutic agents and radiotherapy, has not had any impact on disease progression; therefore, novel chemotherapeutic regimens are necessary. Conroy et al show the marked improvement in survival from metastatic pancreatic cancer in patients treated with oxaliplatin, irinotecan, leucovorin, and fluorouracil (FOL-FIRINOX) compared with gemcitabine. The median survival was increased 4.35 months to 11.15 months for patients treated with FOLFIRINOX, and the objective response rate was 31.6% for the FOLFIRINOX group compared with 9.4% for the gemcitabine-treated patients (Fig 1A). Not surprisingly, the FOLFIRINOX group experienced increased toxicity with neutropenia as the most common side effect. These findings represent a marked departure from multiple previous trials of chemotherapeutic studies that showed modest improvements in survival with new chemotherapeutic regimens. However, the impact of this study may not be immediately transferable to patients with localized pancreatic cancer who are candidates for resection. The role of FOLFIRINOX as an adjuvant regimen to resection will be pursued vigorously. Furthermore, careful studies with FOLFIRINOX as neoadjuvant therapy will be required because the toxicity of the regimen is noteworthy and could potentially limit the number of patients that go on to resection. However, the larger message is that a significant improvement in chemotherapy for pancreatic adenocarcinoma has been achieved, and these findings should lead to a number of studies that hopefully will finally improve the outcome in patients with pancreatic cancer.

K. E. Behrns, MD

Lack of significant liver enzyme elevation and gallstones and/or sludge on ultrasound on day 1 of acute pancreatitis is associated with recurrence after cholecystectomy: A population-based study

Trna J, Vege SS, Pribramska V, et al (Masaryk Univ, Brno, Czech Republic; Mayo Clinic, Rochester, MN)
Surgery 151:199-205, 2012

Background.—In a population-based study, we examined recurrence rates of acute pancreatitis (AP) after cholecystectomy performed to prevent recurrences of AP.

Methods.—We abstracted data from medical records of all Olmsted county residents who underwent cholecystectomy at Mayo Clinic for the management of presumed gallstone or idiopathic AP between 1990 and 2005 ($n = 239$). Based on (i) significantly elevated liver enzymes ($\geq$threefold increase of alanine aminotransferase or aspartate aminotransferase) on day 1 and (ii) the presence of gallstones/sludge in the gall bladder, we categorized patients into 4 groups: A (i + ii), B (i but not ii), C (ii but not i), and D (neither i nor ii). Recurrence rates of AP after cholecystectomy were determined in all groups.

Results.—The median follow-up after cholecystectomy was 99 months (range, 8−220). AP recurred in 13 of 142 patients (9%) in group A, 1 of 17 patients (6%) in group B, 13 of 57 patients (23%) in group C, and 14 of 23 patients (61%) in group D ($P < .0001$ D vs all other groups and $P = .001$ C vs groups A and B). No difference was seen in recurrence rates in groups A vs B ($P = 1.0$). Recurrences were more frequent in patients with normal liver enzymes (A + B vs C + D; $P = .000003$) and in patients without sonographic evidence of gallstones/sludge (A + C vs B + D; $P = .0008$).

Conclusion.—When AP is associated with significantly elevated liver enzymes on day 1, recurrence rates after cholecystectomy are low (9%). However, postcholecystectomy recurrence rates of AP are high in those without such laboratory abnormalities (34%), especially in those without gall bladder stones/sludge (61%) on abdominal ultrasonography. Our results raise doubts about the efficacy of cholecystectomy to prevent recurrent AP in patients with the absence of either a significant elevation of liver tests on day 1 of AP or gallstones and/or sludge in the gall bladder on initial ultrasound examination.

▶ Gallstone pancreatitis is a relatively common and straightforward diagnosis that is often readily managed by timely cholecystectomy in patients with edematous pancreatitis. However, on occasion, the etiology of acute pancreatitis is elusive and sometimes implied by the presence of increased concentrations of serum liver enzymes and/or the presence of gallstones on ultrasonography. This study by Trna et al considers the recurrence rate of acute pancreatitis in the presence or absence of increased liver enzymes on day 1 and gallstones. Not surprisingly, when the diagnosis of gallstone-induced pancreatitis is "soft" (without enzyme elevation and gallstones on ultrasonography), the recurrence rate of pancreatitis is high (61%). Clearly, these data suggest that a misdiagnosis of gallstone-induced pancreatitis occurs with some frequency in patients without enzyme elevation or gallstones, and a cholecystectomy, in this case, will present a high risk/benefit ratio. In addition, surgeons should be wary of the patients who have gallstones on ultrasonography but do not have increased liver enzymes on day 1 because the recurrence rate was 23%. When presented with these 2 scenarios, surgeons often proceed with cholecystectomy because the alternative is to assign the diagnosis of idiopathic pancreatitis and have few therapeutic options for the patient. The results of this study strongly suggest that further evaluation, especially immediately, during repeated attacks of pancreatitis is warranted. Patients should present to their physicians immediately when symptoms arise so liver enzymes can be tested to determine which patients may benefit from cholecystectomy. These data add a new dimension to our treatment of patients with gallstone-induced pancreatitis and suggest that continued refinement of management algorithms is useful.

K. E. Behrns, MD

Laparoendoscopic Rendezvous Versus Preoperative ERCP and Laparoscopic Cholecystectomy for the Management of Cholecysto-Choledocholithiasis: Interim Analysis of a Controlled Randomized Trial

Tzovaras G, Baloyiannis I, Zachari E, et al (Univ of Thessaly Med School, Larissa, Greece)

Ann Surg 255:435-439, 2012

Background.—Although the ideal management of cholecysto-choledo-choli-thiasis is controversial, the 2-stage approach [endoscopic retrograde cholangiopancreatography (ERCP), sphincterotomy, and common bile duct (CBD) clearance followed by laparoscopic cholecystectomy] remains the standard way of management worldwide. One-stage approach using the so-called laparoendoscopic rendezvous (LERV) technique offers some advantages, mainly by reducing the hospital stay and the risk of post-ERCP pancreatitis.

Objective.—To compare the LERV 1-stage approach with the standard 2-stage approach consisting of preoperative ERCP followed by laparoscopic cholecystectomy for the treatment of cholecysto-choledocholithiasis.

Setting.—Controlled randomized trial, University/Teaching Hospital.

Methods.—Patients with cholecysto-choledocholithiasis were randomized either to LERV or to the 2-stage approach. Both elective and emergency cases were included in the study. Primary endpoint was to detect difference in overall hospital stay, whereas secondary endpoints were (i) to detect differences in morbidity (especially post-ERCP pancreatitis) and (ii) success of CBD clearance. This is an interim analysis of the first 100 randomized patients.

Results.—Hospital stay was significantly shorter in the LERV group; median 4 (2−19) days versus 5.5 (3−22) days, $P = 0.0004$. There was no difference in morbidity and success of CBD clearance between the 2

TABLE 3.—Complications

	Group I	Group II
Bile leak	3	1
Cholangitis	2	1
Pulmonary emboli	0	1
Bleeding from sphincterotomy	0	1
Bleeding form drain site	1	0
Collection/biloma	0	1
Wound infection	0	1
Urinary retention (UTI)	1	0

groups. Post-ERCP amylase value was found significantly lower in the LERV group: median 65 (16–1159) versus 91 (30–1846), $P = 0.02$.

Conclusions.—Interim analysis of the results suggests the superiority of the LERV technique in terms of hospital stay and post-ERCP hyperamylasemia (Table 3).

▶ Tzovaras et al conducted a randomized trial of a single-stage laparoscopic-endoscopic procedure compared with the standard 2-stage procedure (endoscopic retrograde cholangiopancreatography followed by laparoscopic cholecystectomy) in patients with suspected choledocholithiasis. The authors hypothesized that this approach would decrease the hospital length of stay (as the primary endpoint) and, presumably, the cost of the procedure. The results showed that the length of stay was indeed decreased in the group of patients undergoing the rendezvous procedure (5.5 days vs 4 days). Costs were not determined in this study. However, the length of stay in both groups of patients appears relatively long. The rendezvous procedure or each individual procedure of the 2-stage approach should be outpatient procedures and thus require no postprocedure hospital stay. Understandably, the diagnosis of choledocholithiasis may require 36 to 48 hours to fully establish, but certainly a major cost savings opportunity appears to exist in both arms of the trial. Importantly, even though a statistical difference between the rate of death and complications was not evident between the groups, the rendezvous group of patients did include a single patient that died versus none in the control group. Furthermore, although the number of complications did not differ (Table 3), 5 significant complications did occur in the rendezvous group. Therefore, the safety of this approach should be scrutinized in follow-up studies because bile leaks and cholangitis may lead to death or permanent disability. Although this article nicely addresses a standardized approach to a single-stage procedure for choledocholithiasis and the results support its use, we should continue to study these patients for unintended consequences and look for further opportunities in efficient delivery of care.

K. E. Behrns, MD

Endoscopic Retrograde Cholangiopancreatography Prior to Laparoscopic Cholecystectomy: A Common and Potentially Hazardous Technique That Can Be Avoided

Alkhaffaf B, Parkin E, Flook D (The Royal Oldham Hosp, England)
Arch Surg 146:329-333, 2011

Objective.—To establish the extent to which preoperative endoscopic retrograde cholangiopancreatography (ERCP) is practiced by a representative group of surgeons in the United Kingdom, and to determine its safety and efficacy when compared with a policy of routine intraoperative cholangiography (RIOC), without preoperative ERCP, employed by a single surgical unit.

Design.—Comparison study between patients undergoing laparoscopic cholecystectomy and patients undergoing laparoscopic cholecystectomy with RIOC.

Setting.—Four hospitals in the Pennine Acute Hospitals NHS Trust in the northwest of England.

Patients.—A total of 1622 patients undergoing laparoscopic cholecystectomy during the period from 2005 to 2007.

Results.—Of the 1622 patients included in our analysis, 463 patients had an RIOC performed by a single surgical unit. Of the remaining 1159 patients, 188 (16.2%) underwent a preoperative ERCP for suspected common bile duct stones, 107 (56.9%) of whom had negative results. Three patients, 2 of whom had no common bile duct stones, developed post-ERCP pancreatitis. The median duration between ERCP and laparoscopic cholecystectomy was 75 days. Of the 463 patients who underwent an RIOC, 36 (7.8%) had common bile duct stones, 18 (50% of common bile duct stone cases, 3.9% of all 436 RIOC cases) of whom had no preoperative markers for common bile duct stones. There were no bile duct injuries among patients who underwent an RIOC.

Conclusions.—Preoperative ERCP is widely used in the United Kingdom, but it frequently results in negative findings and therefore is unnecessary. It is associated with significant morbidity, which can be avoided when a policy of RIOC is employed.

▶ The use of preoperative and intraoperative cholangiography has been debated for decades because we lack sensitive and specific markers of choledocholithiasis. Importantly, because most surgeons have little experience with laparoscopic common bile duct exploration (CBDE) and are hesitant to perform an open CBDE when the gallbladder can be removed laparoscopically, many patients with even a slight suspicion of choledocholithiasis have preoperative common bile duct imaging with either endoscopic retrograde cholangiopancreatography (ERCP) or magnetic resonance cholangiopancreatography (MRCP). Alkhaffaf et al used regional data to assess the use and benefit of ERCP. Not surprisingly, they found overuse of ERCP and properly note that this nontherapeutic procedure is associated with complications, some of which are significant. In lieu of ERCP, the authors advocate routine intraoperative cholangiography, a not uncommon practice. However, their data suggest that 36 of 463 (7.8%) had positive cholangiograms with this approach. Thus, 92.2% percent of the patients had a nontherapeutic cholangiogram, whereas of those patients who underwent preoperative cholangiography by ERCP or MRCP, 38.5% had positive imaging. No doubt, this last group of patients was selected for cholangiography because of a high suspicion of choledocholithiasis. Furthermore, when stones were evident on routine intraoperative cholangiography, they were not treated, but the bile duct was stented and an ERCP was performed nearly 50 days after the diagnosis. Surely, placement of these transcystic catheters is associated with complications and risk of cholangitis, say nothing about patient discomfort. Immediate postoperative ERCP is well tolerated in these cases and should be performed for patient comfort and prompt removal of common bile duct stones. Although ERCP is certainly used too frequently in the preoperative assessment of patients with a low likelihood of choledocholithiasis, routine cholangiography also has a high nontherapeutic rate and can be accompanied by complications, especially when noted choledocholithiasis is not immediately treated.

K. E. Behrns, MD

Forty-Year Experience With Flow-Diversion Surgery for Patients With Congenital Choledochal Cysts With Pancreaticobiliary Maljunction at a Single Institution

Takeshita N, Ota T, Yamamoto M (Tokyo Women's Med Univ, Japan)
Ann Surg 254:1050-1053, 2011

Background.—Congenital choledochal cyst with pancreaticobiliary maljunction (PBM) is known as a high-risk factor for various complications such as cholangitis, pancreatitis, and carcinogenesis of the biliary system by mutual refluxes of bile and pancreatic juice. Furthermore, it is not rare to suffer from postoperative complications if the wrong operative procedure is chosen. Therefore, we sought to review the relationship between operative procedure for types I and IV-A (Todani's classification) congenital choledochal cyst with PBM, and long-term treatment outcome.

Subjects and Methods.—A retrospective review was carried out of 144 patients who underwent flow diversion surgery in our institution during the 40-year period from 1968 to 2008 and who did not have a coexisting malignant tumor at the time of surgery.

Results.—Of these 144 patients, 137 underwent complete cyst excision and 7 underwent pancreas head resection as flow diversion surgery. The follow-up periods ranged from 1 to 345 months and from 1 to 271 months (average, 100.2 and 94.1) in patients with type I and type IV-A cysts, respectively. Regarding surgical treatment outcome, postoperative progress was good in 130 (90.3%) of the 144 patients. Fourteen patients required hospitalization for long-term postoperative complications such as cholangitis, pancreatitis, intrahepatic calculi, pancreatic calculus, and carcinogenesis during postoperative follow-up. Of these, 2 patients who underwent surgery for type IV-A cysts died because of secondary biliary cirrhosis with liver failure and advanced intrahepatic cholangiocarcinoma, respectively.

Conclusions.—The present study shows that flow diversion surgery for congenital choledochal cysts with PBM significantly reduces the risk of subsequent development of malignancy in the biliary tract, and it is vital to choose the appropriate operative procedure to prevent occurrence of these postoperative complications.

▶ Takeshita et al report a large experience of 144 patients with choledochal cysts without malignancy that were treated by cyst excision and hepaticoenterostomy. The series of patients consisted of 110 patients with type I choledochal cysts and 34 patients with type IV-A cysts. Incidentally, an additional 27 patients with type I cysts and 9 patients with type IV-A cysts were excluded from the study because they had a concomitant diagnosis of cancer, primarily in the biliary tree. This report is interesting because generally a choledochal cyst is treated with complete excision of the extrahepatic biliary tree and Roux-en-Y hepaticojejunostomy; however, 16 patients also had hepatectomy or pancreatectomy. Furthermore, 67 of the 144 patients did not have a Roux-en-Y hepaticojejunostomy but a hepaticoduodenostomy with or without a jejunal interposition. The results were good with 6.4% of type I patients experiencing a complication and 20.6% of type IV-A patients developing primarily cholangitis or intrahepatic stones. Clearly, this series shows the need for complete excision of the extrahepatic bile duct with a wide anastomosis. In addition, operative procedures that permit free drainage of bile into the intestine without reflux of enteric content into the bile duct are important. The authors noted that in the later years of this series hepaticojejunostomy has been the procedure of choice to avoid enteric reflux with subsequent cholangitis that complicates a hepaticoduodenostomy. Hopefully, this work, along with other publications, will sound the death knell for hepaticoand choledochoduodenostomy, procedures that do not permit adequate drainage of bile and are complicated by enteric reflux that too frequently results in postoperative cholangitis and secondary biliary cirrhosis.

K. E. Behrns, MD

Specialist Early and Immediate Repair of Post-laparoscopic Cholecystectomy Bile Duct Injuries Is Associated With an Improved Long-term Outcome
Perera MTPR, Silva MA, Hegab B, et al (Univ Hosp Birmingham, UK)
Ann Surg 253:553-560, 2011

Introduction.—A majority of bile duct injuries (BDI) sustained during laparoscopic cholecystectomy require formal surgical reconstruction, and traditionally this repair is performed late. We aimed to assess longterm outcomes after repair, focusing on our preferred early approach.

Methods.—A total of 200 BDI patients [age 54 (20–83); 64 male], followed up for median 60 (5–212) months were assessed for morbidity. Factors contributing to this were analyzed with a univariate and multivariate analysis.

Results.—A total of 112 (56%) patients were repaired by specialist hepatobiliary surgeons [timing of repair: immediate, n = 28; early (<21 days), n = 43; and late (>21 days) n = 41], whereas 45 (22%) underwent repair by nonspecialist surgeons before specialist referral [immediate, n = 16; early, n = 26 and late, n = 03]. Outcomes after immediate and early repairs were comparable to late repairs when performed by specialists [recurrent cholangitis: 11%, 12%, and 10%; $P = 0.96$, NS; re-stricture: 18%, 5%, and 29%; $P = 0.01$; nonsurgical intervention: 14%, 5%, and 24%; $P < 0.03$; redo surgery: 4%, 2%, and 5%; $P = 0.81$, NS; overall morbidity: 21%, 14%, and 39%; $P < 0.02$]. On multivariate analysis, immediate and early repairs done by nonspecialist surgeons were independent risk factors ($P < 0.05$) for recurrent cholangitis [50% and 27%], re-structuring (75% and 61%), redo reconstructions (31% and 61%), and overall morbidity (75% and 84%).

Conclusion.—Immediate and early repair after BDI results in comparable, if not better long-term outcomes compared to late repair when performed by specialists.

▶ Thamara et al studied 200 patients that sustained a bile duct injury during cholecystectomy and found that patients that had a nonhepatobiliary surgeon specialist perform the repair of the injury had an increased risk of recurrent cholangitis and strictures and needed further inventions, such and biliary stenting or revisional surgery. Conversely, hepatobiliary surgeons who performed immediate or early (< 21 days) repair of a bile duct injury had comparatively good results. Patients with a concomitant vascular injury, usually a right hepatic artery transection, had a complicated recovery. These results demonstrate the importance of prompt recognition and immediate repair of the bile duct injury. The highlight of this manuscript is an outreach service whereby hepatobiliary specialist surgeons perform repair at the index hospital when the injury is recognized immediately. This is a unique service that is infrequently, if ever, performed in the United States. This type of service is an outstanding example of patient-centric care that offers timely repair of a bile duct injury with good long-term results. Perhaps this practice should be adopted in the United States.

K. E. Behrns, MD

Complex hepatobiliary surgery in the community setting: is it safe and feasible?
Chamberlain RS, Klaassen Z, Paragi PR (Saint Barnabas Med Ctr, Livingston, NJ)
Am J Surg 202:273-280, 2011

Background.—Complex hepatobiliary surgical procedures for benign and malignant conditions are regularly performed at tertiary academic referral centers with excellent outcomes, but whether similar surgical outcomes are achievable in community hospitals is not well documented.

Methods.—Eighty-four patients underwent complex hepatobiliary surgery between December 2004 and December 2008. Data were prospectively analyzed, including patient demographics, operative procedures, perioperative parameters, pathology, complications up to 30 days postoperatively, and long-term outcomes.

Results.—The most frequent procedures performed were isolated segmentectomy or segmentectomies (n = 41 [49%]). Major hepatic resections (n = 32 [38%]) included 25 lobectomies (30%) and 7 trisegmentectomies (8%). Nine patients (11%) had surgical complications, and the most common indications for surgery was metastatic carcinoma (n = 42 [50%]).

Conclusions.—Complex hepatobiliary surgery can be performed safely at a community-based teaching hospital with excellent outcomes. In the ongoing debate centering on mandatory referral and centralization of complex surgical procedures, tertiary community hospitals with well-determined outcomes should be included.

▶ Regionalization of complex surgical care in patients with disorders of the pancreas and liver has been promoted as a mechanism to concentrate and improve care. Most of the discussions around this topic have centered on hospital volume, while others examine the total processes required to care for these patients. Chamberlain et al published their results on care of patients requiring liver or biliary surgery in a community setting. They present excellent outcomes in 84 patients who had surgery over a 4-year period. Thus, it would appear that they are performing about 20 major resections per year or 1.5 per month. They nicely compared their results with other published results and made a cogent argument for including larger community hospitals with specialized surgical care in the discussions of regionalization. Obviously, regionalization would have a major impact on patient care, and convenience and follow-up of surgical care may prove difficult. This manuscript clearly shows that high-quality complex hepatobiliary surgery can be performed by skilled surgeons and clinicians in a community setting. However, perhaps a more important question not addressed by the data presented is "How many patients did you refer for complex hepatobiliary disease?" While many patients with complex hepatobiliary disorders can be cared for in the community setting, it is important to recognize and refer those patients who may be better served in an academic, tertiary care center. Our collective surgical goal should be to deliver the right care to the right patient at the right time and in the right setting. We should seek data that look at a cross section of patients with hepatobiliary disease who were cared for in multiple settings so we can appropriately care for these complicated patients.

K. E. Behrns, MD

Laparoscopic Liver Resection: An Examination of Our First 300 Patients

Cannon RM, Brock GN, Marvin MR, et al (Univ of Louisville School of Medicine, KY; Univ of Louisville, KY; et al)
J Am Coll Surg 213:501-507, 2011

Background.—Laparoscopic liver resection is a procedure in evolution. In the last decade it has evolved from a novel procedure to a standard part of the hepatic surgeon's armamentarium. Few data exist on the development of a laparoscopic resection program.

Study Design.—With IRB approval, a retrospective review of 300 consecutive laparoscopic liver resections was undertaken. To determine changing results and patterns of practice, the cohort was divided into 3 consecutive groups of 100 patients. Patient demographics, indications for operation, operative factors, and in-hospital outcomes were examined. Continuous variables were analyzed with the Kruskal-Wallis test; continuous variables were compared with Fisher's exact test. Univariate and multivariate analyses of major complications ($\geq$grade 3) were performed using logistic regression.

Results.—Of the 300 patients, 173 (61.6%) were female, with a median age of 54 years. There were 133 (44.3%) major resections. The median number of segments resected increased (3 vs 2, p = 0.015), as did the percentage of repeat hepatectomies (13.0% vs 2.0%, p = 0.001). At the same time, median operative time decreased (2.25 vs 3.0 hours, p < 0.001). and estimated blood loss was similar (150 mL vs 150 mL, p = 0.635). Morbidity was similar (11% vs 14%, p = 0.300), as was mortality (1% vs 3%, p = 0.625).

Conclusions.—Laparoscopic liver resection has evolved from a novel procedure to a vital technique in liver surgery. Our group has demonstrated the ability over time to perform more difficult resections with similar morbidity and decreased operative length (Table 3).

▶ Since the early 1990s, minimally invasive techniques have dramatically changed the approach to intra-abdominal diseases. This revolution in the operative approach to diseases continues today with laparoscopic techniques applied to increasingly complex patients. Routinely, the laparoscopic approach is now used for all types of colon surgery, complex pancreatic surgery including pancreatoduodenectomy, and now, as Cannon et al report, liver resections. The authors nicely chronicled the incremental introduction of laparoscopic approaches to liver resection and the inevitable increase in patient complexity as their experience increased (Table 3). Furthermore, the results are undoubtedly an improvement compared with open surgery with decreased transfusion requirements and a short length of stay. Although laparoscopic hepatectomy is gaining widespread acceptance and the technique results in excellent patient outcomes, a word of caution should be introduced. The data clearly show that less than half of the patients had a malignancy, and therefore, many laparoscopic resections are performed for benign disease. Open operations for benign liver disease are uncommon, and thus, the question of whether patients with benign disease are receiving an operation just because it can be approached laparoscopically is

TABLE 3.—Comparison Between Eras

Factor	Era 1 (n = 100)	Era 2 (n = 100)	Era 3 (n = 100)	p Value
Sex, n (%)				
Male	31 (33.0)	37 (41.6)	40 (40.9)	0.415
Female	63 (67.0)	52 (58.4)	58 (59.2)	
Age, y median	51	56	56.5	0.039
Cirrhosis, n (%)	11 (11.0)	11 (11.0)	20 (20.0)	0.125
Malignancy, n (%)	40 (40.0)	45 (45.0)	47 (47.0)	0.581
Previous abdominal operation, n (%)	24 (24.0)	30 (30.0)	36 (36.0)	0.205
Previous hepatectomy, n (%)	2 (2.0)	2 (2.0)	13 (13.0)	0.001
Major hepatectomy, n (%)	39 (61.0)	42 (42.0)	52 (52.0)	0.154
Segments resected, n, median	2	2	3	0.015
Estimated blood loss, mL, median	150	150	150	0.635
Operating room time, h, median	3.0	2.5	2.25	<0.001
Hand assist, n (%)	79 (79.0)	72 (72.0)	60 (60.0)	0.013
Transfused, n (%)	8 (8.0)	8 (8.0)	5 (5.0)	0.718
Major complication, n (%)	14 (14.0)	7 (7.0)	11 (11.0)	0.300
Mortality, n (%)	3 (3.0)	1 (1.0)	1 (1.0)	0.625
Length of stay, d, median	3	3	3	0.705

raised. Perhaps more patients with benign disease choose to have an operation because a minimally invasive approach is offered, and they deem the risk of the operation as a reasonable trade-off compared with pain or other symptoms. However, we must continually scrutinize our application of new techniques and ensure that we are using them in the appropriate settings.

K. E. Behrns, MD

Risk factors for central bile duct injury complicating partial liver resection
Boonstra EA, de Boer MT, Sieders E, et al (Univ of Groningen, The Netherlands)
Br J Surg 99:256-262, 2012

Background.—Bile duct injury is a serious complication following liver resection. Few studies have differentiated between leakage from small peripheral bile ducts and central bile duct injury (CBDI), defined as an injury leading to leakage or stenosis of the common bile duct, common hepatic duct, right or left hepatic duct. This study analysed the incidence, risk factors and consequences of CBDI in liver resection.

Methods.—Patients undergoing liver resection between 1990 and 2007 were included in this study. Those having resection for bile duct-related pathology or trauma, or after liver transplantation were excluded. Characteristics and outcome variables were collected prospectively and analysed retrospectively.

Results.—There were 19 instances of CBDI in 462 liver resections (4·1 per cent). One-third of patients with CBDI required surgical reintervention and construction of a hepaticojejunostomy. Resection type ($P < 0·001$), previous liver resection ($P = 0·039$) and intraoperative blood loss ($P = 0·002$) were associated with an increased risk of CBDI. Of all resection types, extended left hemihepatectomy was associated with the highest incidence of CBDI (2 of 9 procedures).

Conclusion.—Patients undergoing extended left hemihepatectomy or repeat hepatectomy were at increased risk of CBDI.

▶ Boonstra et al present a relatively small but telling series of patients who had acquired central bile duct injuries during partial hepatectomy. They summarized the findings of 19 patients (4.1% of hepatectomies) and noted that 33% of the patients required operative management. Furthermore, risk factors for bile duct injury included left hemi-hepatectomy, previous hepatectomy, and operative blood loss. Moreover, the stakes were high, as 16% of the patients died. Although the authors nicely summarize the findings of this small series and offer risk factors for central bile duct injury, this type of study raises questions about surgeon familiarity with liver anatomy and the complexities of liver surgery. Today, the surgical community often discusses the need for generalists versus surgical specialists or subspecialists, and the debate is often polarizing and vigorous. However, this article highlights the importance of surgical subspecialists to deal with complex problems. What is a surgical subspecialist? These surgeons devote their career and training in a particular area of study and continually innovate such that this discipline of surgery continues to evolve. Not only are they master surgeons, but they are creative and develop new techniques or procedures that improve patient safety and outcomes. What does it take to become a surgical subspecialist? Studies outside of surgery and medicine estimate that 10 000 hours of practice are required to achieve mastery. Thus, to become a master surgical subspecialist requires years of practice beyond training. Depending on the circumstances, achieving mastery may require 10 years of posttraining experience. This article nicely highlights the complexities of high-end surgery and need for surgical subspecialists in addition to surgical generalists.

K. E. Behrns, MD

Factors associated with delays to emergency care for bowel obstruction
Hwang U, Aufses AH Jr, Bickell NA (Mount Sinai School of Medicine, NY)
Am J Surg 202:1-7, 2011

Background.—Our objective was to determine factors associated with delays to first treatment for emergency department (ED) patients diagnosed with small-bowel obstruction (SBO).

Methods.—This was a retrospective study of ED patients with SBO. Data were collected from medical records, administrative databases, and staffing schedules at an urban, tertiary care medical center from June 1, 2001, to November 30, 2002. Patient-related characteristics and processes of ED and hospital care were evaluated. Outcomes studied were time to first treatment (nasogastric tube or surgery) and risk of surgical resection.

Results.—A total of 193 patients were diagnosed with confirmed intestinal obstruction. Patients with longer times to first treatment arrived during ED clinician hand-offs (adjusted hazard ratio, .40; 95% confidence interval, .17—.98). Patients with longer times to surgery consult (ref. first quartile) had greater odds of surgical resection (second quartile adjusted odds ratio, 6.91; 95% confidence interval, 1.85—24.80).

Conclusions.—Remediable ED and hospital factors were associated with longer times to treatment for patients with bowel obstruction.

▶ The surgical management of small bowel obstruction is often guided by the adage "the sun should not set on a patient with a bowel obstruction," which implies surgical treatment should occur within hours rather than days. Hwang et al studied the time to first treatment of patients who presented to an emergency department with a diagnosis of bowel obstruction. They found patients that experienced delays in treatment were often diagnosed around the time of clinician hand-offs. Furthermore, a delay in surgical consult was associated with an increased risk of bowel resection at the time of surgery. Both of these data points highlight the competency of communication—how can we communicate in a more timely fashion and more effectively to improve the care of our patients? Certainly, intradepartmental rounds among the emergency department physicians at the time of hand-off could be facilitated by face-to-face contact between physicians and patients at risk, like those requiring a disposition related to the diagnosis of acute bowel obstruction. Furthermore, rounds with the surgical team could lead to a more rapid diagnosis and treatment. Importantly, the authors do not discuss in detail the surgical team responsible for these patients. The recent introduction of an acute care surgical service, which is designed to render rapid care to patients in the emergency department, may have a team member who spends the majority of his or her time in the emergency department and facilitates the care of patients with a small bowel obstruction.

K. E. Behrns, MD

Appendicitis outcomes are better at resident teaching institutions: a multi-institutional analysis
Yaghoubian A, de Virgilio C, Lee SL (Harbor-UCLA Med Ctr, Torrance, CA; Kaiser Permanente Los Angeles Med Ctr, CA)
Am J Surg 200:810-813, 2010

Background.—This study compared the outcomes of appendicitis between teaching and nonteaching institutions.

Methods.—A retrospective review was performed of all appendicitis patients aged >18 years from 1998 to 2007. The outcomes from 2 teaching institutions (each with its own general surgery residency program) were compared with those from 11 nonteaching institutions. Study outcomes included postoperative morbidity and length of hospitalization.

Results.—A total of 3,242 patients were treated at the teaching institutions (mean age, 41 years; 61% men) and 14,483 at the nonteaching institutions (mean age, 38 years; 54% men). The perforated appendicitis rate was 29%

at the teaching institution and 28% at the nonteaching institutions ($P = .20$). For nonperforated appendicitis, there was no difference in the incidence of wound infection between the teaching and nonteaching institutions (2.7% vs 2.3%, $P = .30$). There was a lower rate of abscess drainage (.4% vs 1%, $P = .02$), a lower readmission rate (1.7% vs 3.5%, $P < .0001$), and shorter lengths of stay (1.7 ± 1.5 vs 1.8 ± 1.6 days, $P = .002$) at teaching institutions. For perforated appendicitis, there were also lower rates of wound infection (4.8% vs 7%, $P = .03$), abscess drainage (4.9% vs 10%, $P < .0001$), and need for readmission (4.2% vs 8.4%, $P < .0001$) at the teaching hospitals. The lengths of stay were similar (5.0 ± 4.2 vs 5.2 ± 3.1 days, $P = .30$). Use of laparoscopy was lower and nonoperative management of perforated appendicitis higher at the teaching hospitals.

Conclusions.—Teaching institutions were more likely to perform appendectomy using an open technique and to manage perforated appendicitis nonoperatively. Infectious complications and readmission rates for both perforated and nonperforated appendicitis were lower at teaching institutions.

▶ The quality of patient care is receiving the high level of observation that it deserves, and as such, patient outcomes are increasingly scrutinized. Short-term surgical outcomes may be receiving more attention than other specialty results because the outcomes are readily quantifiable and surgeons have a long history of self-examination through media such as morbidity and mortality conference. It is generally accepted that surgical outcomes for common procedures performed in the teaching institution are not as good as outcomes obtained in a community setting. Yaghoubian et al dispel this notion by comparing the outcome of appendectomy in 2 teaching institutions to the results in 11 private groups. The results demonstrated that appendectomy for nonperforated appendicitis performed at a teaching institution was associated with decreased need for postoperative abscess drainage, lower readmission rate, and slightly decreased length of stay. Surprisingly, laparoscopic appendectomy was used less frequently in the teaching environment. For patients who had a perforated appendix, the rate of wound infection, abscess drainage, and readmission were all lower in the teaching hospital. Although the reasons for these results are not obvious, experience has taught us that processes of care are most important. It may be that the built-in redundancy in a teaching institution provides another set of eyes that questions the processes of care that in turn results in improved outcomes. Although not impossible to study, it would be difficult to determine whether redundancy leads to improved outcomes. However, there is little doubt that a team of care providers that continues to ask questions leads to thoughtful reflection of our care pathways and, it is hoped, improved outcomes.

K. E. Behrns, MD

Amoxicillin plus clavulanic acid versus appendicectomy for treatment of acute uncomplicated appendicitis: an open-label, non-inferiority, randomised controlled trial

Vons C, Barry C, Maitre S, et al (Hôpital Antoine Béclère (Assistance Publique-Hôpitaux de Paris and Université Paris XI), Clamart, France; Hôpital Paul Brousse, Villejuif, France; Hôpital Lariboisière (Assistance Publique-Hôpitaux de Paris and Université Paris VII), France; et al)

Lancet 377:1573-1579, 2011

Background.—Researchers have suggested that antibiotics could cure acute appendicitis. We assessed the efficacy of amoxicillin plus clavulanic acid by comparison with emergency appendicectomy for treatment of patients with uncomplicated acute appendicitis.

Methods.—In this open-label, non-inferiority, randomised trial, adult patients (aged 18—68 years) with uncomplicated acute appendicitis, as assessed by CT scan, were enrolled at six university hospitals in France. A computer-generated randomisation sequence was used to allocate patients randomly in a 1:1 ratio to receive amoxicillin plus clavulanic acid (3 g per day) for 8—15 days or emergency appendicectomy. The primary endpoint was occurrence of postintervention peritonitis within 30 days of treatment initiation. Non-inferiority was shown if the upper limit of the two-sided 95% CI for the difference in rates was lower than 10 percentage points. Both intention-to-treat and per-protocol analyses were done. This trial is registered with ClinicalTrials.gov, number NCT00135603.

Findings.—Of 243 patients randomised, 123 were allocated to the antibiotic group and 120 to the appendicectomy group. Four were excluded from analysis because of early dropout before receiving the intervention, leaving 239 (antibiotic group, 120; appendicectomy group, 119) patients for intention-to-treat analysis. 30-day postintervention peritonitis was significantly more frequent in the antibiotic group (8%, n = 9) than in the appendicectomy group (2%, n = 2; treatment difference 5·8; 95% CI 0·3—12·1). In the appendicectomy group, despite CT-scan assessment, 21 (18%) of 119 patients were unexpectedly identified at surgery to have complicated appendicitis with peritonitis. In the antibiotic group, 14 (12% [7·1—18·6]) of 120 underwent an appendicectomy during the first 30 days and 30 (29% [21·4—38·9]) of 102 underwent appendicectomy between 1 month and 1 year, 26 of whom had acute appendicitis (recurrence rate 26%; 18·0—34·7).

Interpretation.—Amoxicillin plus clavulanic acid was not non-inferior to emergency appendicectomy for treatment of acute appendicitis. Identification of predictive markers on CT scans might enable improved targeting of antibiotic treatment (Table 2).

▶ In the past few years, several studies have suggested that acute appendicitis can be treated with antibiotic therapy. The rationale for this approach may be likened to the treatment of uncomplicated sigmoid diverticulitis. Because the appendix is a large diverticulum of the colon and the pathophysiology of appendicitis

TABLE 2.—Incidence of Primary Endpoint Events and Complicated Appendicitis With Peritonitis and Postoperative Peritonitis Within 30 days After the Start of Treatment in Both Groups (intention-to-treat population)

	Appendicectomy Group (n=119)	Antibiotic-Treatment Group (n=120)	Difference (95% CI)
Primary endpoint events			
30-day post-therapeutic peritonitis	2 (2%)*	9 (8%)†	5·8 (0·3 to 12·1)
Incidence of peritonitis			
Complicated appendicitis with peritonitis identified at surgery	21 (18%)‡	9 (8%)†	−10·1 (−18·7 to −1·7)
Postoperative peritonitis	2 (2%)‡	2 (2%)§	0 (−4·4 to 4·4)

Data are number unless otherwise stated.
*In the appendicectomy group, two cases of postoperative peritonitis occurred; these patients had postoperative localised peritonitis successfully treated with antibiotics.
†In the antibiotic group, complicated appendicitis with peritonitis was identified during appendicectomy performed within 30 days of treatment initiation in nine of 14 patients who did not show improvement.
‡Discovery of a complicated appendicitis with peritonitis in the appendicectomy group was not a primary endpoint.
§Two patients in the antibiotic group, who underwent secondary appendicectomy, had postoperative peritonitis.

(obstruction) mimics that of sigmoid diverticulitis, the initial treatment with antibiotics appears justified. Vons et al conducted a randomized, noninferiority, controlled trial of amoxicillin plus clavulanic acid versus appendectomy for the treatment of uncomplicated appendicitis. The results convincingly demonstrate that antibiotic treatment is inferior to appendectomy in the treatment of appendicitis, as assessed by the primary end point of 30-day occurrence of peritonitis (Table 2). In addition, the complications associated with antibiotic treatment were significant. The authors justly conclude that improved diagnostic criteria may enable improved selection of patients with appendicitis who can be treated by antibiotics alone; however, this study demonstrates that appendectomy remains the gold-standard treatment.

K. E. Behrns, MD

Is Colonoscopy Still Mandatory After a CT Diagnosis of Left-Sided Diverticulitis: Can Colorectal Cancer be Confidently Excluded?
Lau KC, Spilsbury K, Farooque Y, et al (Fremantle Hosp, Western Australia, Australia; Curtin Univ, Perth, Western Australia, Australia)
Dis Colon Rectum 54:1265-1270, 2011

Background.—It is routine practice to perform colonoscopy as a follow-up after an attack of diverticulitis, with the main aim to exclude any underlying malignancy.

Purpose.—This study aimed to determine whether colonoscopy is necessary and what additional information is gained from this procedure.

Design.—This is a study of a retrospective cohort.

Settings and Patients.—From January 2003 to June 2009, patients in whom left-sided diverticulitis was diagnosed on CT scan were matched with colonoscopy reports within 1 year from the date of CT by the use of radiology and endoscopy databases. Patients who had colonoscopy within 1 year before the CT scan were excluded. The Western Australian Cancer Registry was cross-referenced to identify patients who subsequently received diagnoses of cancers for whom colonoscopy reports were unavailable.

Main Outcome Measures.—The main outcome measures were the number of patients in whom colorectal cancers were diagnosed and other incidental findings, eg, polyps, colitis, and stricture.

Results.—Left-sided diverticulitis was diagnosed in 1088 patients on CT scan, whereas follow-up colonoscopy reports were available for 319 patients. Eighty-two (26%) patients had incidental findings of polyps (9 polyps >1 cm), and 9 patients (2.8%) received diagnoses of colorectal cancers on colonoscopy. After cross-referencing with the cancer registry, the overall prevalence of colorectal cancer among the cohort within 1 year of CT scan was 2.1% (23 cases). The odds of a diagnosis of colorectal cancer were 6.7 times (95% CI 2.4−18.7) in patients with an abscess reported on CT, 4 times (95% CI 1.1−14.9) in patients with local perforation, and 18 times (95% CI 5.1−63.7) in patients with fistula compared with patients with uncomplicated diverticulitis.

Limitations.—This study was limited by the unavailability of data for private/interstate hospitals, and the relatively small number of cancer cases reduced the statistical power of the study.

Conclusions.—We recommend routine colonoscopy after an attack of presumed left-sided diverticulitis in patients who have not had recent colonic luminal evaluation. The rate of occult carcinoma is substantial

TABLE 3.—Demographic Factors and Additional CT Findings Associated with Increased Odds of Colorectal Cancer in the Diverticulitis Cohort with and without Simultaneous Covariate Adjustment in Logistic Regression Models

| | | Unadjusted[a] | | | Adjusted[b] | |
	OR[c]	95% CI	P	OR[c]	95% CI	P
Age[d]	**1.2**	1.1−1.4	.007	**1.2**	1.1−1.4	.012
Sex						
Male	1.00	—		1.00	—	—
Female	1.5	0.7−3.5	.334	1.2	0.5−3.0	.664
Local perforation on CT						
No	1.00	—	—	1.00	—	—
Yes	1.9	0.5−6.5	.241	**4.0**	1.1−14.9	.040
Abscess on CT						
No	1.00	—	—	1.00	—	—
Yes	**4.6**	1.8−12.0	.002	**6.7**	2.4−18.7	<.001
Fistula on CT						
No	1.00	—	—	1.00	—	—
Yes	**12.2**	3.8−38.9	<.001	**18.0**	5.1−63.7	<.001

[a]Each variable entered into separate logistic regression models.
[b]All variables entered simultaneously into a single logistic regression model.
[c]Odds ratios in bold have P values of <.05.
[d]Age entered into the model as a continuous variable in 5-year age groups.

in this patient population, in particular, when abscess, local perforation, and fistula are observed (Table 3).

▶ Lau et al performed an interesting retrospective analysis of patients that had a computed tomography (CT) diagnosis of left-sided diverticulitis to determine the frequency of colon cancer diagnosed on a subsequent colonoscopy. The results were quite intriguing in that 2.8% of the patients had a colon cancer with a cancer prevalence of 2.1%. Impressively, the presence of an abscess, local perforation, or fistula markedly increased the risk of colorectal cancer with odds ratios of 6.7, 4, and 18, respectively (Table 3). This study provides the important message that patients with complicated diverticulitis on CT must have a subsequent endoscopy. However, what about the patients with uncomplicated diverticulitis? The authors concluded that colonoscopy should be performed on all patients with a CT diagnosis of diverticulitis, but the challenge for all surgeons will be to limit the number of investigations. Were there any distinguishing features in the patients that did not have colorectal cancer? Are there parameters that would allow us to withhold a colonoscopy in a group of patients? With increasing emphasis on decreasing cost, we must not only ask questions about which patients need further investigation but also which groups of patients do not need additional evaluation.

K. E. Behrns, MD

Outcome of patients with acute sigmoid diverticulitis: Multivariate analysis of risk factors for free perforation

Ritz J-P, Lehmann KS, Frericks B, et al (Charité—Universitätsmedizin Berlin, Germany)

Surgery 149:606-613, 2011

Background.—Sigmoid diverticulitis (SD) is common in the West; its incidence is increasing as the average age of the population increases. The aim of this study was to assess the clinical outcomes of patients with acute SD and to determine whether emergency operation was associated more often with previous episodes of acute diverticulitis.

Methods.—All consecutive patients admitted for acute SD were recruited prospectively over an 11-year period from January 1998 to December 2008. Multiple logistic regression was used to identify risk factors for free perforation.

Results.—We included 934 patients (490 men and 444 women; median age, 59.2 years): 450 (48.2%) presented for their first SD episode and 484 (51.8%) had a prior history of SD. Free perforation occurred in 152 patients: during the first episode of SD in 114 patients (25.3%), during the second in 29 (12.7%), during the third in 8 (5.9%), and during the fifth in 1 patient (0.9%; $P < .001$). No patient with >5 previous episodes of SD had free perforation. All 152 patients with free perforation required emergent operative intervention. After initial conservative therapy in 782 patients, 82 required early elective operative intervention owing to exacerbation of infection under antibiotic treatment. Late elective colectomy was performed in 299 patients during the inflammation-free interval, and operative intervention was recommended in 345 patients owing to complicated diverticulitis. Uncomplicated SD in 56 patients was managed conservatively. Comorbidity (>1 disorder) and the first episode of SD were identified as risk factors for free perforation on multiple logistic regression.

Conclusion.—The risk of free perforation in acute SD decreases with the number of previous episodes of SD. The first episode thus is the most dangerous for a free perforation. The indication for colectomy should not be made based on the potential risk of free perforation.

▶ The indications for surgical treatment of sigmoid diverticulitis have recently come under heavy scrutiny. The traditional dogma that a second episode of diverticulitis warrants elective operative therapy has been challenged, and, indeed, many surgeons and institutions have backed away from this approach. However, a watchful-waiting approach raises anxiety that the next episode of diverticulitis for any given patient will present with a free perforation with the attendant increased mortality, morbidity, and need for multiple operations. Ritz et al performed an important retrospective study examining a large (N = 934 patients) number of patients who presented to their institution over an 11-year period. The data convincingly demonstrate that perforation is more common in the first presentation than in subsequent bouts of diverticulitis (25% vs 8%). These findings provide some solace to the surgeon who follows a patient who has had multiple episodes of diverticulitis. Conversely, the data show that 120 patients (13%) had more than 3 episodes of diverticulitis and that CT findings demonstrated sigmoid colon thickening, inflammation, stricture, and fistula. Although operative therapy for diverticulitis need not be instituted with the first or second episode, the development of multiple complications from diverticulitis may result in difficult operations that lead to increased morbidity. Although this study provides direct evidence that patients are unlikely to present with a perforation with recurrent diverticulitis, it also demonstrates that in a subset patients, nonoperative therapy is likely overutilized and may result in poorer outcomes.

K. E. Behrns, MD

Sigmoidectomy Syndrome? Patients' Perspectives on the Functional Outcomes Following Surgery for Diverticulitis
Levack MM, Savitt LR, Berger DL, et al (Massachusetts General Hosp and Harvard Med School, Boston; et al)
Dis Colon Rectum 55:10-17, 2012

Background.—Bowel function following surgery for diverticulitis has not previously been systematically described.

Objective.—This study aimed to document the frequency, severity, and predictors of suboptimal bowel function in patients who have undergone sigmoid colectomy for diverticulitis.

Design.—This study is a retrospective analysis.

Setting.—This study was conducted at a large, academic medical center.

Patients.—Three hundred twenty-five patients who underwent laparo-scopic or open sigmoid colectomy with restoration of intestinal continuity for diverticulitis were included in the study population. Of these, 249 patients (76.6%) returned a 70-question survey incorporating the Fecal Incontinence Severity Index, the Fecal Incontinence Quality of Life Scale, and the Memorial Bowel Function Instrument.

Main Outcome Measures.—Survey responders and nonresponders were compared with the use of χ^2 and *t* tests. Responders with suboptimal bowel function (fecal incontinence, urgency and/or incomplete emptying) were then compared with those with good outcomes by the use of logistic regression analysis to determine the predictors of poor function.

Results.—Of the responders, 24.8% reported clinically relevant fecal incontinence (Fecal Incontinence Severity Index ≥ 24), 19.6% reported fecal urgency (Memorial Bowel Function Instrument Urgency Subscale ≥ 4), and 20.8% reported incomplete emptying (Memorial Bowel Function Instrument Emptying Subscale ≥ 4). On logistic regression analysis, fecal incontinence was predicted by female sex (OR $= 2.3$, $p = 0.008$) and the presence of a preoperative abscess (OR $= 1.4$, $p < 0.05$). Fecal urgency was associated with female sex (OR $= 1.3$, $p < 0.05$) and a diverting ileostomy (OR $= 2.1$, $p < 0.001$). Incomplete emptying was associated with female sex (OR $= 1.4$, $p < 0.05$) and postoperative sepsis (OR $= 1.9$, $p < 0.05$).

Limitations.—This study was limited by the fact that we did not use a nondiverticulitis control group and we had limited preoperative data on the history of bowel impairment symptoms.

Conclusion.—One-fifth of patients reported fecal urgency, fecal incontinence, or incomplete emptying after surgery for diverticulitis. Despite the limitations of our study, these results are concerning and should be investigated further prospectively.

▶ A common postoperative instruction to patients who undergo colon resection would generally include a statement that bowel movements may be irregular in frequency and content for a period of a few weeks, but following this period of adjustment, the bowel habits should return to near normal. Clearly, this article by Levack et al debunks this generality. In fact, the survey outcomes from this study indicate that more than 20% of patients will experience fecal urgency, incontinence, or incomplete emptying of stool. Why are these findings relatively new? Simply put, we have failed to systematically look at the functional bowel outcomes for multiple groups of patients. Sure, this study is limited because there is no control group and perhaps bowel function after a right colectomy is associated with a 20% incidence of dysfunction. Furthermore, these results may or may not be specifically related to patients with diverticulitis. Nonetheless, this work clearly demonstrates a significant proportion of patients have functional outcomes that fall short of anticipated results. The authors rightly call for a prospective study to confirm the published findings, and this should be performed on a large group of patients with subgroup analysis so we can assess variables associated with less than desired functional outcome. The recent focus on patient satisfaction has resulted in increased awareness of the need to assess patient outcomes from multiple perspectives. Clearly, this is an important focal point that will help us continually improve patient care.

K. E. Behrns, MD

The Efficacy of Nonoperative Management of Acute Complicated Diverticulitis

Dharmarajan S, Hunt SR, Birnbaum EH, et al (Washington Univ School of Medicine, St Louis, MO)
Dis Colon Rectum 54:663-671, 2011

Background.—The surgical management of acute complicated diverticulitis has evolved to avoid emergency surgery in favor of elective resection. The optimal manner to accomplish this goal remains debatable.

Objective.—The purpose of this study was to examine the efficacy of nonoperative management of acute diverticulitis with abscess or perforation.

Design.—A retrospective review was performed of an institutional review board-approved database of patients admitted with a diagnosis of acute complicated diverticulitis from 1995 to 2008. Patient demographics, disease manifestation, management, and outcomes were collected.

Settings.—This study was conducted at a tertiary care hospital/referral center.

Patients.—Patients were included who presented with complicated diverticulitis defined as having an associated abscess or free air diagnosed by CT scan.

Main Outcome Measures.—Primary end points were the success of nonoperative management and need for surgery during the initial admission.

Results.—One hundred thirty-six patients were identified with perforated diverticulitis: 19 had localized free air, 45 had abscess <4 cm or distant free air measuring <2 cm, 66 had abscess >4 cm or distant free air <2 cm, and 6 had distant free air with free fluid. Thirty-eight patients (28%) required percutaneous abscess drains and 37 (27%) required parenteral nutrition. Only 5 patients (3.7%) required urgent surgery at the time of admission, and 7 (5%) required urgent surgery for failed nonoperative management. Thus, the overall success rate of nonoperative management was 91%. One hundred twenty-four of 131 (95%) patients were treated with nonoperative management successfully. Twenty-five of 27 (92.5%) patients with free air remote from the perforation site were successfully treated nonoperatively.

Conclusions.—Nonoperative management of acute complicated diverticulitis is highly effective. For patients with free air remote from the site of perforation, nonoperative management is able to convert an emergent situation into an elective one in 93% of cases. The decision to attempt

TABLE 2.—Nonoperative Interventions for Perforated Diverticulitis by CT Grade

CT Grade	Total No. of Patients	Length of Stay (Days)	No. (%) Requiring Percutaneous Abscess Drainage	No. (%) Requiring TPN	Total No. (%) Requiring Nonoperative Intervention
1	19	5.8 ± 6.1	0 (0)	1 (5)	1 (5)
2 — Total	45[a]	5.7 ± 4.5	1 (2)	12 (27)	13 (29)
Abscess ≤4 cm	38	5.6 ± 4.8	1 (3)	11 (29)	11 (29)
Distant free air ≤2 cm	11	8.2 ± 5.8	0 (0)	3 (27)	3 (27)
3 — Total	66[b]	10.7 ± 11.2	37 (56)	24 (36)	47 (71)
Abscess >4 cm	60	10.3 ± 11.5	37 (62)	21 (35)	45 (75)
Distant free air >2 cm	16	12.9 ± 17.7	10 (63)	6 (38)	12 (75)
4	6[c]	8	0 (0)	0 (0)	0 (0)
Total: all grades	136	8.0 ± 8.9	38 (28)	37 (27)	61 (45)
p[d]		<.001	<.001	.02	<.001

TPN = total parenteral nutrition.
[a]Four patients had both abscess <4 cm and distant free air <2 cm.
[b]Ten patients had both abscess >4 cm and distant free air >2 cm.
[c]Five of 6 patients with CT grade 4 diverticulitis underwent emergent operation.
[d]P values compare proportion of total patients with CT grades 1 to 3.

nonoperative therapy must be made based on the patient's physiologic state and associated comorbidities (Table 2).

▶ Dharmarajan et al present a novel approach to the treatment of complicated acute diverticulitis. These 136 patients had free air or abscesses located in either the pericolonic area or distant to the perforation, and these were graded according to size. Using this grading system, 91% of patients were treated nonoperatively using bowel rest, antibiotics, percutaneous drainage, and total parental nutrition (Table 2). Although this approach has been described, in part, previously, the approach in this series was well defined and methodical. Only 5% of the patients required an emergency operation because of physiologic parameters. This study shows that a nonoperative approach to colonic perforation can be successful in a large proportion of patients. However, although the data are quite convincing, too few details regarding patient comorbidities are relayed. This is important because surgeons must know when they should not use a nonoperative approach. Certainly, as pointed out by the authors, this would be a high-risk approach in an immunosuppressed patient. Furthermore, should diabetic patients be treated nonoperatively? This study is important in that it defines a new, well-outlined approach to nonoperative treatment of acute complicated diverticular disease. Perhaps a study comparing the value (outcomes/costs) of this approach should be conducted.

K. E. Behrns, MD

Diverting Loop Ileostomy and Colonic Lavage: An Alternative to Total Abdominal Colectomy for the Treatment of Severe, Complicated Clostridium difficile Associated Disease

Neal MD, Alverdy JC, Hall DE, et al (Univ of Pittsburgh School of Medicine, PA; Univ of Chicago, IL)
Ann Surg 254:423-429, 2011

Objective.—To determine whether a minimally invasive, colon-preserving approach could serve as an alternative to total colectomy in the treatment of severe, complicated *Clostridium difficile*—associated disease (CDAD).

Background.—C. *difficile* is a significant cause of morbidity and mortality worldwide. Most cases will respond to antibiotic therapy, but 3% to 10% of patients progress to a severe, complicated, or "fulminant" state of life-threatening systemic toxicity. Although the advocated surgical treatment of total abdominal colectomy with end ileostomy improves survival in severe, complicated CDAD, outcomes remain poor with associated mortality rates ranging from 35% to 80%.

Methods.—All patients who were diagnosed with severe, complicated ("fulminant") CDAD and were treated at the University of Pittsburgh Medical Center or VA Pittsburgh Healthcare System between June 2009 and January 2011 were treated with this novel approach. The surgical approach involved creation of a loop ileostomy, intraoperative colonic lavage with warmed polyethylene glycol 3350/electrolyte solution via the ileostomy and postoperative antegrade instillation of vancomycin flushes via the ileostomy. The primary end point for the study was resolution of CDAD. The matching number of patients treated with colectomy for CDAD preceding the initiation of this current treatment strategy was analyzed for historical comparison.

Results.—Forty-two patients were treated during this time period. There was no significant difference in age, sex, pharmacologic immunosuppression, and Acute Physiology and Chronic Health Evaluation-II scores between our current cohort and historical controls. The operation was accomplished laparoscopically in 35 patients (83%). This treatment strategy resulted in reduced mortality compared to our historical population (19% vs 50%; odds ratio, 0.24; $P = 0.006$). Preservation of the colon was achieved in 39 of 42 patients (93%).

Conclusions.—Loop ileostomy and colonic lavage are an alternative to colectomy in the treatment of severe, complicated CDAD resulting in reduced morbidity and preservation of the colon.

▶ Neal et al propose a new method of treatment of patients with severe, complicated *Clostridium difficile*—associated disease (CDAD). Heretofore, severe CDAD has been treated by total abdominal colectomy and end ileostomy. However, this group has demonstrated that laparoscopic loop ileostomy with 8-L colonic, polyethylene glycol lavage followed by vancomycin instillation in the colon results in decreased mortality compared with historical controls. In 42 matched patients, the mortality rate decreased from 50% to 20% using this novel approach.

Only 3 patients had a subsequent colectomy, and the colonic resection was required in retrospect in only 2 patients. This work is exciting not only because it is novel but because it is rooted in the basic physiology of colonocytes, bacteriology, and sepsis. As the investigative group aptly describes, because the colonic injury is related to a toxin, rather than invasion of an organism, the injurious agent and the accompanying neutrophils that incite the systemic inflammatory response system can be flushed through the colon. The remaining unanswered question is when this procedure should be performed in the spectrum of CDAD. The authors address this question in part by proposing an unvalidated scoring system to assess the severity of disease. However, whether patients with mild-moderate, severe, or severe-complicated disease should undergo this operative approach remains to be determined. Undoubtedly, this is the first study of many that will continue to change the surgical treatment of patients with severe CDAD.

K. E. Behrns, MD

Management of Malignant Colonic Polyps: A Population-Based Analysis of colonoscopic Polypectomy Versus surgery

Cooper GS, Xu F, Barnholtz Sloan JS, et al (Univ Hosps Case Med Ctr, Cleveland, OH; Case Comprehensive Cancer Ctr, Cleveland, OH)
Cancer 118:651-659, 2012

Background.—The management of colon polyps containing invasive carcinoma includes surgical resection or colonoscopic polypectomy. To date, there are very limited population-based data comparing outcomes with the 2 management approaches.

Methods.—Using the linked Surveillance Epidemiology and End Results–Medicare database, we identified 2077 patients aged ≥66 years with an initial diagnosis of stage T1N0M0 malignant polyp from 1992-2005. Patients were categorized as surgical or polypectomy depending on the most invasive treatment. To adjust for potential selection bias in treatment assignment, using multivariate analysis, patients were divided into quintiles of likelihood of polypectomy (propensity scores), and outcomes were compared in each quintile.

Results.—Surgical resection was performed in 1340 (64.5%) patients and polypectomy was performed in 737 (35.5%) patients. Predictors for undergoing polypectomy ($P<.001$) included older age, greater comorbidity, no history of polyps, diagnosis in 2002 or later, left colon site of cancer, well-differentiated tumors, and colonoscopy performed in an outpatient setting. Both 1-year and 5-year survival were higher in the surgical group (92% and 75%, respectively) than in the polypectomy group (88% and 62%, respectively). The unadjusted hazard ratio was 1.15 (95% confidence interval [CI], 1.31-1.74). After adjusting for propensity quintile, the hazard ratio was 1.15 (95% CI, 0.98-1.33). Within each propensity quintile, the risk of death was similar between the 2 groups (interaction test $P = .96$).

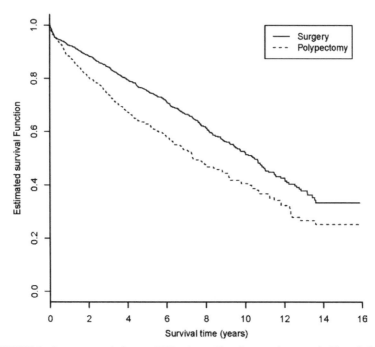

FIGURE 1.—Long-term survival among 2077 patients with malignant polyps treated with surgical resection or colonoscopic polypectomy is shown. In unadjusted analysis, survival was improved among patients treated surgically (*P*<.001 [log-rank test]). (Reprinted from Cooper GS, Xu F, Barnholtz Sloan JS, et al. Management of malignant colonic polyps: a population-based analysis of colonoscopic polypectomy versus surgery. *Cancer.* 2012;118:651-659. Copyright 2012 American Cancer Society. This material is reproduced with permission of Wiley-Liss, Inc., a subsidiary of John Wiley & Sons, Inc.)

Conclusions.—In this large, population-based sample, more than one-third of patients with malignant polyps were treated with colonoscopic polypectomy. Outcomes were similar to surgical patients with comparable clinical characteristics and could be offered to patients who meet appropriate clinical criteria (Fig 1).

▶ The definitive oncologic treatment of T1 adenocarcinomas of the colon arising in an adenomatous polyp is controversial. These minimally invasive cancers can generally easily be removed by colonoscopic polypectomy and thus spare patients a major operation. However, removal of the polyp and surrounding mucosa obviously provides no information about potential lymph node metastases or lymphovascular space invasion. For these reasons, there has been considerable debate about the optimal approach and case series have not provided convincing data. Cooper et al tackled this dilemma using a population database, the Surveillance Epidemiology and End-Results (SEER) Medicare database, to study the outcomes of 2077 patients with colonic polyps with T1 cancers treated either by colonoscopic polypectomy or surgical resection. Thirty-five percent of the patients had colonoscopic removal. The unadjusted data (Fig 1) show that patients treated surgically had improved survival compared with those patients treated endoscopically. However, when the data were adjusted for selection bias for treatment by propensity scoring, the difference in survival was not apparent. Likely the survival following either treatment approach is quite good, and therefore small differences are difficult to discern. However, do propensity scores adequately assign bias? In this study, all variables, and not just those that were statistically different on multivariate analysis, were included in the propensity scoring. Perhaps this approach should be compared with propensity scoring in which only statistically significant selection factors are included. Importantly, we must be careful to base major treatment decisions on data that are derived from population databases that are further manipulated. Although these statistical approaches may be valid, we are confronted with a data set that shows that patients fare better with surgery unless the data are adjusted. Does it make sense clinically to resect only the polyp and not surrounding lymph nodes in a potentially curable patient?

K. E. Behrns, MD

Optimizing Surgical Care of Colon Cancer in the Older Adult Population
Kennedy GD, Rajamanickam V, O'Connor ES, et al (Univ of Wisconsin School of Medicine and Public Health, Madison)
Ann Surg 253:508-514, 2011

Objective.—We have undertaken the current study to evaluate factors that correlate with postoperative complications in older patients undergoing surgery for colon cancer.

Patients and Methods.—The database of the American College of Surgeons (ACS) National Surgical Quality Improvement Program (NSQIP) from years 2005 to 2008 was accessed. Patients age 65 and older were included according to Current Procedural Terminology and International Classification of Disease-9 codes. Preoperative and operative variables were examined and postoperative complications assessed using a combination of univariate and multivariate statistical models. Propensity score matching was used to control for nonrandomization of the database.

Results.—We found that patients undergoing laparoscopic (n = 2113) and open (n = 3801) surgery for the diagnosis of colon cancer were similar in age and gender. However, patients undergoing laparoscopic surgery were generally at lower risk for developing postoperative complications (16.1% vs. 25.4%, $P < 0.005$). Statistical models controlling for preoperative and operative variables demonstrated patients with elevated body mass index (odds ratio [OR] = 1.26), a history of chronic obstructive pulmonary disease (OR = 1.63), over age 85 (OR = 1.35), a surgery lasting longer than 4 hours (OR = 1.48), or having undergone an open operation (OR = 1.53) to have increased risk for developing postoperative complications. Propensity score match analysis confirmed these results.

Conclusions.—Identification of preoperative factors that predispose patients to postoperative complications could allow for the institution of protocols that may decrease these events. Furthermore, expanding the role of laparoscopy in the treatment of older patients with colon cancer may decrease rates of postoperative complications.

▶ The elderly population in the United States will occupy an increasing proportion of patients that require surgical treatment, especially for colon cancer. Therefore, examination of variables that will improve the outcome of elderly patients with colon cancer is pertinent and timely. Kennedy et al used the American College of Surgeons National Surgical Quality Improvement Program to examine outcome variables in almost 6000 elderly patients (N = 2113 laparoscopic; N = 3801 open) undergoing surgery for colon cancer. They used 3 statistical approaches to assess predictors of outcome and found that the laparoscopic surgical approach was associated with fewer complications (16.1% vs 25.4%). Furthermore, postoperative complications were more likely in patients with an increased body mass index, chronic obstructive pulmonary disease, age over 85 years, surgery duration greater than 4 hours, and an open operation. This is one of several recent studies that assess risk factors in elderly patients. Several previous studies have suggested that the elderly, usually defined as greater than 65 years of age, have similar outcomes to young patients. However, recent analyses contest this finding. Perhaps, as we operate on more elderly patients, our anecdotal experience suggests that the outcome of this subset of patients does not match that of the accompanying literature. Furthermore, the costs associated with the often prolonged hospital stay of these patients are likely having a great influence on hospitals' bottom lines. More importantly, several articles like this one provide risk factors for selecting patients or operative approaches. Will we continue to offer operations to elderly patients with known risk factors for complications? We need to take these findings a step further and compare the outcomes of elderly patients that have operative therapy versus those who chose nonoperative therapy and assess not only duration of life but quality of life.

K. E. Behrns, MD

Identification of a Biomarker Profile Associated With Resistance to Neoadjuvant Chemoradiation Therapy in Rectal Cancer

Garcia-Aguilar J, Chen Z, Smith DD, et al (City of Hope, Duarte, CA; et al)
Ann Surg 254:486-493, 2011

Objective.—To identify a biomarker profile associated with tumor response to chemoradiation (CRT) in locally advanced rectal cancer.

Background.—Rectal cancer response to neoadjuvant CRT is variable. Whereas some patients have a minimal response, others achieve a pathologic complete response (pCR) and have no viable cancer cells in their surgical specimens. Identifying biomarkers of response will help select patients more likely to benefit from CRT.

Methods.—This study includes 132 patients with locally advanced rectal cancer treated with neoadjuvant CRT followed by surgery. Tumor DNA from pretreatment tumor biopsies and control DNA from paired normal surgical specimens was screened for mutations and polymorphisms in 23 genes. Genetic biomarkers were correlated with tumor response to CRT (pCR vs non-pCR), and the association of single or combined biomarkers with tumor response was determined.

Results.—Thirty-three of 132 (25%) patients achieved a pCR and 99 (75%) patients had non-pCR. Three individual markers were associated with non-pCR; v-Ki-ras2 Kirsten rat sarcoma viral oncogene homolog muta-tion ($P = 0.0145$), *cyclin D1* G870A (AA) polymorphism ($P = 0.0138$), and *methylenetetrahydrofolate reductase (NAD(P)H)* C677T (TT) polymor-phism ($P = 0.0120$). Analysis of biomarker combinations revealed that none of the 27 patients with both *tumor protein p53 (p53)* and *v-Ki-ras2 Kirsten rat sarcoma viral oncogene homolog* mutations had a pCR. Further, in patients with both *p53* and *v-Ki-ras2 Kirsten rat sarcoma viral oncogene homolog* mutations or the *cyclin D1* G870A (AA) polymorphism or the *methylenetetrahydrofolate reductase (NAD(P)H)* C677T (TT) polymor-phism (n = 52) the association with non-pCR was further strengthened; 51 of 52 (98%) of patients were non-pCR. These biomarker combinations had a validity of more than 70% and a positive predictive value of 97% to 100%, predicting that patients harboring these mutation/polymorphism profiles will not achieve a pCR.

Conclusions.—A specific biomarker profile is strongly associated with non-pCR to CRT and could be used to select optimal oncologic therapy in rectal cancer patients. ClinicalTrials.org Identifier: NCT00335816.

▶ The era of personalized medicine is upon us, and the work of Garcia-Aguilar et al takes a major step into this epoch. Responsiveness to treatment for either benign or malignant disease will be shaped by a patient's genetic profile. In this article, individual genes and combinations of genes that predicted lack of responsiveness to neoadjuvant therapy for rectal cancer were identified. The study was likely designed to find biomarkers that were associated with respon-siveness to preoperative chemoradiation therapy, but nonetheless, a group of patients who do not respond to a treatment will be spared the toxicity. Obvi-ously, a limitation of this study, as noted in the discussion, is the relatively small group of patients. Large numbers of patients will need to be studied and validated to determine the individual or combined genetic signatures that will predict response to treatment. This will be a Herculean task that will demand surgeons take a different approach to patients and disease manage-ment. In addition, the workforce in medicine must undergo change since treat-ment decisions will be made on large volumes of genetic data, which physicians are not prepared to interpret at this point. Will a biostatistician become the decision-maker in the health care team? Although personalization of medicine is exciting and potentially hugely beneficial to the patient and society, who will pay for it in times of major economic difficulties facing health care? This excellent article is thought-provoking and makes one wonder how the future of medicine will progress. We must stand ready to adapt to significant change in the care of our patients.

K. E. Behrns, MD

Morbidity Risk Factors After Low Anterior Resection With Total Mesorectal Excision and Coloanal Anastomosis: A Retrospective Series of 483 Patients

Bennis M, Parc Y, Lefevre JH, et al (Univ Paris VI (Pierre and Marie Curie), France)

Ann Surg 255:504-510, 2012

Objective.—To report postoperative morbidity after low anterior resection (LAR) and coloanal anastomosis (CAA) for rectal cancer and identify possible risk factors of complications.

Background.—Coloanal anastomosis after total mesorectal excision (TME) is associated with significant morbidity. Precise data on the specific morbidity and the risk factors are lacking.

Methods.—We analyzed retrospectively 483 consecutive LARs with TME and CAA carried out in a single center between 1996 and 2005. All complications occurring up to 3 months after LAR and up to 3 months after closure of the diverting stoma were graded according to the Dindo classification.

Results.—Of 483 patients, 164 (33.9%) suffered at least 1 complication, leading to death in 2 (0.4%) patients. Grade III/IV complications occurred in 69 of 483 (14.2%) patients. Thirty-four (7.0%) patients developed leakage of the CAA and 3 patients had leakage of the small bowel anastomosis after stoma closure. Ileostomy closure was carried out after a mean of 88.7 days (36−630) after LAR. The stoma was not closed in 4 of 456 (0.6%) patients. In multivariate analysis, male sex ($P = 0.0216$) and postoperative transfusion ($P = 0.0025$) were associated with complications. Medical complications were furthermore associated with previous thromboembolic events ($P = 0.0012$) and associated surgery at the time of LAR ($P = 0.0010$). Circumferential tumor localization was predictive of surgical complications ($P = 0.0015$). The only factor associated with a risk of leakage was transfusion ($P = 0.0216$).

Conclusions.—In this series morbidity occurred in 34% and dehiscence of the CAA in 7.0%. Transfusion requirement was an independent risk factor for postoperative complications and anastomotic leakage.

▶ The treatment of rectal cancer has evolved significantly in the last 2 decades largely because of the introduction of neoadjuvant therapy for T3 tumors and transanal excision for T1 and possibly T2 tumors. However, this study by Bennis et al demonstrates that surgical treatment of rectal cancer treated by low anterior resection with total mesorectal excision and coloanal anastomosis has improved significantly in the last 15 years. The findings of this retrospective study of 483 patients found that the mortality rate was 0.4% and the morbidity rate was 34%. Furthermore, the overall leak rate, including that of the diverting stoma, was 7%, and surprisingly, the rate of permanent stoma was an incredibly low 0.87%. Notably, however, the rate of a permanent stoma was 10.8% in patients that experienced an anastomotic leak. Risk factors for postoperative complications were male sex and blood transfusion, whereas the latter was also predictive of anastomotic leak. These results were likely the product of a standardized system of care that had excellent compliance by all practitioners. However, of note, 179 patients received neoadjuvant therapy, but 235 patients were ypT3, indicating that 56 patients (11.6%) either had tumors that were untreated with neoadjuvant therapy or grew in the face of treatment. This is an important subset of patients that deserve elaboration. However, overall, the authors should be congratulated for outstanding results with a coloanal anastomosis that often carries great risk. Clearly, their standardized approach has yielded excellent results that serve as a benchmark.

K. E. Behrns, MD

Surgery for Locally Recurrent Rectal Cancer in the Era of Total Mesorectal Excision: Is There Still a Chance for Cure?

Rahbari NN, Ulrich AB, Bruckner T, et al (Univ of Heidelberg, Germany)
Ann Surg 253:522-533, 2011

Objective.—To evaluate the perioperative outcome and long-term survival of patients who underwent surgical resection for recurrent rectal cancer within a multimodal approach in the era of total mesorectal excision (TME).

Background.—Introduction of TME has reduced local recurrence and improved oncological outcome of patients with rectal cancer. Local recurrence after TME still occurs in 2% to 8% of patients and presents a challenge to surgical and medical oncologists. However, there has been very limited data on the perioperative and long-term outcome of patients who are operated for local recurrence in the era of TME.

Methods.—A total of 107 patients who were identified from a prospective rectal cancer database underwent surgical exploration for recurrent rectal cancer after previous TME between October 2001 and April 2009. Risk factors of perioperative morbidity were analyzed using a multivariate logistic regression model. Independent predictors of disease-specific survival were identified by a Cox proportional hazards regression model, as were those of local recurrence and disease recurrence at any site.

Results.—Surgical resection was performed in 92 patients and negative resection margins were achieved in 54 (58.7%) of these. Recurrent disease was located intraluminally and extraluminally in 35 (38.0%) patients and 57 (62.0%) patients, respectively. A total of 19 (20.6%) patients had metastatic extrapelvic disease at the time of surgery. Perioperative surgical morbidity and in-hospital mortality accounted for 42.4% and 3.3%, respectively. On multivariate analysis, partial sacrectomy was associated with surgical morbidity ($P = 0.004$). Three- and 5-year disease-specific survival rates were 61% and 47%. Three-year survival rate of patients with extrapelvic disease who underwent R0 resection was 42%. On multivariate analysis, surgical morbidity ($P = 0.001$), presence of extrapelvic disease ($P = 0.006$), and noncurative (R1; R2) resection ($P < 0.0001$) were identified as independent adverse predictors of disease-specific survival, whereas a transabdominal resection (as opposed to an abdominoperineal resection/pelvic exenteration) was associated with a more favorable prognosis ($P = 0.04$).

Conclusions.—Surgical resection of local recurrence from rectal cancer in the era TME can be carried out with acceptable morbidity and curative resection rates. Curative resection remains the major prognostic factor and may enable long-term survival even in patients with extrapelvic disease.

▶ Rahbari et al question whether recurrent rectal cancer following total mesorectal excision can be cured. In 92 of 107 patients, surgical resection of recurrent rectal disease was performed, and in nearly 60% of these patients, negative margins were achieved. These operations were undertaken in the setting of multimodality therapy using various combinations of chemotherapy and radiotherapy. The mortality rate was 3.3%, and the morbidity rate was 42%. Three- and 5-year disease-specific survival rates were 61% and 47%, respectively. Even in patients with extrapelvic disease, the 3-year survival rate of R0 resections was 42%. These data convincingly demonstrate that there is indeed a chance for cure of recurrent rectal disease, but the cost, in terms of morbidity, is relatively high. Furthermore, complex operations associated with the need for sacral resection and blood products were associated with surgical morbidity. This study provides pertinent data that provide surgeons with information allowing an open discussion with patients about the chance for cure from recurrent rectal cancer. However, a caveat must be introduced—the median follow-up was relatively short at 23 months. In addition, because the morbidity of surgery was relatively high, the value of the treatment would be best assessed with quality-of-life data. Clinical cancer studies that examine the results of treatment should be accompanied by data that demonstrate the delivery of quality life to the patients. It is only in this context that we will be able to fully assess our treatment regimens.

K. E. Behrns, MD

Pathologic Complete Response of Primary Tumor Following Preoperative Chemoradiotherapy for Locally Advanced Rectal Cancer: Long-term Outcomes and Prognostic Significance of Pathologic Nodal Status (KROG 09-01)
Yeo S-G, Kim DY, Kim TH, et al (Natl Cancer Ctr, Goyang, Korea; et al)
Ann Surg 252:998-1004, 2010

Objective.—To investigate long-term outcomes of locally advanced rectal cancer (LARC) patients with postchemoradiotherapy (post-CRT) pathologic complete response of primary tumor (ypT0) and determine prognostic significance of post-CRT pathologic nodal (ypN) status.

Background.—LARC patients with post-CRT pathologic complete response were suggested to have favorable long-term outcomes, but prognostic significance of ypN status has never been specifically defined in ypT0 patients.

Methods.—The Korean Radiation Oncology Group collected clinical data for 333 LARC patients with ypT0 following preoperative CRT and curative radical resections between 1993 and 2007. Sphincter preservation surgery and abdominoperineal resection were performed in 283 (85.0%) and 50 (15.0%) patients, respectively. Postoperative chemotherapy was given to 285 (85.6%) patients. Survival was estimated by the Kaplan-Meier method, and the Cox proportional hazard model was used in multivariate analyses.

Results.—After median follow-up of 43 (range = 14–172) months, 5 year disease-free survival (DFS) was 84.6% and overall survival (OS) was 92.8%. The ypN status was ypT0N0 in 304 (91.3%), ypT0N1 in 22 (6.6%), and ypT0N2 in 7 (2.1%) patients. The ypN status was the most relevant independent prognostic factor for both DFS and OS in

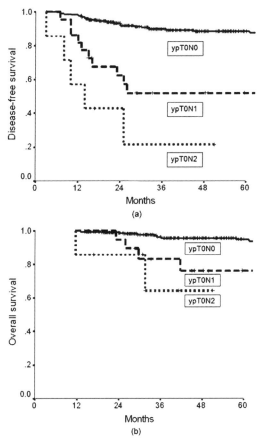

FIGURE 1.—Disease-free survival (A) and overall survival (B) by ypN status in 333 ypT0N0–2 patients. The 5-year DFS rates were 88.5%, 51.9%, and 21.4%, and the 5-year OS rates were 94.8%, 76.2%, and 64.3% in ypT0N0 (n = 304), ypT0N1 (n = 22), and ypT0N2 (n = 7) patients, respectively. (Reprinted from Yeo S-G, Kim DY, Kim TH, et al. Pathologic complete response of primary tumor following preoperative chemoradiotherapy for locally advanced rectal cancer: long-term outcomes and prognostic significance of pathologic nodal status (KROG 09-01). *Ann Surg.* 2010;252:998-1004. © Southeastern Surgical Congress.)

ypT0 patients. The 5-year DFS and OS was 88.5% and 94.8% in ypT0N0 patients, and 45.2% and 72.8% in ypT0N+ patients (both, $P < 0.001$).

Conclusions.—LARC patients achieving ypT0N0 after preoperative CRT had favorable long-term outcomes, whereas positive ypN status had a poor prognosis even after total regression of primary tumor (Fig 1).

▶ Yeo et al significantly advance our understanding of patient outcomes following neoadjuvant chemoradiotherapy for locally advanced rectal cancer. This multi-institutional trial retrospectively analyzed the outcome of patients who had a variety of chemotherapeutic regimens and varying doses of radiation therapy followed by anal sphincter—preserving surgery (85%) or abdominoperineal resection (15%). Patients who had a complete clinical primary tumor response (n = 333) were followed for a median of 43 months. As demonstrated in Fig 1, patients without lymph node involvement on pathologic assessment had a significantly increased disease-free survival (85%) and overall survival (93%); however, patients with new or persistent nodal involvement had a significantly worse outcome. Although several studies have demonstrated the improved survival after a complete clinical response, this study clearly shows that posttreatment lymph node involvement portends a poor prognosis. Furthermore, most of these patients also had postoperative chemotherapy. These results clearly show that postoperative chemotherapy regimens in patients with N1 or N2 lymph node status need to be altered and studied. This study demonstrates the value of refining our approach to treatment protocols by continually assessing our data not only for the successes of treatment but for the areas where treatment must be improved.

K. E. Behrns, MD

What Is the Risk for a Permanent Stoma After Low Anterior Resection of the Rectum for Cancer? A Six-Year Follow-Up of a Multicenter Trial
Lindgren R, Hallböök O, Rutegård J, et al (Örebro Univ Hosp, Sweden; Linköping Univ Hosp, Sweden; Umeå Univ, Sweden)
Dis Colon Rectum 54:41-47, 2011

Purpose.—The aim of this study was to assess the risk for permanent stoma after low anterior resection of the rectum for cancer.

Methods.—In a nationwide multicenter trial 234 patients undergoing low anterior resection of the rectum were randomly assigned to a group with defunctioning stomas (n = 116) or a group with no defunctioning stomas (n = 118). The median age was 68 years, 45% of the patients were women, 79% had preoperative radiotherapy, and 4% had International Union Against Cancer cancer stage IV. The patients were analyzed with regard to the presence of a permanent stoma, the type of stoma, the time point at which the stoma was constructed or considered as permanent, and the reasons for obtaining a permanent stoma. Median follow-up was 72 months (42–108). One patient with a defunctioning stoma who died within 30 days after the rectal resection was excluded from the analysis.

Results.—During the study period 19% (45/233) of the patients obtained a permanent stoma: 25 received an end sigmoid stoma and 20 received a loop ileostomy. The end sigmoid stomas were constructed at a median of 22 months (1−71) after the low anterior resection of the rectum, and the loop ileostomies were considered as permanent at a median of 12.5 months (1−47) after the initial rectal resection. The reasons for loop ileostomy were metastatic disease (n = 6), unsatisfactory anorectal function (n = 6), deteriorated general medical condition (n = 3), new noncolorectal cancer (n = 2), patient refusal of further surgery (n = 2), and chronic constipation (n = 1). Reasons for end sigmoid stoma were unsatisfactory anorectal function (n = 22) and urgent surgery owing to anastomotic leakage (n = 3). The risk for permanent stomas in patients with symptomatic anastomotic leakage was 56% (25/45) compared with 11% (20/188) in those without symptomatic anastomotic leakage (P < .001).

Conclusion.—One patient of 5 ended up with a permanent stoma after low anterior resection of the rectum for cancer, and half of the patients with a permanent stoma had previous symptomatic anastomotic leakage (Fig 2).

▶ Using data gathered from a previously published multicenter trial, Lindgren et al found that 1 in 5 patients who underwent a low anterior resection for cancer had a permanent ostomy at 6 years of follow-up. This finding was regardless of

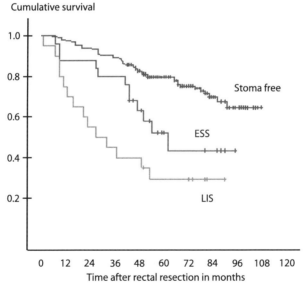

FIGURE 2.—Kaplan-Meier curve demonstrating crude survival in 233 patients undergoing LAR from December 1999 to June 2005 at a median follow-up of 72 months (42−108) in patients who were stoma free (n = 188), had permanent LIS (n = 20), or who had permanent ESS (n = 25). LAR = low anterior resection; LIS = permanent loop ileostomy; ESS = permanent end sigmoid stoma. (Reprinted from Lindgren R, Hallböök O, Rutegård J, et al. What is the risk for a permanent stoma after low anterior resection of the rectum for cancer? A six-year follow-up of a multicenter trial. *Dis Colon Rectum.* 2011;54:41-47, with permission from The ASCRS.)

the intent for an ostomy with 16% of those patients primarily diverted requiring a permanent stoma, whereas 22% of those patients not diverted requiring a stoma. The primary risk factor for a permanent stoma was a symptomatic anastomotic leak. In addition, age greater than 75 years was an independent predictor for a permanent stoma. This study highlights the necessity of a water-tight low anastomosis in the performance of a low anterior resection because more than half of the patients who had a permanent stoma had a postoperative leak. These data beg the question, "Should all patients with a low anterior resection have a diverting ostomy in an attempt to prevent a leak?" The authors correctly point out that the mere presence of an ostomy will increase the likelihood of having a permanent ostomy. However, the data confirm that a leak is the primary factor in the necessity of a permanent stoma. Fig 2 is also important because it clearly demonstrates that freedom from a stoma results in improved long-term survival. Certainly, there are numerous factors that affect survival, but the presence of a stoma indicates an overall poor medical condition from a variety of causes. The authors should be congratulated for the use of a multicenter trial to address pertinent questions about anorectal function and the risk of a permanent stoma.

K. E. Behrns, MD

Enhanced recovery pathways optimize health outcomes and resource utilization: A meta-analysis of randomized controlled trials in colorectal surgery

Adamina M, Kehlet H, Tomlinson GA, et al (Univ Hosps Case Med Ctr Cleveland, OH; Copenhagen Univ, Denmark; Univ of Toronto, Ontario, Canada; et al)
Surgery 149:830-840, 2011

Background.—Health care systems provide care to increasingly complex and elderly patients. Colorectal surgery is a prime example, with high volumes of major procedures, significant morbidity, prolonged hospital stays, and unplanned readmissions. This situation is exacerbated by an exponential rise in costs that threatens the stability of health care systems. Enhanced recovery pathways (ERP) have been proposed as a means to reduce morbidity and improve effectiveness of care. We have reviewed the evidence supporting the implementation of ERP in clinical practice.

Methods.—Medline, Embase, and the Cochrane library were searched for randomized, controlled trials comparing ERP with traditional care in colorectal surgery. Systematic reviews and papers on ERP based on data published in major surgical and anesthesiology journals were critically reviewed by international contributors, experienced in the development and implementation of ERP.

Results.—A random-effect Bayesian meta-analysis was performed, including 6 randomized, controlled trials totalizing 452 patients. For patients adhering to ERP, length of stay decreased by 2.5 days (95% credible interval [CrI] -3.92 to -1.11), whereas 30-day morbidity was halved (relative risk, 0.52; 95% CrI, 0.36$-$0.73) and readmission was not increased (relative risk, 0.59; 95% CrI, 0.14—1.43) when compared with patients undergoing traditional care.

Conclusion.—Adherence to ERP achieves a reproducible improvement in the quality of care by enabling standardization of health care processes. Thus, while accelerating recovery and safely reducing hospital stay, ERPs optimize utilization of health care resources. ERPs can and should be routinely used in care after colorectal and other major gastrointestinal procedures.

▶ The rapid increase in health care costs over the last several years has prompted payers to seek models of reimbursement that move from paying for quantity to paying for quality. Surgical benchmarks for quality include length of stay, readmission rates, and morbidity. Multiple colorectal surgery groups have addressed this issue by instituting enhanced recovery pathways (ERP) that clearly define the preoperative, intraoperative, and postoperative proscriptive care plans that delineate the perioperative management. Adamina et al report here a meta-analysis that examined the collective results of 6 published studies using ERP. They found that use of these pathways was associated with a 2.5-day decrease in length of stay and a 50% reduction in morbidity without increasing the readmission rate. Clearly, this article and the component studies show the effectiveness of ERP, so why are these patient care plans so infrequently adopted? First and foremost, physicians, and especially surgeons, were trained to be independent practitioners rather than group participants. Adherence to ERP requires relinquishing freedom of care and following an agreed-upon, evidence-based care plan that may deviate significantly from previously used care. Thus, compliance with such care plans is low. Second, surgeons often suggest that the patients they care for are more complicated than others and therefore cannot be managed by an ERP. Obviously, patients come with different comorbidities, but for a large group of patients having a particular operation (colectomy), we can measure and predict the patients that have additional comorbidities and require a modified care plan. The time for implementation of ERP for many types of operative procedures is now, before we are forced to alter patient care and receive lower compensation without input.

K. E. Behrns, MD

Randomized clinical trial of fluid restriction in colorectal surgery
Abraham-Nordling M, Hjern F, Pollack J, et al (Danderyd Hosp, Stockholm, Sweden; et al)
Br J Surg 99:186-191, 2012

Background.—Perioperative fluid therapy can influence postoperative hospital stay and complications after elective colorectal surgery. This trial was designed to examine whether an extremely restricted perioperative fluid protocol would reduce hospital stay beyond the existing fast-track hospital time of 7 days after surgery.

Methods.—Patients were randomized to restricted or standard perioperative intravenous fluid regimens in a single-centre trial. Randomization was stratified for colonic, rectal, open and laparoscopic surgery. Patients were all treated within a fast-track protocol (careful preoperative preparation, optimal analgesia, early oral nutrition and early mobilization). The primary endpoint was length of postoperative hospital stay. The secondary endpoint was complications within 30 days.

Results.—Seventy-nine patients were randomized to restricted and 82 to standard fluid therapy. Patients in the restricted group received a median of 3050 ml fluid on the day of surgery compared with 5775 ml in the standard group ($P < 0\cdot001$). There was no difference between groups in primary hospital stay (median $6\cdot0$ days in both groups; $P = 0\cdot194$) or stay including readmission (median $6\cdot0$ days in both groups; $P = 0\cdot158$). The proportion of patients with complications was significantly lower in the restricted group (31 of 79 *versus* 47 of 82; $P = 0\cdot027$). Vasopressors were more often required in the restricted group (97 *versus* 80 per cent; $P < 0\cdot001$).

Conclusion.—Restricted perioperative intravenous fluid administration does not reduce length of stay in a fast-track protocol.

▶ Several investigators have examined outcomes with restricted perioperative fluid regimens to decrease complications and shorten the postoperative length of stay. Abraham-Nordling et al conducted a well-designed clinical trial to address the role of fluid restriction after colorectal surgery with the primary endpoint of length of stay. The results noted no difference in length of stay, but important differences in the groups are notable. First, the restricted group had significantly fewer complications, especially anastomotic problems, even though this variable did not achieve statistical significance. However, the restricted group tended to have more cardiovascular and renal complications than the standard group. What factors may explain these outcomes? Likely, patient variability is an important factor, and the definitions of standard therapy may also have an impact. For instance, it is unusual for colorectal surgery patients in the United States to be treated with vasopressors in the perioperative period. Even in the standard therapy group, 80% of patients received vasopressors, whereas 97% in the restricted group received this treatment. How this may influence the complications and outcomes is not clear. Finally, the fluid regimens in this and other studies are dichotomous, either restricted or standard therapy, but our patients do not belong to dichotomous groups. Therefore, fluid regimens that account for patient-specific factors such as cardiac disease are needed. This is the judgment and art of medicine. Although we may use a restricted fluid regimen as a foundation of treatment, modifications of such regimens for individual patients may be necessary. Standardization of care is desirable, but we must allow flexibility of care that permits optimal treatment of the individual patient.

K. E. Behrns, MD

Randomized clinical trial of perioperative selective decontamination of the digestive tract *versus* placebo in elective gastrointestinal surgery
Roos D, Dijksman LM, Oudemans-van Straaten HM, et al (Onze Lieve Vrouwe Gasthuis, Amsterdam, The Netherlands; et al)
Br J Surg 98:1365-1372, 2011

Background.—This randomized clinical trial analysed the effect of perioperative selective decontamination of the digestive tract (SDD) in elective gastrointestinal surgery on postoperative infectious complications and leakage.

Methods.—All patients undergoing elective gastrointestinal surgery during a 5-year period were evaluated for inclusion. Randomized patients received either SDD (polymyxin B sulphate, tobramycin and amphotericin) or placebo in addition to standard antibiotic prophylaxis. The primary endpoint was postoperative infectious complications and anastomotic leakage during the hospital stay or 30 days after surgery.

Results.—A total of 289 patients were randomized to either SDD (143) or placebo (146). Most patients (190, 65·7 per cent) underwent colonic surgery. There were 28 patients (19·6 per cent) with infectious complications in the SDD group compared with 45 (30·8 per cent) in the placebo group ($P = 0·028$). The incidence of anastomotic leakage in the SDD group was 6·3 per cent *versus* 15·1 per cent in the placebo group ($P = 0·016$). Hospital stay and mortality did not differ between groups.

Conclusion.—Perioperative SDD in elective gastrointestinal surgery combined with standard intravenous antibiotics reduced the rate of postoperative infectious complications and anastomotic leakage compared with standard intravenous antibiotics alone. Perioperative SDD should be considered for patients undergoing gastrointestinal surgery. Registration number: P02.1187L (Dutch Central Committee on Research Involving Human Subjects).

▶ Selective decontamination of the digestive tract (SDD) has been studied multiple times previously, dating back to the 1970s. However, this strategy to reduce infectious complications following gastrointestinal surgery or in immuno-compromised patients has not been popular. Roos et al showed in this study that indeed SDD can decrease the rate of infectious complications following gastrointestinal surgery, but SDD still has several pitfalls that need to be addressed before its widespread adoption. Because SDD administration is associated with a reduced rate of infectious complications (these complications are costly), the approach is worthwhile, but we must take time to definitively address the issues with medication compliance and efficacy. First, the issue of compliance with medication intake needs to be considered. Patients will not comply with this awful-tasting combination of medicines. A partnership with industry or payers, who wish to decrease the costs of infectious complications, should be able to assist with rectifying this problem. Second, it is clear that 2 days of preparation is inadequate. Assuming we improve the taste of the medicine, could this regimen not be administered at home for 3 to 5 days preoperatively? Finally, it is clear that even though patients took the medications, only 45% of patients seemed to achieve the benefit of rectal decontamination. Presumably, the low rate of decontamination occurred because of the short 2-day preparation; however, this shortcoming needs to be addressed up front to truly determine whether the gastrointestinal tract can be decontaminated. SDD is a worthwhile approach, but we must cease studying SDD in clinical trials, which continue to show promise, until we address the basic defects with the approach. Too often we restudy approaches without clearly addressing the fundamental issues with a treatment strategy.

K. E. Behrns, MD

The Effect of Alvimopan on Recovery After Laparoscopic Segmental Colectomy
Obokhare ID, Champagne B, Stein SL, et al (Univ Hosps Case Med Ctr, Cleveland, OH)
Dis Colon Rectum 54:743-746, 2011

Background.—Alvimopan, a peripherally acting μ-opioid receptor antagonist, was recently approved for the reduction of postoperative ileus after open colectomy. No data are available regarding the use of alvimopan following laparoscopic segmental colectomy.

Objective.—This study was designed to evaluate the effectiveness of alvimopan in patients undergoing laparoscopic segmental colectomy.

Design.—A retrospective review of segmental laparoscopic colectomy was conducted in a population of patients using an accelerated postcolectomy care pathway. Patients that received alvimopan were identified from an institutional review board-approved database and matched with nonalvimopan patients for age, sex, procedure, and diagnosis. Patients with a diverting ileostomy or with contraindications for alvimopam were excluded.

Results.—One hundred patients undergoing laparoscopic colectomy received alvimopan perioperatively and were matched with a similar group of nonalvimopan patients. Although patients on alvimopan were significantly less likely to develop postoperative ileus (4% vs 12%; $P=.04$), there was no difference in length of hospital stay (3.63 days in the alvimopan group vs 3.78 in the nonalvimopan group; $P=.84$) or 30-day readmission rate (4.0% vs 4.2%; $P=.95$).

Conclusions.—As the cost of providing health care continues to increase, reductions in perioperative complications and hospital stay are important to hospital efficiency and patient care. Alvimopan effectively reduces the incidence of postoperative ileus in patients undergoing open colectomy; however, hospital stay and readmission rates were not altered in this laparoscopic group. Further study is required before alvimopan can be routinely used in patients undergoing laparoscopic colectomy (Table 1).

▶ In the last decade, significant emphasis has been placed on prompt discharge of patients following surgery. This is complicated in patients undergoing gastrointestinal surgery because of the unpredictable nature of postoperative ileus.

TABLE 1.—Patient Demographics and Surgical Characteristics

	Alvimopan (ALC)	No Alvimopan (NLC)	P
No. of patients	100	100	
Mean age, y	62	61	
Female, n	55	51	.57
Male, n	45	49	.57
POI	4%	12%	.04[a]
LOS (mean days)	3.63	3.78	.84[a]
Diagnosis			
Crohn's	12%	9%	.49
Diverticulitis	20%	20%	1.00
Colon cancer	61%	68%	.30
Other[b]	7%	3%	.19
Readmission rates, n (%)	4 (4)	6 (4.17)	.95[a]

ALC = alvimopan laparoscopic colectomy; NLC = nonalvimopan laparoscopic colectomy; POI = postoperative ileus; LOS = length of stay.
[a]P value of <.05 was considered significant.
[b]Other includes ulcerative colitis, rectal prolapse, and volvulus.

However, with the administration of the opioid antagonist, alvimopan, postoperative ileus has decreased in patients who have had an open segmental colectomy. The value of alvimopan in laparoscopic colectomy, however, has not been demonstrated. Obokhare et al addressed this question by retrospectively comparing the outcome of patients undergoing laparoscopic segmental colectomy with perioperative alvimopan compared with a matched group of patients that underwent colectomy without alvimopan. The results showed that fewer patients with alvimopan experienced postoperative ileus compared with patients without alvimopan administration (Table 1). Importantly, however, the length of stay was not influenced by alvimopan. The length of stay was 3.63 days with alvimopan versus 3.78 without alvimopan. This group of experienced authors has obviously worked diligently to decrease the length of stay by implementing standardized postoperative care pathways, as the control group length of stay is less than 4 days, which is substantially less than the typical 4.5 days. Therefore, demonstration of alvimopan effectiveness in this group of patients may be difficult given the already short length of stay. The authors are on the right track, however, in recommending a randomized trial to determine if further decreases in length of stay are possible.

K. E. Behrns, MD

Long-term Results After Stapled Hemorrhoidopexy: A Prospective Study With a 6-Year Follow-Up

Ommer A, Hinrichs J, Möllenberg H, et al (Evang. Huyssens-Stiftung, Essen, Germany; et al)

Dis Colon Rectum 54:601-608, 2011

Background.—Stapled hemorrhoidopexy was introduced in 1998 as a new technique for treating advanced hemorrhoidal disease. Despite a clear perioperative advantage regarding pain and patient comfort, literature reviews indicate a higher recurrence rate for stapled hemorrhoidopexy than for conventional techniques.

Objective.—Our aim was to present long-term on the use of this technique.

Design.—Observational study.

Setting and Patients.—Consecutive patients with hemorrhoid prolapse treated at a regional surgical center from May 27, 1999, through December 31, 2003.

Intervention.—Stapled hemorrhoidopexy with accompanying resection of residual hemorrhoidal nodules if necessary.

Main Outcome Measures.—Standardized patient questionnaire regarding satisfaction, resolution of symptoms, and performance of further interventions.

Results.—Of 257 patients (82 female, 175 male, mean age 53 ± 13 years) undergoing stapled hemorrhoidopexy, follow-up data were available for 224 patients (87.2%) with a mean duration of 6.3 ± 1.2 years. Of these, 195 patients (87.1%) were satisfied or very satisfied with the operation outcome; 19 patients (8.5%) were moderately satisfied; and 10 (4.5%) were not satisfied. Regarding preoperative anal symptoms, complete relief was observed in 179 patients (80.6%) for prolapse, 172 (77.5%) for bleeding, 139 (85.3%) for mucus discharge, 139 (78.5%) for burning sensation, and 115 (75.5%) for itching. Considering all recorded symptoms, 194 patients (86.6%) reported absence and or an improvement at follow-up. Twelve patients (5.4%) reported newly developed incontinence in the sense of urge symptoms; 42 patients out of 51 patients (82.4%) with preexisting incontinence reported an improvement. Local or topical retreatment (ointment, suppositories, sclerotherapy) was performed in 48 patients (21.4%). Reoperation for residual or newly developed hemorrhoidal nodules was needed in 8 patients (3.6%).

Limitations.—Lack of a comparative group.

Conclusion.—Our long-term results show that this strategy for stapled hemorrhoidopexy can achieve a high level of patient satisfaction and symptom control, with a low rate of reoperation for recurrent hemorrhoidal symptoms.

▶ Ommer et al present the first long-term follow-up of patients who underwent stapled hemorrhoidectomy. Two hundred twenty-four patients were followed for more than 6 years; nearly 90% of the patients were satisfied, and only 3.6% of patients required repeat surgery for recurrent or persistent hemorrhoidal tissue. Less than 5% of patients retrospectively assessed postoperative pain as intolerable. Moreover, patients returned to work less than 3 weeks after the operation—truly remarkable. These findings represent a drastic improvement compared with conventional hemorrhoidectomy, which is associated with substantial postoperative pain and anal and bowel dysfunction. In addition, the word on the street suggests that data reported for postoperative pain from traditional hemorrhoidectomy was often obtained 4 weeks or more after the operation—that is, after the pain improved. Follow-up was not conducted earlier because of the severity of pain the patients exhibited and the lack of adequate therapy for this pain. Major advances in postoperative pain control are not common, which altered the surgical technique (with a low rate of complications and recurrences) with markedly decreased post-operative pain as a major advance in the care of patients with hemorrhoids.

K. E. Behrns, MD

Topical Diltiazem Cream Versus Botulinum Toxin A for the Treatment of Chronic Anal Fissure: A Double-Blind Randomized Clinical Trial

Samim M, Twigt B, Stoker L, et al (Diakonessenhuis Hosp, Utrecht, The Netherlands)
Ann Surg 255:18-22, 2012

Objective.—A double-blind randomized clinical trial to compare topical diltiazem with botulinum toxin A (BTA) in the treatment of chronic anal fissure.

Background.—Chronic anal fissures remain a challenging condition. Topical diltiazem and BTA are promising agents in the treatment of anal fissure. As to date diltiazem and BTA were never compared in a solid randomized trial, which is the purpose of this study.

Methods.—One hundred thirty-four patients were randomized to receive either diltiazem cream and placebo injection or BTA injection and placebo cream. The primary end point was fissure healing after 3 months.

Results.—After 3 months healing of the fissure was noted in 32 of 74 (43%) patients in the diltiazem group and 26 of 60 (43%) patients in the BTA group. Reduction >50% in mean pain score was noted in 58 of 74 (78%) patients in the diltiazem group and 49 of 60 (82%) patients in the BTA group. Perianal itching was the only side effect reported and was noted in 15% of patients in the diltiazem group, and this difference was statistically significant ($P = 0.012$).

Conclusions.—BTA yields higher healing rates in the short term, though after 3 months diltiazem and BTA resulted in equal healing rates. Also no significant difference in pain reduction was observed for both treatments. This study shows no significant advantage of one treatment compared to the other. This randomized clinical trial is registered by the Dutch Trial Register as NTR1012 (Fig 2).

▶ Chronic anal fissure remains a vexing problem for the colorectal and general surgeon because of the significant pain and debility caused by the break of the anal mucosa and exposure of the underlying sphincter muscle. The last decade has witnessed the introduction of several nonoperative treatments because of the risk of incontinence for flatus or stool with lateral internal sphincterotomy. Injection of botulinum A toxin and administration of diltiazem cream are 2 of the recently studied nonoperative treatments. Samin et al conducted a double-blind trial of these 2 agents to compare them head to head and found equivalency in

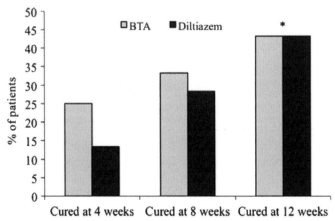

FIGURE 2.—Cumulative percentages of patients cured after treatment with BTA or Diltiazem. *$P = 0.992$ (X^2 test). (Reprinted from Samim M, Twigt B, Stoker L, et al. Topical diltiazem cream versus botulinum toxin a for the treatment of chronic anal fissure: a double-blind randomized clinical trial. *Ann Surg.* 2012;255:18-22. © Southeastern Surgical Congress.)

results after 12 weeks (Fig 2). The healing rate with both treatments was a disappointing 43%, although both were relatively free of major side effects. Factors that may be involved in choosing one treatment over another include (1) cost, which is higher for botulinum A toxin unless 4 patients are treated in the same day; (2) treatment compliance, which is better for botulinum A toxin because it is injected and does not require twice-daily application like diltiazem cream; and (3) side effects such as perianal itching that may accompany diltiazem use. Though this well-designed trial answers an important question, it does leave one contemplating where lateral internal sphincterotomy resides in the management of anal fissure. The results tend to be excellent, but the treatment may result in incontinence, which is obviously devastating to the patient. Hopefully, the authors will conduct another study that compares lateral internal sphincterotomy with either botulinum A toxin or diltiazem cream so we can definitively determine the role of sphincterotomy in this disease.

K. E. Behrns, MD

Cessation of Clopidogrel Before Major Abdominal Procedures

Chernoguz A, Telem DA, Chu E, et al (Mount Sinai School of Medicine, NY)
Arch Surg 146:334-339, 2011

Objective.—To determine whether timing of clopidogrel bisulfate cessation influences outcome after abdominal operations.

Methods.—A review was performed of 104 patients receiving clopidogrel who underwent abdominal operations between March 2003 and March 2009. Patients were grouped by last clopidogrel use: group A (<7 days) and group B (≥7 days).

Results.—Of 104 patients, 43 were in group A and 61 were in group B. Overall, 6 deaths occurred (group A, 5 patients [12%] vs group B, 1 [2%]; $P=.03$) and 27 patients required intensive care unit admission (group A, 16 patients [37%] vs group B, 11 [18%]; $P=.03$). Twenty-one patients developed a postoperative bleeding complication; 19 complications were managed by blood transfusion and 2 required reoperation. Group A vs group B had significantly increased rates of postoperative bleeding requiring blood transfusion (13 patients [30%] vs 8 [13%]; $P=.03$). No significant difference in postoperative bleeding resulting in reoperation or mortality was demonstrated. Timing of clopidogrel cessation within 7 days did not affect postoperative bleeding risk. Eighty-nine patients (86%) underwent elective operations (group A, 30 patients [70%] vs group B, 59 [97%]; $P<.001$). While elective patients in group A vs those in group B demonstrated a trend toward increased risk of postoperative bleeding requiring transfusion (7 patients [23%] vs 8 [14%]; $P=.25$), no significant difference in intensive care unit admission (group A, 6 patients [20%] vs group B, 9 [15%]; $P=.31$) or mortality (1 [3%] vs 1 [2%]; $P=.62$) was demonstrated.

Conclusions.—While clopidogrel use within 7 days of an operation significantly increased the risk of postoperative bleeding, most bleeding episodes were successfully managed by transfusion without an increase in bleeding-related mortality or necessity for reoperation. After controlling for operative urgency, no significant difference in mortality or intensive care unit admission was demonstrated in patients undergoing elective procedures. High-risk patients undergoing elective operations may not require preoperative clopidogrel cessation. When clopidogrel cessation is warranted, 7 days before the procedure is recommended. Perioperative risk does not vary by timing of cessation within 7 days of an operation.

▶ On occasion, the management of complex patients requires that the surgeon choose between 2 or more treatment strategies that have significant risk. For example, should antiplatelet therapy for a coronary stent be ceased prior to an operation to decrease the risk of bleeding even though it may put the patient at risk for coronary thrombosis? Neither choice is attractive, but coronary thrombosis is potentially lethal, whereas bleeding likely would be controlled through blood or blood component transfusion or potentially reoperation. Chernoguz et al provide us with data regarding the use of clopidogrel around the time of a major operation. They found that patients that stopped their medication within 7 days of the operation had an increased risk of postoperative hemorrhage. However, when controlled for the health status of the patient and the urgency of the operation, cessation of clopidogrel before or after 7 days was not an independent factor predicting postoperative bleeding. The authors conclude the cessation of clopidogrel 7 days or more may not be necessary. However, this conclusion accepts that some patients will require blood transfusion, which is not without short-term and long-term consequences. Blood transfusion reactions and immunologic effects, especially in cancer patients, associated with the transfusion of blood products, may create substantial harm to patients. In fact, postoperative bleeding is an important patient safety indicator in the University Health Consortium Quality Measures Report, presumably because it has an adverse effect on patient outcome. The authors should be congratulated on providing data that permits optimal patient care in complex scenarios, but we must all be cognizant of the need to decrease all risks to our patients rather than accepting trade-offs.

K. E. Behrns, MD

Readmission Rates After Abdominal Surgery: The Role of Surgeon, Primary Caregiver, Home Health, and Subacute Rehab
Martin RCG, Brown R, Puffer L, et al (Univ of Louisville School of Medicine, KY)
Ann Surg 254:591-597, 2011

Objective.—To prospectively evaluate predictive factors of hospital readmission rates in patients undergoing abdominal surgical procedures.

Background.—Recommendations from MedPAC that the Centers for Medicare and Medicaid Services (CMS) report upon and determine payments based in part on readmission rates have led to an attendant interest by payers, hospital administrators and far-sighted physicians.

Methods.—Analysis of 266 prospective treated patients undergoing major abdominal surgical procedures from September 2009 to September 2010. All patients were prospectively evaluated for underlying comorbidities, number of preop meds, surgical procedure, incision type, complications, presence or absence of primary and/or secondary caregiver, their education level, discharge number of medications, and discharge location. Univariate and multivariate analyses were performed.

Results.—Two hundred twenty-six patients were reviewed with 48 (18%) gastric-esophageal, 39 (14%) gastrointestinal, 88 (34%) liver, 58 (22%) pancreas, and 33 (12%) other. Seventy-eight (30%) were readmitted for various diagnoses the most common being dehydration (26%). Certain preoperative and intraoperative factors were not found to be significant for readmission being, comorbidities, diagnosis, number of preoperative medications, patient education level, type of operation, blood loss, and complications. Significant predictive factors for readmission were age (≥ 69 years), number of discharged (DC) meds (≥ 9 medications), $\leq 50\%$ oral intake (52% vs. 23%), and DC home with a home health agency (62% vs. 11%).

Conclusion.—Readmission rates for surgeons WILL become a quality indicator of performance. Quality parameters among Home Health agencies are nonexistent, but will reflect on surgeon's performance. Greater awareness regarding predictors of readmission rates is necessary to demonstrate improved surgical quality.

▶ Over the past several years, potential financial rewards incurred by hospitals have encouraged timely discharge of patients. This practice has led surgeons to discharge patients when indicators of independent living are first apparent, and thus the readmission rate for patients has increased. The conflict between early discharge and an increased likelihood of readmission is particularly difficult to resolve in patients who have gastrointestinal operations. Return of bowel function is often an indicator for discharge in these patients, and bowel function is notoriously erratic following abdominal operations. Thus, the criteria for discharge that will lead to a lower readmission rate are nebulous. Martin et al studied 266 patients who had abdominal operations to determine the rate of readmission and factors associated with readmission. They found that 30% of the patients were readmitted; factors predictive of readmission were age over 69 years, greater than 9 discharge medications, poor oral intake, and discharge with home health agency assistance. Most of these factors are not surprising; however, employment of a home health agency, in theory, should permit early identification of medical issues that may be addressed with an outpatient visit that will avoid readmission. Personal experience would suggest that too frequently, home health agencies send patients too late to the emergency room, where readmission becomes de facto. Surgeons and hospitals need to work closely with home health agencies to establish goals for patient care and criteria for outpatient visits and hospital readmission. Health care systems need to become more invested in the entire cycle of patient care, and postdischarge care with integration of home health agencies will be necessary to decrease the readmission rate.

K. E. Behrns, MD

Risk Factors for Mortality in Major Digestive Surgery in the Elderly: A Multicenter Prospective Study

Duron J-J, Duron E, Dugue T, et al (Univ Hosp Pitie-Salpêtrière, Paris, France; Univ Hosp Broca, Paris, France; Saint Philibert Hosp, Lomme, France; et al)
Ann Surg 254:375-382, 2011

Objective.—To identify the mortality risk factors of elderly patients ($\geq$65 years old) during major digestive surgery, as defined according to the complexity of the operation.

Background.—In the aging populations of developed countries, the incidence rate of major digestive surgery is currently on the rise and is associated with a high mortality rate. Consequently, validated indicators must be developed to improve elderly patients' surgical care and outcomes.

Methods.—We acquired data from a multicenter prospective cohort that included 3322 consecutive patients undergoing major digestive surgery across 47 different facilities. We assessed 27 pre-, intra-, and postoperative demographic and clinical variables. A multivariate analysis was used to identify the independent risk factors of mortality in elderly patients (n = 1796). Young patients were used as a control group, and the end-point was defined as 30-day postoperative mortality.

Results.—In the entire cohort, postoperative mortality increased significantly among patients aged 65−74 years, and an age $\geq$65 years was by itself an independent risk factor for mortality (odds ratio [OR], 2.21; 95%

confidence interval [CI], 1.36–3.59; $P = 0.001$). The mortality rate among elderly patients was 10.6%. Six independent risk factors of mortality were characteristic of the elderly patients: age ≥85 years (OR, 2.62; 95% CI, 1.08–6.31; $P = 0.032$), emergency (OR, 3.42; 95% CI, 1.67–6.99; $P = 0.001$), anemia (OR, 1.80; 95% CI, 1.02–3.17; $P = 0.041$), white cell count > 10,000/mm³ (OR, 1.90; 95% CI, 1.08–3.35; $P = 0.024$), ASA class IV (OR, 9.86; 95% CI, 1.77–54.7; $P = 0.009$) and a palliative cancer operation (OR, 4.03; 95% CI, 1.99–8.19; $P < 0.001$).

Conclusion.—Characterization of independent validated risk indicators for mortality in elderly patients undergoing major digestive surgery is essential and may lead to an efficient specific workup, which constitutes a necessary step to developing a dedicated score for elderly patients (Fig 1).

▶ The surgical literature is peppered with articles that examine patient age as a factor predictive of mortality. Heretofore, a number of reports cited by Duron et al suggest that age in and of itself is not predictive of mortality. How can this difference be reconciled? First, many of the previous studies examined age as a factor in site-specific surgery, such as pancreas surgery. Second, the authors of many of these studies are international experts in their particular fields and thus may have not only better results, but a referral bias that favors healthier elderly patients. This article represents a balanced cross-section of practice, including academic surgery, community surgery, and private surgery. Furthermore, the number of patients (N = 3322) included in the study is large, and numerous potential factors were critically examined using rigorous statistical analysis. The study clearly shows that age (Fig 1) is an independent risk factor for death. In addition, 6 factors—age greater than 85, anemia, emergency, leukocytosis, American Society of Anesthesiologists class IV, and palliative cancer surgery—were independently predictive of death following digestive surgery. Emergency surgery was particularly noteworthy with a mortality rate of 33%. The authors nicely address each of these risk factors and strategies to ameliorate the effects, such as early diagnosis and intervention or less invasive treatments. However, the more difficult question may be "Should we offer any invasive therapy for elderly patients with digestive disease who have one or more of

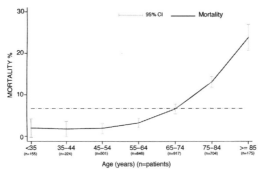

FIGURE 1.—Mortality according to age. (Reprinted from Duron J-J, Duron E, Dugue T, et al. Risk factors for mortality in major digestive surgery in the elderly: a multicenter prospective study. *Ann Surg.* 2011;254:375-382. © Southeastern Surgical Congress.)

these risk factors?" It would be intriguing to know the proportion of elderly patients with these risk factors who were engaged in a discussion of nonoperative palliative care. Likely these discussions do not occur on a frequent basis, and I for one am guilty as charged.

K. E. Behrns, MD

General surgery training without laparoscopic surgery fellows: The impact on residents and patients

Linn JG, Hungness ES, Clark S, et al (Northwestern Univ, Chicago, IL)
Surgery 150:752-758, 2011

Background.—To evaluate resident case volume after discontinuation of a laparoscopic surgery fellowship, and to examine disparities in patient care over the same time period.

Methods.—Resident case logs were compared for a 2-year period before and 1 year after discontinuing the fellowship, using a 2-sample *t* test. Databases for bariatric and esophageal surgery were reviewed to compare operative time, length of stay (LOS), and complication rate by resident or fellow over the same time period using a 2-sample *t* test.

Results.—Increases were seen in senior resident advanced laparoscopic (Mean Fellow Year = 21 operations vs Non Fellow Year = 61, $P < 0.01$), esophageal (1 vs 11, $P < .01$) and bariatric volume (9 vs 36, $P < .01$). Junior resident laparoscopic volume increased ($P < 0.05$). No difference in LOS or complication rate was seen with resident vs fellow assistant. Operative time was greater for gastric bypass with resident assistant (152 ± 51 minutes vs 138 ± 53, $P < .05$).

Conclusion.—Discontinuing a laparoscopic fellowship significantly increases resident case volume in laparoscopic surgery. Operative time for complex operations may increase in the absence of a fellow. Other patient outcomes are not affected by this change.

▶ Linn et al performed an interesting study that compared general surgery resident experience in minimally invasive surgery in the presence and absence of a laparoscopic surgery fellowship training program. The results demonstrated that resident volume increased significantly in laparoscopic esophageal surgery and bariatric surgery in the absence of a minimally invasive surgery fellow. The increased surgery volume was noted for junior and senior residents, and importantly, this change did not alter patient length of stay or complications. This article nicely points out that minimally invasive surgery is general surgery and vice versa. Undoubtedly, the introduction of laparoscopic surgery has changed the landscape for training not only general surgery residents and minimally invasive surgery fellows but also surgical oncology, thoracic surgery, colorectal surgery, pediatric surgery fellows, and others. In surgical training programs and academic surgery departments, the focus has been on the specialty and trainee that teaches and learns a specific operation. However, should our priority not be focused on providing the best training so that the credentialed surgeon provides the best care? If so, then we should bring all our educational resources together to collectively train young surgeons. We should break down vertical barriers to surgical care and have trainees learn from experts who work together to provide care for the patient with esophageal cancer. For example, an esophageal cancer surgery program should include a surgical oncologist, a minimally invasive surgeon, and a thoracic surgeon who collectively evaluate and manage patients to provide the best possible care. This shift will require major changes in training programs, but also departmental infrastructure and referral patterns. Without a doubt, surgery is rapidly becoming a team sport, and we should embrace this change to provide the best quality care for our patients.

K. E. Behrns, MD

Prospective, Comparative Study of Postoperative Quality of Life in TEP, TAPP, and Modified Lichtenstein Repairs
Belyansky I, Tsirline VB, Klima DA, et al (Carolinas Med Ctr, Charlotte, NC)
Ann Surg 254:709-715, 2011

Introduction.—The purpose of this study was to compare postoperative quality of life (QOL) in patients undergoing laparoscopic totally extraperitoneal (TEP), transabdominal preperitoneal (TAPP), or modified Lichtenstein (ML) hernia repairs.

Methods.—The International Hernia Mesh Registry (2007–2010) was interrogated. 2086 patients who underwent 2499 inguinal hernia repairs were identified. A Carolinas Comfort Score was self-reported at 1-, 6-, 12-months and results were compared. Subgroups analysis and logistic regression were used to identify confounders and to control for significant variables.

Results.—One hundred seventy-two patients met the exclusion criteria. The distribution of unilateral procedures was TEP (n = 217), TAPP (n = 331), and ML (n = 953). Average follow-up was 12 months. Use of >10 tacks, lack of prostate pathology, recurrent hernia repairs, and bilateral hernia repairs were significant predictors of postoperative pain. One month after surgery 8.9%, 16.6%, and 16.5% were symptomatic for TEP ($P = 0.038$ vs. ML), TAPP and ML, respectively. At 6 months and 1 year no differences were observed. The number of tacks used varied significantly, with 18.1% of TAPP and 2.3% of TEP with >10 tacks ($P = 0.005$). The incidence of hernia recurrences were equivalent: TEP (0.42%), TAPP (1.34%), and ML (1.27%). The number or type of tacks utilized did not impact recurrence rates.

Conclusion.—Use of >10 tacks doubles the incidence of early postoperative pain while having no effect on rates of recurrence. There was no difference in chronic postoperative pain comparing ML, TEP, and TAPP including when controlled for tack use.

▶ Inguinal hernia repair is one of the most common operations performed worldwide, yet the optimal operation remains a matter of debate. Laparoscopic approaches to inguinal hernia repair have provided another less invasive approach to these hernias, but the laparoscopic approaches have not clearly superseded an open approach using mesh fixation of the hernia defect. Belyansky et al hypothesized that the laparoscopic approaches of totally extraperitoneal (TEP) and transabdominal preperitoneal (TAPP) hernia repairs would result in less postoperative pain and, therefore, would be the preferred methods of repair. However, the results from this database of self-reported pain scores suggest that only at 1 month postoperatively is the TEP associated with less pain than a modified Lichtenstein repair. Furthermore, it appears that the use of more than 10 tacks per side to secure the mesh and/or the peritoneum with the laparoscopic approach to hernia repairs has introduced other variables that require study: the number of tacks used, the placement of tacks, material composition of tacks, etc. Advances in science are accompanied by new questions, and undoubtedly we do not have the final answer for the inguinal hernia operation that causes the least amount of pain. One question that was not addressed in this study or in the discussion is whether the TAPP operation has a long shelf life given the use of multiple tacks and increased early pain. Further studies should explore the potential benefits of the TAPP over the TEP repair as a laparoscopic approach; however, the benefits of TAPP repair appear to be waning, with increasing evidence showing the superiority of TEP repair.

K. E. Behrns, MD

A Clinician's Guide to Patient Selection for Watchful Waiting Management of Inguinal Hernia

Sarosi GA Jr, Wei Y, Gibbs JO, et al (Univ of Florida College of Medicine, Gainesville; Hines VA Hosp, IL; Northwestern Univ, Chicago, IL; et al)
Ann Surg 253:605-610, 2011

Objective.—The goal of this study was to assist surgeons in managing patients with minimally symptomatic inguinal hernia by identifying characteristics that predict crossover to surgery or worsening of hernia symptoms.

Background.—Randomized trials have suggested that watchful waiting management of minimally symptomatic inguinal hernia is an acceptable alternative to surgical repair. However, these trials found that roughly a quarter of patients would elect for repair in the first 2 years, suggesting that not all patients are good candidates for watchful waiting.

Methods.—The 336 patients randomized to watchful waiting in the American College of Surgeons Watchful Waiting Hernia Trial constituted the study population. Preoperative patient characteristics were used to predict 2 outcomes, either crossover to surgery or the development of hernia pain limiting activities and/or crossover to surgery. Patients in our study were part of a previously registered randomized trial: NCT00263250.

Results.—At 2 years, 72 patients crossed over to surgery, with pain with strenuous activities [odds ratio (OR), 1.3 per 10-mm visual analog scale pain scale], chronic constipation (OR, 4.9), prostatism (OR, 2.9), being married (OR, 2.3), and good health [OR, 3.0 American Society of

Anesthesiologists Class (ASA) 1 vs 2], predicting crossover. An additional 28 patients developed pain, limiting their activities, with pain during strenuous activities (OR, 1.3 per 10-mm visual analog scale) and chronic constipation (OR, 4.5), predicting the combined outcome of pain limiting activities and/or crossover to surgery. Higher levels of activity reduced the risk (OR, 0.95) of this combined outcome.

Conclusions.—Readily identifiable patient characteristics can predict those patients with minimally symptomatic inguinal hernia who are likely to "fail" watchful waiting hernia management. Consideration of these factors will allow surgeons to optimally tailor hernia management.

▶ Over the last several years, the American College of Surgeons hernia trial has provided insightful data regarding the management of inguinal hernia. This report by Sarosi et al is no exception in that it addresses the role of watchful waiting in patients with minimally symptomatic hernias. This study examined the rate of crossover to surgery and the factors associated with this alteration in management. In addition, they analyzed a larger group of patients who did not cross over to surgery but were limited in activities. The results demonstrate that pain with strenuous activity, chronic constipation, prostatism, and marital status were predictive of likelihood of success of the watchful waiting approach. Importantly, a simple worksheet with answers to these 4 questions and an accompanying probability table allow the surgeon or physician to more accurately counsel the patient regarding the likely success of a watchful waiting approach (Appendix in the original article). This important work demonstrates the power of a well-designed randomized trial that addresses a seemingly straightforward problem and provides an efficient, simple management tool. Although the findings are applicable to many patients, as the authors point out, the findings should not be generalized to all patients with inguinal hernias. The patients in this trial were relatively young with few comorbidities and generally represent an acceptable operative group, so crossover to surgery was an acceptable alternative. However, what is the appropriate treatment for patients who are not as healthy? Are the risks of surgery or the complication rates in a less healthy group of patients prohibitive? These are important questions to address since the patients seen in the surgical clinic often have multiple comorbidities and may therefore have higher risks.

K. E. Behrns, MD

A prospective study on elective umbilical hernia repair in patients with liver cirrhosis and ascites

Eker HH, van Ramshorst GH, de Goede B, et al (Erasmus Univ Med Ctr, Rotterdam, The Netherlands)
Surgery 150:542-546, 2011

Background.—Patients with both cirrhosis and ascites have a 20% risk of developing umbilical hernia. A retrospective study from our center comparing conservative management of umbilical hernia with elective repair in these patients showed a significant risk of mortality as a result of hernia incarceration in conservatively treated patients. The goal of this study was to assess the safety and efficacy of elective umbilical hernia repair in these patients prospectively.

Methods.—Patients with liver cirrhosis and ascites presenting with an umbilical hernia were included in this study. For all patients, the expected time to liver transplantation was more than 3 months, and they did not have a patent umbilical vein in the hernia sac. The following data were collected prospectively for all patients: Child-Pugh-Turcotte (CPT) classification, model for end-stage liver disease (MELD) score, kidney failure, cardiovascular comorbidity, operation-related complications, and duration of hospital stay. Mortality rates were registered in hospital records and verified in government records during follow-up. Mortality rates were registered in hospital records and verified in government records during follow-up. On completion of the study, a retrospective survey was performed to search for any patients who met the study inclusion criteria but were left out of the study cohort.

Results.—In total, 30 patients (25 males) underwent operation at a mean age of 58 years (standard deviation [SD] ± 9 years). Of these 30 patients, 6 were classified as CPT grade A (20%), 19 (63%) as grade B, and 5 (17%) as grade C. The patients' median MELD score was 12 (interquartile range [IQR], 8—16). In 10 (33%) of the 30 patients hernia repair was performed with mesh. The median duration of hospital stay was 3 days (IQR, 2—4). None of the patients were admitted to the intensive care unit. Postoperative complications included pneumonia and decompensation of cirrhosis (1 case each), resulting in prolonged hospital stay for those 2 patients. After a median follow-up period of 25 months (IQR, 14—34), 2 (7%) of the 30 patients died; neither of the deaths were attributable to the umbilical hernia repair. A total of 2 patients suffered recurrence.

Conclusion.—Elective umbilical hernia repair is safe and the preferred approach in cirrhotic patients with ascites.

▶ The presence of a symptomatic umbilical hernia in a patient with liver cirrhosis and ascites has perplexed general surgeons for years. Because of the high risks of operating on this patient population with significant comorbidities, a watchful waiting approach has been used. The obvious risks associated with this approach are skin breakdown over the hernia with leakage of ascites and strangulation of the hernia. Eker et al have carefully studied these patients and initially performed a retrospective study of hernia repair that was necessary for complications. This approach had a complication rate of 43%. The authors subsequently performed a prospective study in which patients with cirrhosis, ascites, and an umbilical hernia underwent repair unless liver transplant was anticipated in 3 months or a patent umbilical vein was evident at the hernia site. This approach in 30 patients was associated with the complication rate of 7%, and only 2 patients had recurrent hernias. Importantly, the patients underwent preoperative management of ascites with dual diuretic therapy and nutritional supplementation. Undoubtedly, this thoughtful approach improved the patient outcome.

The authors have made seminal clinical observations in a group of patients that many surgeons would avoid. However, through a series of studies, they have refined the approach to umbilical hernia repair in patients with cirrhosis and ascites and made a substantial improvement in outcome. These reports represent excellent comparative effectiveness studies that address a difficult surgical issue.

K. E. Behrns, MD

Effects of Nuclear Factor-κB Inhibitors on Colon Anastomotic Healing in Rats

Bedirli A, Salman B, Pasaoglu H, et al (Gazi Univ Med School, Ankara, Turkey)
J Surg Res 171:355-360, 2011

Background.—Nuclear factor (NF)-κB plays an essential role in inflammation. We tested this role by administering NF-κB-inhibitors into rats undergoing a well-established model of colonic anastomotic healing.

Methods.—Wistar rats underwent laparotomy, descending colonic transection, and handsewn reanastomosis. The animals were randomized to receive either a selective NF-κB inhibitor (parthenolide 0.5 mg/kg or resveratrol 0.5 mg/kg) or an equal volume of water by gavages before operation and then daily after surgery. Animals were sacrificed either immediately after anastomotic construction (d 0) or at the third, fifth, or seventh postoperative day.

Results.—Both parthenolide and resveratrol treatment led to early significant increases in plasma levels of IL-6. On d 7, hydroxyproline levels were significantly higher in the parthenolide and resveratrol groups. A similar pattern was observed with the bursting pressure. In contrast, gelatinase activity (MMP-2 and MMP-9 expression) was significantly higher in the control group on postoperative d 3. On d 3, expression of NF-κB activity was up-regulated in the anastomotic area. Both parthenolide and resveratrol completely attenuated NF-κB activity. Study groups also developed more marked inflammatory cell infiltration and collagen deposition on histology analysis.

Conclusions.—Parthenolide and resveratrol significantly improved healing and mechanical stability of colonic anastomoses in rats during the early postoperative period. Both agents may be acting to accelerate the host reparative process as well as to enhance protection of the anastomotic wound bed.

▶ Animal studies provide an important methodology to study wound healing. Although results cannot be directly applied to humans, they offer opportunities to study biochemical mechanisms of healing and then study methods to either inhibit or accelerate the healing process. This report evaluated laparotomy and colon anastomoses with and without nuclear factor (NF)-κB inhibition. Animals who were gavaged with the specific NF-κB inhibitor demonstrated a decrease in NF-κB activity in the area of the colon anastomosis and a significant improvement in mean wound bursting strength at day 7. A significant improvement in collagen deposition in the area of the colon anastomosis was also noted in the NF-κB—inhibited animals.

NF-κB is upregulated in areas of rapid cell proliferation, which occurs in the region of a wound that is healing. However, NF-κB is an essential factor in the enzymatic pathways of almost all cells. It would be important for the authors to evaluate NF-κB activity in other tissues and circulating cells. They noted an increase in the inflammatory response systemically (mean interleukin-6 levels) and in the area of the wound, and this might also result in an increase in the underlying inflammatory status, for example, in the lung. Thus, NF-κB inhibition an animal model studying healing could also be tested to see whether there is an increase in pulmonary dysfunction, for example, during sepsis in this same animal model. Nevertheless, this study is valuable in that it evaluates underlying biochemical processes in the healing wound and suggests one alternative, inhibition of NF-κB, to enhance wound healing in colon anastomoses.

J. M. Daly, MD

The Use of Silver Nylon in Preventing Surgical Site Infections Following Colon and Rectal Surgery

Krieger BR, Davis DM, Sanchez JE, et al (Univ of South Florida, Tampa, FL)
Dis Colon Rectum 54:1014-1019, 2011

Background.—Patients who undergo colorectal surgery have up to a 30% chance of developing a surgical site infection postoperatively. Silver-lon is a silver nylon dressing designed to prevent surgical site infections, but only anecdotal evidence has previously supported its efficacy.

Objective.—The aim of this study was to evaluate the effect of silver nylon dressings in patients undergoing colorectal surgery.

Design.—We performed a prospective, randomized, controlled trial comparing a silver nylon dressing with gauze dressings in patients undergoing elective colorectal surgery.

Setting.—The study was performed at a university-based, tertiary referral center.

Patients.—We studied patients undergoing elective colorectal surgery with an abdominal skin incision of at least 3 cm.

Intervention.—Patients were randomly assigned to receive either a silver nylon or a gauze dressing.

Main Outcome Measures.—The primary end point was surgical site infection occurring within 30 days of surgery.

Results.—One hundred ten patients were enrolled in the study and were randomly assigned to 1 of 2 treatment groups. After a 30-day follow-up period, the incidence of surgical site infection was lower in the silver nylon group compared with the control group (13% vs 33%, $P = .011$). Twenty-five patients in the study developed superficial surgical site infections, 5 in the silver nylon group and 14 in the control group ($P = .021$). Two patients in the study group developed deep wound infections compared with 4 in the control group ($P = .438$). Multivariate analysis revealed that patients in the control group had a 3-fold increase in risk of infection compared with patients in the silver nylon group ($P = .013$).

Limitations.—A limitation of this study is that the members of the surgical team were not blinded to the treatment groups.

Conclusion.—Silver nylon is safe and effective in preventing surgical site infection following colorectal surgery.

▶ This prospective trial randomized 110 patients who underwent colorectal surgery to receive either a standard gauze dressing or a silver nylon dressing at the conclusion of the operation. There was a significant reduction in the incidence of both superficial and deep wound infections in the treated group compared with the control group. Interestingly, the mean duration of hospitalization was similar between groups despite the differences in wound infection rates. This is an interesting paradox but may simply reflect our ability to better use home services liberally whenever a minor complication occurs. It would be interesting to understand the absorptive capacity at the wound for the silver in the dressing and the antibacterial levels of tissue silver. At an approximate cost of $100 per patient, it would appear the use of silver nylon dressings is cost-effective.

J. M. Daly, MD

10 Oncology

Breast

A Novel Automated Assay for the Rapid Identification of Metastatic Breast Carcinoma in Sentinel Lymph Nodes

Feldman S, for the US One Step Nucleic Acid Amplification Clinical Study Group (Columbia Univ College of Physicians and Surgeons, NY; et al)
Cancer 117:2599-2607, 2011

Background.—The authors prospectively evaluated the performance of a proprietary molecular testing platform using one-step nucleic acid amplification (OSNA) for the detection of metastatic carcinoma in sentinel lymph nodes (SLNs) in a large multicenter trial and compared the OSNA results with the results from a detailed postoperative histopathologic evaluation (reference pathology) and from intraoperative imprint cytology (IC).

Methods.—In total, 1044 SLN samples from 496 patients at 11 clinical sites were analyzed. Alternate 1-mm sections were subjected to either detailed histopathologic evaluation with hematoxylin and eosin and pan-cytokeratin immunostaining or the OSNA Breast Cancer System, which was calibrated to detect tumor deposits >0.2 mm by measuring cytokeratin 19 messenger RNA. At 7 sites, IC was performed before permanent section. The OSNA results were classified as negative (<250 copies/μL), micrometastases (from ≥250 to <5000 copies/μL), or macrometastases (≥5000 copies/μL).

Results.—The sensitivity and specificity of the OSNA breast cancer system compared with reference pathology were 77.5% (95% confidence interval, 69.7%-84.2%) and 95.8% (95% confidence interval, 94.3%-97.0%), respectively, before discordant case analyses (DCA). Sensitivity and specificity after DCA were 82.7% and 97.7%, and final concordance was 95.8%. Performance for invasive lobular carcinoma demonstrated 88.2% sensitivity (95% confidence interval, 63.6%-98.5%) and 98.5% specificity (95% confidence interval, 92%-100%). The sensitivity of OSNA was significantly better than that of IC (80% vs 63%; $P=.0229$).

Conclusions.—The OSNA breast cancer system proved to be highly accurate for the detection of metastatic breast cancer in axillary SLNs. Sensitivity was comparable to that predicted for conventional postoperative histologic examination at 2-mm intervals and was significantly more sensitive than IC. Automation, semiquantitative results enabling the differentiation of macrometastasis and micrometastasis, and rapid results

TABLE 7.—Performance Values for the One Step Nucleic Acid Amplification Breast Cancer System and Imprint Cytology[a]

		Performance Value % (95% CI)			
		Before DCA		After DCA	
Variable	OSNA	Imprint Cytology	P	OSNA	P
Agreement	93.4 (91.0-95.4)	93.8 (91.4-95.7)	NS	95.8 (93.7-97.3)	NS
Sensitivity	80.2 (69.9-88.3)	63.0 (51.5-73.4)	.0229	85.5 (75.6-92.6)	.0018
Specificity	95.8 (93.5-97.4)	99.3 (98.1-99.9)	.0007	97.5 (95.6-98.8)	.0324
PPV	77.4 (67.0-85.8)	94.4 (84.6-98.8)	.0082	85.5 (75.6-92.6)	.1519
NPV	96.4 (94.3-97.9)	93.7 (91.2-95.7)	.0691	97.5 (95.6-98.8)	.0061

CI indicates confidence interval; DCA, discordant case analyses; OSNA, the One Step Nucleic Acid Amplification Breast Cancer System; NS, nonsignificant; PPV, positive predictive value; NPV, negative predictive value.

[a]Agreement with reference pathology, assay sensitivity, specificity, PPV, and NPV, together with 95% CIs, were calculated both for the OSNA Breast Cancer System and imprint cytology and were compared with reference pathology. Values are before and after DCA.

render the assay suitable for intraoperative and/or permanent evaluation of SLNs (Table 7).

▶ Rapid identification of positive sentinel lymph nodes, particularly during the anesthetic for the primary treatment, has been difficult. Performing frozen sections can be time consuming and even misleading. This is a prospective multi-center study of 11 clinical sites who evaluated a new testing platform using a 1-step nucleic acid amplification for the detection of metastatic carcinoma in sentinel lymph nodes.

As seen in Table 7, the sensitivity of this new assay was significantly better than the reference pathology, especially after evaluation for discordant case analysis (Table 7). Unfortunately, if there are 1, 2, or 3 sentinel lymph nodes, it takes approximately 33 to 39 to 45 minutes, respectively.

One of the other unresolved controversies in this area is what to do with micrometastatic disease in a sentinel lymph node. In my own practice, I rarely perform an axillary lymph node dissection if there is only minimal microscopic disease in the sentinel lymph node, and then, include the low axilla in the radiation port.

T. J. Eberlein, MD

Association of Occult Metastases in Sentinel Lymph Nodes and Bone Marrow With Survival Among Women With Early-Stage Invasive Breast Cancer
Giuliano AE, Hawes D, Ballman KV, et al (John Wayne Cancer Inst at Saint John's Health Ctr, Santa Monica; Univ of Southern California Norris Comprehensive Cancer Ctr, Los Angeles; Mayo Clinic, Rochester, MN; et al)
JAMA 306:385-393, 2011

Context.—Immunochemical staining of sentinel lymph nodes (SLNs) and bone marrow identifies breast cancer metastases not seen with routine pathological or clinical examination.

Objective.—To determine the association between survival and metastases detected by immunochemical staining of SLNs and bone marrow specimens from patients with early-stage breast cancer.

Design, Setting, and Patients.—From May 1999 to May 2003, 126 sites in the American College of Surgeons Oncology Group Z0010 trial enrolled women with clinical T1 to T2N0M0 invasive breast carcinoma in a prospective observational study.

Interventions.—All 5210 patients underwent breast-conserving surgery and SLN dissection. Bone marrow aspiration at the time of operation was initially optional and subsequently mandatory (March 2001). Sentinel lymph node specimens (hematoxylineosin negative) and bone marrow specimens were sent to a central laboratory for immunochemical staining; treating clinicians were blinded to results.

Main Outcome Measures.—Overall survival (primary end point) and disease-free survival (a secondary end point).

Results.—Of 5119 SLN specimens (98.3%), 3904 (76.3%) were tumor-negative by hematoxylin-eosin staining. Of 3326 SLN specimens examined by immunohistochemistry, 349 (10.5%) were positive for tumor. Of 3413 bone marrow specimens examined by immunocytochemistry, 104 (3.0%) were positive for tumors. At a median follow-up of 6.3 years (through April 2010), 435 patients had died and 376 had disease recurrence. Immunohistochemical evidence of SLN metastases was not significantly associated with overall survival (5-year rates: 95.7%; 95% confidence interval [CI], 95.0%-96.5% for immunohistochemical negative and 95.1%; 95% CI, 92.7%-97.5% for immunohistochemical positive disease; $P = .64$; unadjusted hazard ratio [HR], 0.90; 95% CI, 0.59-1.39; $P = .64$). Bone marrow metastases were associated with decreased overall survival (unadjusted HR for mortality, 1.94; 95% CI, 1.02-3.67; $P = .04$), but neither immunohistochemical evidence of tumor in SLNs (adjusted HR, 0.88; 95% CI, 0.45-1.71; $P = .70$) nor immunocytochemical evidence of tumor in bone marrow (adjusted HR, 1.83; 95% CI, 0.79-4.26; $P = .15$) was statistically significant on multivariable analysis.

Conclusion.—Among women receiving breast-conserving therapy and SLN dissection, immunohistochemical evidence of SLN metastasis was not associated with overall survival over a median of 6.3 years, whereas occult bone marrow metastasis, although rare, was associated with decreased survival.

Trial Registration.—clinicaltrials.gov Identifier: NCT00003854.

▶ This is an observational study that is a part of the American College of Surgeons Oncology Group Z0010 trial of early-stage invasive breast cancer. The authors underwent immunochemical staining by a central laboratory, and treating clinicians were blinded to the results. As is seen in Fig 2 in the original article, whether a sentinel lymph node had immunohistochemical-positive cells had no impact on mortality, recurrence, or death. However, if the patient had occult metastases in the bone marrow, this had significantly higher recurrence, as well as risk of death (Fig 3 in the original article).

This study has important implications for clinical practice in patients with early-stage breast cancer. It appears that occult metastases are not associated with survival differences. However, a longer follow-up may show some impact from micrometastatic disease in a sentinel lymph node.

With respect to bone marrow examination, this is an invasive procedure, and we do not have enough experience to determine whether this should be done more routinely. However, it appears that micrometastatic disease in the bone marrow is associated with higher risk of recurrence and higher risk of death due to metastatic disease.

T. J. Eberlein, MD

Sentinel Node Biopsy Alone for Node-Positive Breast Cancer: 12-Year Experience at a Single Institution
Spiguel L, Yao K, Winchester DJ, et al (Univ of Chicago, IL; NorthShore Univ HealthSystem, Evanston, IL; et al)
J Am Coll Surg 213:122-128, 2011

Background.—Complete node dissection for a tumor-positive sentinel node (SN) is becoming more controversial. We report our institution's 12-year experience with sentinel node biopsy (SNB) alone for a tumor-positive SN.

Study Design.—This was a retrospective review from 1998 to 2009. Of 3,806 patients who underwent SNB, 2,139 underwent SNB alone, of which 1,997 were tumor-negative and 123 were tumor-positive. SNs were staged node-positive (N1mic or N1) according to American Joint Committee on Cancer criteria.

Results.—One hundred and twenty-three node-positive patients underwent SNB alone with no completion axillary dissection for invasive breast cancer. Mean age was 57 years (range 32 to 92 years) and stage distribution was as follows: stage IIA: 76 (62%) patients; stage IIB: 40 (33%) patients; and stage III: 4 patients (3%). Mean size of the tumors was 1.9 cm (range 0.1 to 9 cm). Eighty-nine (72%) underwent lumpectomy and 34 (28%) underwent mastectomy. Ninety-three percent of patients underwent some form of adjuvant therapy. Forty-two patients (34%) did not undergo radiation and there were no axillary recurrences in this group. At median follow-up of 95 months, there has been 1 axillary recurrence (0.8%) and 13 deaths, 4 of which were attributed to metastatic breast cancer and the rest to non—breast-related causes.

Conclusions.—Axillary recurrence is rare after SN biopsy alone. This might be related to favorable tumor and patient characteristics and frequent use of adjuvant therapy (Tables 4 and 5).

▶ This retrospective series is from a large university-related institution near Chicago. The authors have a large series of patients who underwent sentinel lymph node biopsy that was then analyzed retrospectively. As is seen in Table 4,

TABLE 4.—Outcome Data

Outcome	n	%
Alive NED	104	85
Alive AWD	3	2
Expired	13	11
Metastatic breast cancer	5	41
Other cancer	1	1.0
Axillary recurrence	1	0.8
In breast recurrence	2	1.7
Unknown	3	2

AWD, alive with disease; NED, no evidence of disease.

TABLE 5.—Studies on Sentinel Lymph Node Dissection Alone for Node-Positive Disease

First Author	Year	n	Follow-Up, Mo, Mean (Range)	Axillary Recurrence, %
Guenther[8]	2003	46	32 (4−61)	0
Fant[9]	2003	31	28 (21−48)	0
Naik[7]	2004	210	31 (1−75)	1.4
Chagpar[22]	2005	15	40 (1−54)	0
Swenson[17]	2005	67	33 (2−73)	1.5
Langer[23]	2005	27	42 (12−64)	0
Jeruss[6]	2005	73	27 (1−98)	0
Fan[16]	2005	38	29 (6−76)	2.6
Haid[21]	2006	10	47 (7−90)	0
Pejavar[20]	2006	16	24−60	0
Schulze[14]	2006	6	39 (32−66)	0
Park[19]	2007	287	23 (6−87)	2.1
Hwang[18]	2007	196	30 (1−62)	0
Takei1[5]	2007	120	34 (2−83)	0
Bilimoria[5]	2009	1988	64 (60−72)	0.6−1.2
Bulte[13]	2009	20	46 (11−64)	0

Editor's Note: Please refer to original journal article for full references.

with a median follow-up of 95 months, only 1 patient had axillary recurrence. There may be several explanations for this low axillary recurrence rate. Up to 50% of the patients had 3 or more sentinel lymph nodes removed. Yet only 2 of the patients had 3 or more histologically positive sentinel lymph nodes. Thus, the authors likely excluded patients with large axillary lymph node tumor burden from this series. Additionally, 93% of the patients received some form of adjuvant systemic therapy—either chemotherapy, hormone therapy, or radiation therapy. For sure, the fact that these authors tended to remove a larger number of sentinel lymph nodes at the time of sentinel lymph node biopsy may account for some of the very low axillary recurrence rates.

These authors believed omitting completion axillary lymph dissection in early-stage breast cancer patients with tumor-positive sentinel lymph nodes is acceptable, but not if the patient has clinically positive lymph nodes or neoadjuvant therapies or if the tumor burden is such that 3 or more sentinel lymph nodes have tumors in them. Finally, in Table 5, there is a summary of axillary recurrence rates following sentinel lymph node dissection alone; these numbers are relatively small, which supports the authors' recommendations.

T. J. Eberlein, MD

Adjuvant Docetaxel for High-Risk, Node-Negative Breast Cancer
Martín M, for the GEICAM 9805 Investigators (Hosp General Universitario Gregorio Marañón, Madrid, Spain; et al)
N Engl J Med 363:2200-2210, 2010

Background.—A regimen of docetaxel, doxorubicin, and cyclophospha-mide (TAC) is superior to a regimen of fluorouracil, doxorubicin, and

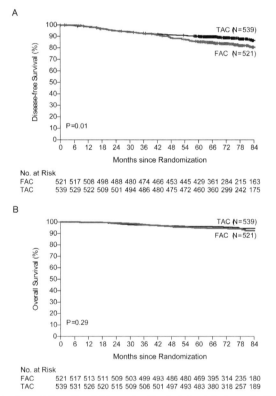

FIGURE 1.—Analyses of Overall and Disease-free Survival. Panel A shows the Kaplan—Meier esti-mates of the probability of diseasefree survival for the 1060 patients included in the intention-to-treat analysis who were randomly assigned to receive TAC or FAC. The unadjusted hazard ratio for disease recurrence in the TAC group as compared with the FAC group was 0.68 (95% CI, 0.49 to 0.93; P = 0.01). The tick marks on the curves denote censored data. Panel B shows the Kaplan—Meier estimates of the probability of overall survival. The unadjusted hazard ratio for death in the TAC group as compared with the FAC group was 0.76 (95% CI, 0.45 to 1.26; P = 0.29). FAC denotes fluorouracil, doxorubicin, and cyclophosphamide; and TAC docetaxel, doxorubicin, and cyclophosphamide. (Reprinted from Martín M, for the GEICAM 9805 Investigators. Adjuvant docetaxel for high-risk, node-negative breast cancer. *N Engl J Med*. 2010;363:2200-2210. © 2010 Massachusetts Medical Society.)

cyclophosphamide (FAC) when used as adjuvant therapy in women with node-positive breast cancer. The value of taxanes in the treatment of node-negative disease has not been determined.

Methods.—We randomly assigned 1060 women with axillary-node–negative breast cancer and at least one high-risk factor for recurrence (according to the 1998 St. Gallen criteria) to treatment with TAC or FAC every 3 weeks for six cycles after surgery. The primary end point was disease-free survival after at least 5 years of follow-up. Secondary end points included overall survival and toxicity.

Results.—At a median follow-up of 77 months, the proportion of patients alive and disease-free was higher among the 539 women in the TAC group (87.8%) than among the 521 women in the FAC group (81.8%), representing a 32% reduction in the risk of recurrence with TAC (hazard ratio, 0.68; 95% confidence interval [CI], 0.49 to 0.93; P=0.01 by the log-rank test). This benefit was consistent, regardless of hormonereceptor status, menopausal status, or number of high-risk factors. The difference in survival rates (TAC, 95.2%; FAC, 93.5%) was not significant (hazard ratio, 0.76; 95% CI, 0.45 to 1.26); however, the number of events was small (TAC,

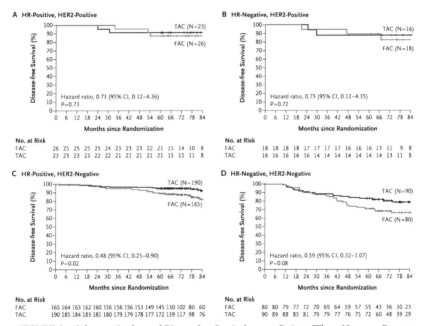

FIGURE 3.—Subgroup Analyses of Disease-free Survival among Patients Whose Hormone-Receptor Status and HER2 Status Were Determined Centrally. Disease-free survival was analyzed for patients with the following tumor characteristics: positive hormone-receptor (HR) status and positive HER2 status (Panel A, 49 patients), negative HR status and positive HER2 status (Panel B, 34 patients), positive HR status and negative HER2 status (Panel C, 355 patients), and negative HR status and negative HER2 status (Panel D, 170 patients). The tick marks on the curves denote censored data. FAC denotes fluorouracil, doxorubicin, and cyclophosphamide; and TAC docetaxel, doxorubicin, and cyclophosphamide. (Reprinted from Martín M, for the GEICAM 9805 Investigators. Adjuvant docetaxel for high-risk, node-negative breast cancer. *N Engl J Med.* 2010;363:2200-2210. © 2010 Massachusetts Medical Society.)

26; FAC, 34). Rates of grade 3 or 4 adverse events were 28.2% with TAC and 17.0% with FAC (P<0.001). Toxicity associated with TAC was diminished when primary prophylaxis with granulocyte colony-stimulating factor was provided.

Conclusions.—As compared with adjuvant FAC, adjuvant TAC improved the rate of disease-free survival among women with high-risk, node-negative breast cancer. (Funded by GEICAM and Sanofi-Aventis; ClinicalTrials.gov number, NCT00121992.) (Figs 1 and 3).

▶ This is a randomized prospective trial in women with axillary node—negative breast cancer but with high risk for recurrence (tumor size greater than 2 cm, estrogen receptor negative/progesterone receptor negative, age younger than 35 years, or histologic grade 2 or 3). The patients were randomized to docetaxel, doxorubicin, and cyclophosphamide or fluorouracil, doxorubicin, and cyclophosphamide.

As seen in Fig 1, there is a significant increase in disease-free survival for the docetaxel regimen. However, there is still not a corresponding increase in overall survival.

When subgroup analysis was performed as seen in Fig 3, there was a more significant improvement in disease-free survival for the docetaxel group in patients who were hormone receptor positive but human epidermal growth factor receptor type 2 (HER2) negative and even more dramatic in the hormone-negative HER2/neu—negative patients. The acute toxic effects of this regimen are manageable using granulocyte colony-stimulating factor prophylaxis.

T. J. Eberlein, MD

Axillary Dissection vs No Axillary Dissection in Women With Invasive Breast Cancer and Sentinel Node Metastasis: A Randomized Clinical Trial
Giuliano AE, Hunt KK, Ballman KV, et al (John Wayne Cancer Inst at Saint John's Health Ctr, Santa Monica, CA; M D Anderson Cancer Ctr, Houston, TX; Mayo Clinic Rochester, MN; et al)
JAMA 305:569-575, 2011

Context.—Sentinel lymph node dissection (SLND) accurately identifies nodal metastasis of early breast cancer, but it is not clear whether further nodal dissection affects survival.

Objective.—To determine the effects of complete axillary lymph node dissection (ALND) on survival of patients with sentinel lymph node (SLN) metastasis of breast cancer.

Design, Setting, and Patients.—The American College of Surgeons Oncology Group Z0011 trial, a phase 3 noninferiority trial conducted at 115 sites and enrolling patients from May 1999 to December 2004. Patients were women with clinical T1-T2 invasive breast cancer, no palpable adenopathy, and 1 to 2 SLNs containing metastases identified by frozen section, touch preparation, or hematoxylin-eosin staining on permanent section.

Targeted enrollment was 1900 women with final analysis after 500 deaths, but the trial closed early because mortality rate was lower than expected.

Interventions.—All patients underwent lumpectomy and tangential whole-breast irradiation. Those with SLN metastases identified by SLND were randomized to undergo ALND or no further axillary treatment. Those randomized to ALND underwent dissection of 10 or more nodes. Systemic therapy was at the discretion of the treating physician.

Main Outcome Measures.—Overall survival was the primary end point, with a non-inferiority margin of a 1-sided hazard ratio of less than 1.3 indicating that SLND alone is noninferior to ALND. Disease-free survival was a secondary end point.

Results.—Clinical and tumor characteristics were similar between 445 patients randomized to ALND and 446 randomized to SLND alone. However, the median number of nodes removed was 17 with ALND and 2 with SLND alone. At a median follow-up of 6.3 years (last follow-up, March 4, 2010), 5-year overall survival was 91.8% (95% confidence interval [CI], 89.1%-94.5%)with ALND and 92.5% (95% CI, 90.0%-95.1%) with SLND alone; 5-year disease-free survival was 82.2% (95% CI, 78.3%-86.3%) with ALND and 83.9% (95% CI, 80.2%-87.9%) with SLND alone. The hazard ratio for treatment-related overall survival was 0.79 (90% CI, 0.56-1.11) without adjustment and 0.87 (90% CI, 0.62-1.23) after adjusting for age and adjuvant therapy.

Conclusion.—Among patients with limited SLN metastatic breast cancer treated with breast conservation and systemic therapy, the use of SLND alone compared with ALND did not result in inferior survival.

Trial Registration.—clinicaltrials.gov Identifier: NCT00003855. (Fig 2).

▶ This article is a multicenter American College of Surgeons Oncology Group Z0011 trial. All patients underwent breast conservation and whole-breast irradiation. Patients who had a sentinel lymph metastasis were randomized to undergo

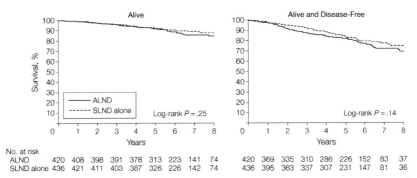

FIGURE 2.—Survival of the ALND Group Compared with SLND-Alone Group. ALND indicates axillary lymph node dissection; SLND, sentinel lymph node dissection. (Reprinted from Giuliano AE, Hunt KK, Ballman KV, et al. Axillary dissection vs no axillary dissection in women with invasive breast cancer and sentinel node metastasis: a randomized clinical trial. *JAMA.* 2011;305:569-575. Copyright 2011 American Medical Association. All rights reserved.)

axillary lymph node dissection or no further axillary treatment. Systemic therapy was at the discretion of the treating physician.

As can be seen in Fig 2, there is no difference between patients treated with sentinel lymph node dissection alone or axillary lymph dissection with respect to survival or disease-free survival.

It is unlikely, even with longer follow-up, there would be any difference in the parameters detected.

Axillary lymph node dissection does provide prognostic information by identifying the number of lymph nodes containing metastatic disease. However, in most practical situations, this will not significantly change systemic therapy decisions.

T. J. Eberlein, MD

Ductal Carcinoma In Situ Treated With Breast-Conserving Surgery and Accelerated Partial Breast Irradiation: Comparison of the MammoSite Registry Trial With Intergroup Study E5194

Goyal S, Vicini F, Beitsch PD, et al (Cancer Inst of New Jersey and UMDNJ/ Robert Wood Johnson Med School, New Brunswick; William Beaumont Hosp, Royal Oak, MI; Dallas Breast Ctr, TX; et al)
Cancer 117:1149-1155, 2011

Background.—The purpose of this study was to determine the ipsilateral breast tumor recurrence (IBTR) in ductal carcinoma in situ (DCIS) patients treated in the American Society of Breast Surgeons MammoSite Breast Brachytherapy Registry Trial who met the criteria for E5194 treated with local excision and adjuvant accelerated partial breast irradiation (APBI).

Methods.—A total of 194 patients with DCIS were treated between 2002 and 2004 in the MammoSite registry trial; of these, 70 patients met the enrollment criteria for E5194: 1) low to intermediate grade (LIG)—pathological size >0.3 but <2.5 cm and margins ≥3 mm (n = 41) or 2) high grade (HG)—pathological size <1 cm and margins ≥3 mm (n = 29). All patients were treated with lumpectomy followed by adjuvant APBI using MammoSite. Median follow-up was 52.7 months (range, 0-88.4). SAS (version 8.2) was used for statistical analysis.

Results.—In the LIG cohort, the 5-year IBTR was 0%, compared with 6.1% at 5 years in E5194. In the HG cohort, the 5-year IBTR was

---

TABLE 3.—Comparison of IBTR Rates—Present Study Versus ECOG 5194

	5-Year IBTR
LIG-E5194	6.1%
LIG—present study	0%
HG—E5194	15.3%
HG—present study	5.3%

5.3%, compared with 15.3% at 5 years in E5194. The overall 5-year IBTR was 2%, and there were no cases of elsewhere or regional failures in the entire cohort. The 5-year contralateral breast event rate was 0% and 5.6% in LIG and HG patients, respectively (compared with 3.5% and 4.2%, respectively, in E5194).

Conclusions.—This study found that patients who met the criteria of E5194 treated with APBI had extremely low rates of recurrence (0% vs 6.1% in the LIG cohort and 5.3% vs 15.3% in the HG cohort) (Table 3).

▶ As mammography is improving, the diagnosis of ductal carcinoma in situ is increasing. In the past, ductal carcinoma in situ was frequently treated with mastectomy. As an invasive breast cancer, treatment with whole-breast irradiation reduces the risk of recurrence following breast conservation. The purpose of this study was to determine if accelerated partial breast irradiation could be used as an alternative. This is a multi-institutional trial.

Here the authors showed that they were able to achieve very low ipsilateral breast recurrence using accelerated partial breast irradiation. Of note, however, more than half of the patients also received tamoxifen.

Thus, in patients who meet the very strict criteria established in this trial, adjuvant accelerated partial breast radiation may be an option (Table 3).

T. J. Eberlein, MD

Ductal Carcinoma In Situ Treated With Breast-Conserving Surgery and Radiotherapy: A Comparison With ECOG Study 5194

Motwani SB, Goyal S, Moran MS, et al (The Cancer Inst of New Jersey, New Brunswick; Yale Univ School of Medicine, New Haven, CT; et al)
Cancer 117:1156-1162, 2011

Background.—Recent data from Eastern Cooperative Oncology Group (ECOG) Study 5194 (E5194) prospectively defined a low-risk subset of ductal carcinoma in situ (DCIS) patients where radiation therapy was omitted after lumpectomy alone. The purpose of the study was to determine the ipsilateral breast tumor recurrence (IBTR) in DCIS patients who met the criteria of E5194 treated with lumpectomy and adjuvant whole breast radiation therapy (RT).

Methods.—A total of 263 patients with DCIS were treated between 1980 and 2009 who met the enrollment criteria for E5194: 1) low to intermediate grade (LIG) with size >0.3 cm but <2.5 cm and margins >3 mm (n = 196), or 2) high grade (HG), size <1 cm and margins >3 mm (n = 67). All patients were treated with lumpectomy and whole breast RT with a boost to a median total tumor bed dose of 6400 cGy. Standard statistical analyses were performed with SAS (v. 9.2).

Results.—The average follow-up time was 6.9 years. The 5-year and 7-year IBTR for the LIG cohort in this study was 1.5% and 4.4% compared with 6.1% and 10.5% in E5194, respectively. The 5-year and 7-year IBTR

TABLE 2.—Comparison of IBTRs in the Current Study Versus ECOG 5194

	LIG: E5194	LIG: Current Study	HG: E5194	HG: Current Study
5-Year IBTR	6.1%	1.5%	15.3%	2%
7-Year IBTR	10.5%	4.4%	18%	2%

IBTR indicates ipsilateral breast tumor recurrence; ECOG, Eastern Cooperative Oncology Group; LIG, low to intermediate grade; HG, high grade.

for the HG cohort was 2.0% and 2.0% in this study compared with 15.3% and 18% in E5194, respectively.

Conclusions.—Adjuvant whole breast radiation therapy reduced the rate of local recurrence by more than 70% in patients with DCIS who met the criteria of E5194 (6.1% to 1.5% in the LIG cohort and 15.3% to 2% in the HG cohort). Additional follow-up is necessary given that 70% of IBTRs occurred after 5 years (Table 2).

▶ This is a multicenter prospective study looking at breast-conserving surgery and external beam radiation therapy but in comparison with patients who were eligible for the Eastern Cooperative Oncology Group (ECOG) 5194. This is a prospective study of observation after breast-conserving surgery. As seen in Table 2, radiation therapy conferred substantial benefit to patients when compared with observation alone.

There are several caveats with this study. The patient population in this particular study did not undergo as rigorous a pathologic assessment as was done in the ECOG 5194 study. Although this might bias current studies' population toward a higher relapse rate, the benefit of risk reduction in ipsilateral recurrence is larger in this study than seen in some other studies and may be explained because of the rigor of uniform radiotherapy as well as a boost dose. Finally, this study is retrospective in nature and therefore could be vulnerable to patient selection bias. In the future, genomic evaluation of these patients should help select which ones would be best treated with observation, partial breast radiation, or whole breast radiation (Table 2).

T. J. Eberlein, MD

Effect of Occult Metastases on Survival in Node-Negative Breast Cancer
Weaver DL, Ashikaga T, Krag DN, et al (Univ of Vermont College of Medicine and Vermont Cancer Ctr, Burlington; et al)
N Engl J Med 364:412-421, 2011

Background.—Retrospective and observational analyses suggest that occult lymph-node metastases are an important prognostic factor for disease recurrence or survival among patients with breast cancer. Prospective data on clinical outcomes from randomized trials according to sentinel-node involvement have been lacking.

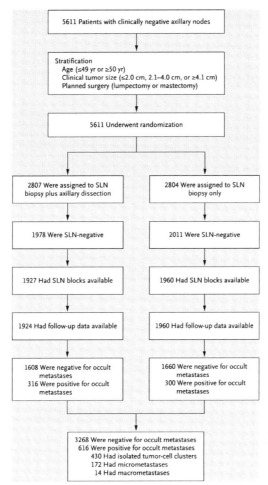

FIGURE 1.—Randomization and Results of Evaluation for Occult Metastases. The patients who underwent sentinel-lymph-node (SLN) biopsy plus axillary dissection and the patients who underwent SLN biopsy alone were combined into two analytic cohorts: patients in whom occult metastases were detected and patients in whom occult metastases were not detected. The categories for metastasis size (isolated tumor-cell clusters, micrometastases, and macrometastases) were used for subgroup analysis. (Reprinted from Weaver DL, Ashikaga T, Krag DN, et al. Effect of occult metastases on survival in node-negative breast cancer. *N Engl J Med.* 2011;364:412-421. Copyright © 2011 Massachusetts Medical Society. All rights reserved.)

Methods.—We randomly assigned women with breast cancer to sentinel-lymph-node biopsy plus axillary dissection or sentinel-lymph-node biopsy alone. Paraffin-embedded tissue blocks of sentinel lymph nodes obtained from patients with pathologically negative sentinel lymph nodes were centrally evaluated for occult metastases deeper in the blocks. Both routine staining and immunohistochemical staining for cytokeratin were used at two widely spaced additional tissue levels. Treating physicians were unaware

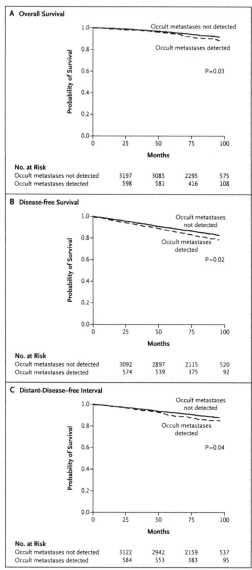

FIGURE 2.—Kaplan–Meier Survival Estimates According to the Presence or Absence of Occult Metastases Detected in Initially Negative Sentinel Lymph Nodes. Panel A shows the probability of overall survival. The Kaplan–Meier estimate of overall survival at 60 months among patients in whom occult metastases were not detected was 95.8%; among patients in whom occult metastases were detected, it was 94.6%. Panel B shows the probability of disease-free survival. The Kaplan–Meier estimate of disease-free survival at 60 months among patients in whom occult metastases were not detected was 89.2%; among patients in whom occult metastases were detected, it was 86.4%. Panel C shows the probability of distant-disease–free survival. The Kaplan–Meier estimate of distant-disease-free survival at 60 months among patients in whom occult metastases were not detected was 92.5%; among patients in whom occult metastases were detected, it was 89.7%. (Reprinted from Weaver DL, Ashikaga T, Krag DN, et al. Effect of occult metastases on survival in node-negative breast cancer. *N Engl J Med.* 2011;364:412-421. Copyright © 2011 Massachusetts Medical Society. All rights reserved.)

of the findings, which were not used for clinical treatment decisions. The initial evaluation at participating sites was designed to detect all macrometastases larger than 2 mm in the greatest dimension.

Results.—Occult metastases were detected in 15.9% (95% confidence interval [CI], 14.7 to 17.1) of 3887 patients. Log-rank tests indicated a significant difference between patients in whom occult metastases were detected and those in whom no occult metastases were detected with respect to overall survival (P=0.03), disease-free survival (P=0.02), and distant-disease-free interval (P=0.04). The corresponding adjusted hazard ratios for death, any outcome event, and distant disease were 1.40 (95% CI, 1.05 to 1.86), 1.31 (95% CI, 1.07 to 1.60), and 1.30 (95% CI, 1.02 to 1.66), respectively. Five-year Kaplan-Meier estimates of overall survival among patients in whom occult metastases were detected and those without detectable metastases were 94.6% and 95.8%, respectively.

Conclusions.—Occult metastases were an independent prognostic variable in patients with sentinel nodes that were negative on initial examination; however, the magnitude of the difference in outcome at 5 years was small (1.2 percentage points). These data do not indicate a clinical benefit of additional evaluation, including immunohistochemical analysis, of initially negative sentinel nodes in patients with breast cancer. (Funded by the National Cancer Institute; ClinicalTrials.gov number, NCT00003830.) (Figs 1 and 2).

▶ Fig 1 in the article demonstrates the randomization schema for this study. Fig 2 shows that occult metastases in patients with sentinel nodes that were negative on initial examination did have a statistically significant reduction in overall survival, disease-free survival, and distant disease—free interval. However, as seen in Fig 2A, the overall survival difference was 1.2% at 5 years.

The authors concluded that additional tissue levels or routine immunohistochemical analysis for sentinel lymph node evaluation is not needed. Although the difference in survival in patients with micrometastatic disease in sentinel lymph node is very small, continued follow-up and analysis of this and other trials will be important to detect whether the difference becomes larger.

T. J. Eberlein, MD

Local, Regional, and Systemic Recurrence Rates in Patients Undergoing Skin-Sparing Mastectomy Compared With Conventional Mastectomy
Yi M, Kronowitz SJ, Meric-Bernstam F, et al (The Univ of Texas M D Anderson Cancer Ctr, Houston)
Cancer 117:916-924, 2011

Background.—Although the use of SSM is becoming more common, there are few data on long-term, local-regional, and distant recurrence rates after treatment. The purpose of this study was to examine the rates of local, regional, and systemic recurrence, and survival in breast cancer

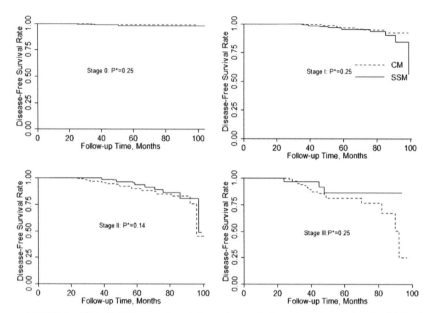

FIGURE 3.—Clinical TNM stage adjusted disease-free survival rates in patients undergoing SSM and CM (*P values were calculated by stratified log-rank test). (Reprinted from Yi M, Kronowitz SJ, Meric-Bernstam F, et al. Local, regional, and systemic recurrence rates in patients undergoing skin-sparing mastectomy compared with conventional mastectomy. *Cancer.* 2011;117:916-924. Copyright 2011 American Cancer Society. This material is reproduced with permission of Wiley-Liss, Inc., a subsidiary of John Wiley & Sons, Inc.)

TABLE 6.—Multivariate Stratified Cox Proportional Hazards Model of Breast Cancer Disease-Specific Survival

	HR[a]	P[a]	95% CI[a]
Local-Regional recurrence			
No	Referent		
Yes	10.2	<.0001	4.1-25.3
Surgery type			
CM	Referent		
SSM	0.6	.1	0.3-1.2
Estrogen receptor status			
Positive	Referent		
Negative	4.0	<.0001	2.1-7.8
Positive lymph node			
No	Referent		
Yes	2.4	.007	1.3-4.4

HR, hazard ratio; CI, confidence interval; CM, conventional mastectomy; SSM, skin-sparing mastectomy.
[a]Stratified by clinical TNM stage and age.

patients who underwent skin-sparing mastectomy (SSM) or conventional mastectomy (CM) at our institution.

Methods.—Patients with stage 0 to III unilateral breast cancer who underwent total mastectomy at our center from 2000 to 2005 were included in this study. Kaplan-Meier curves were calculated, and the log-rank test was used to evaluate the differences between overall and disease-free survival rates in the 2 groups.

Results.—Of 1810 patients, 799 (44.1%) underwent SSM and 1011 (55.9%) underwent CM. Patients who underwent CM were older (58.3 vs 49.3 years, *P*<.0001) and were more likely to have stage IIB or III disease (53.0% vs 31.8%, *P*<.0001). Significantly more patients in the CM group received neoadjuvant chemotherapy and adjuvant radiation therapy (*P*<.0001). At a median follow-up of 53 months, 119 patients (6.6%) had local, regional, or systemic recurrences. The local, regional, and systemic recurrence rates did not differ significantly between the SSM and CM groups. After adjusting for clinical TNM stage and age, disease-free survival rates between the SSM and CM groups did not differ significantly.

Conclusions.—SSM is an acceptable treatment option for patients who are candidates for immediate breast reconstruction. Local-regional recurrence rates are similar to those of patients undergoing CM (Fig 3, Table 6).

▶ This is a retrospective analysis of a prospective database comparing skin-sparing mastectomy with conventional mastectomy at the MD Anderson Cancer Center.

Patients who have undergone conventional mastectomy tended to be older, have later-stage disease, and receive neoadjuvant chemotherapy or adjuvant radiation therapy. As seen in Fig 3, when TNM stage was evaluated, disease-free survival rates were no different. Using multivariate analysis (Table 6), local-regional recurrence, estrogen receptor status, and positive lymph nodes all predicted for impact on survival but surgery type did not. Thus, skin-sparing mastectomy does not seem to increase the risk of recurrence. Any surgeon should develop a comfort level with the technical challenges of skin-sparing mastectomies to provide this option to their patients (Fig 3, Table 6).

T. J. Eberlein, MD

Radiation Therapy for Ductal Carcinoma In Situ: A Decision Analysis
Punglia RS, Burstein HJ, Weeks JC (Harvard Med School, Boston, MA)
Cancer 118:603-611, 2012

Background.—The benefit of adding radiation therapy after excision of ductal carcinoma in situ (DCIS) is widely debated. Randomized clinical trials are underpowered to delineate long-term outcomes after radiation.

Methods.—The authors of this report constructed a Markov decision model to simulate the clinical course of DCIS in a woman aged 60 years who received treatment with either of 2 breast-conserving strategies: excision alone or excision plus radiation therapy. Sensitivity analyses were used to study the influence of risk of local recurrence, likelihood of invasive disease at recurrence, surgical choice at recurrence, and patient age at diagnosis on treatment outcomes.

Results.—The addition of radiation therapy was associated with slight improvements in invasive disease-free and overall survival. However, radiation therapy decreased the chance of having both breasts intact over a patient's lifetime. Radiation therapy improved survival by 2.1 months for women who were diagnosed with DCIS at age 60 years but decreased the chance of having both breasts by 8.6% relative to excision alone. The differences in outcomes between the treatment strategies became smaller with increasing age at diagnosis. Sensitivity analyses revealed a greater benefit for radiation with an increased likelihood of invasive recurrence. The decrement in breast preservation with radiation therapy was mitigated by an increased likelihood of mastectomy at the time of recurrence or new breast cancer diagnosis.

Conclusions.—The current analysis quantified the benefits of radiation after excision of DCIS but also revealed that radiation therapy may increase the likelihood of eventual mastectomy. Therefore, the authors concluded that patient age and preferences should be considered when making the decision to add or forgo radiation for DCIS (Fig 2, Table 2).

▶ This is a very nice article by the group at the Dana Farber Cancer Institute. They constructed a Markov decision model to simulate the clinical course of

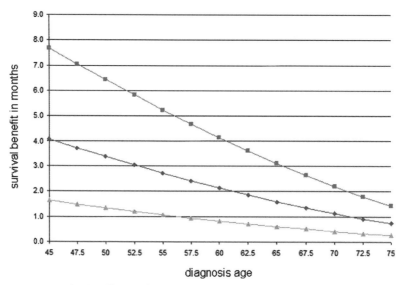

FIGURE 2.—This chart illustrates the overall survival benefit with radiation therapy according to age at diagnosis using baseline estimates and maximum and minimum benefit estimates. The benefit to survival with radiation therapy is plotted against age at diagnosis. The blue line represents the benefit using baseline assumptions (a 10-year risk of local recurrence without radiation therapy of 0.2495 and 50% of recurrences consisting of noninvasive disease), the pink line represents the maximum possible radiation benefit (a 10-year risk of local recurrence of 0.35 and 70% of recurrences consisting of invasive disease), and the green line represents the minimum possible radiation benefit (a 10-year risk of local recurrence of 0.15 and 30% of recurrences consisting of invasive disease). For interpretation of the references to color in this figure legend, the reader is referred to web version of this article. (Reprinted from Punglia RS, Burstein HJ, Weeks JC. Radiation therapy for ductal carcinoma in situ: a decision analysis. *Cancer.* 2012;118:603-611. Copyright 2012, American Cancer Society. This material is reproduced with permission of Wiley-Liss, Inc., a subsidiary of John Wiley & Sons, Inc.)

TABLE 2.—One-Way Sensitivity Analyses for the Addition of Radiation Therapy in Women Aged 60 Years

Variable	Range Studied Baseline Δ	Invasive DFS 11.7 mo Δ of Range, mo	OS 2.1 mo Δ of Range, mo	Percentage With Both Breasts During Lifetime −8.6% Δ of Range, %
LR at 10 y	0.2495 0.15-0.35	7.0-16.7	1.3-3.0	−7.6 to −9.6
Reduction in LR with RT	0.46 0.30-0.70	8.0-17.4	1.4-3.1	−11.6 to −4.1
Proportion of invasive LR	0.50 0.30-0.70	9.0-15.9	1.4-2.9	−9 to −8.2
Proportion of invasive new cancer	0.69 0.30-0.80	11.2-11.9	2.1-2.2	−9 to −8.5
Contralateral breast cancer/y	0.008 0.004-0.010	12.1-11.6	2.1-2.2	−10 to −8.1
Proportion mastectomy at recurrence or new cancer if no previous RT	0.32[a] 0.20-0.48	11.7-11.5	2.1-2.1	−11.7 to −4.3

Abbreviations: Delta (Δ), difference with the addition of radiation therapy; DFS, disease-free survival; LR, local recurrence; OS, overall survival; RT, radiation therapy.
[a]In baseline analysis, this variable is a function of the stage of recurrence or new diagnosis; on average, it is 0.32.

ductal carcinoma in situ (DCIS) in a woman 60 years of age who received breast-conserving surgery alone or breast-conserving surgery plus radiation therapy.

As is seen in Table 2, addition of radiation therapy to surgical primary treatment for DCIS improves survival by 2.1 months. However, there was an 8.6% decrease in the chance of the patient keeping both breasts during her lifetime. As seen in Fig 2, the benefit of treatment actually diminishes as the patient ages.

Therefore, any surgeon treating DCIS should read this article and include patient age and patient preferences before making a definitive recommendation of intervention in this patient population.

T. J. Eberlein, MD

Colon

Association of *CHFR* Promoter Methylation with Disease Recurrence in Locally Advanced Colon Cancer
Tanaka M, Chang P, Li Y, et al (The Univ of Texas MD Anderson Cancer Ctr, Houston)
Clin Cancer Res 17:4531-4540, 2011

Purpose.—This study was designed to determine whether DNA methylation biomarkers are associated with recurrence and survival in colon cancer patients.

Experimental Design.—A retrospective analysis of 82 patients who received curative surgical resection for American Joint Committee on Cancer (AJCC) high-risk stage II or III colon cancer (1999—2007) was conducted. DNA methylation status was quantitatively evaluated by the pyrosequencing method. We preselected three tumor suppressor genes and one locus of interest; *CHFR, ID4, RECK,* and *MINT1.* Mean methylation levels of multiple CpG sites in the promoter regions were used for analysis; 15% or more was defined as methylation positive. The association of recurrence-free survival (RFS) and overall survival (OS) with methylation status was analyzed by the log-rank test, Kaplan—Meier method, and Cox proportional hazards model.

Results.—Methylation levels of *ID4, MINT1,* and *RECK* did not correlate with RFS or OS. *CHFR* was methylation positive in 63% patients. When methylation status was dichotomized (negative or low: <30%, high: ≥30%), patients with *CHFR* methylation-high (44%) had worse RFS (*P* = 0.006) and reduced OS (*P* = 0.069). When stratified by stage, *CHFR* methylation-high was associated with reduced RFS (*P* = 0.004) and OS (*P* = 0.010) in stage III patients. *CHFR* methylation-high was commonly associated with N2 disease (*P* = 0.04) and proximal tumors (*P* = 0.002). Multivariate analysis indicated AJCC T4 disease and *CHFR* methylation-high (*P* = 0.001 and *P* = 0.015, respectively) were independent predictors for recurrence.

Conclusions.—The extent of *CHFR* promoter methylation correlates with RFS, indicating it is a promising epigenetic marker for recurrence.

▶ This is a retrospective analysis of stage 2 and 3 colon cancer patients from the MD Anderson Cancer Center. The authors looked at tumor suppressor genes and relapse-free survival and overall survival. As seen in Fig 1 in the original article, high methylation levels of *CHFR* promoter region was associated with a reduced recurrence-free survival in all patients that were analyzed in this study, but this effect was dramatic in stage 3 patients and not significant in stage 2 patients. Further multivariate analysis found that high levels of *CHFR* methylation were commonly associated with advanced nodal disease in proximal tumors. This marker may be an excellent marker for recurrence of tumor. This promoter may have an important role in tumor metastasis and may be a marker that requires more aggressive adjuvant systemic therapy as well as a potential for research to identify specific targeted therapies for this promoter.

T. J. Eberlein, MD

Hepatic Colorectal

A Randomized Trial of *Ex vivo* CD40L Activation of a Dendritic Cell Vaccine in Colorectal Cancer Patients: Tumor-Specific Immune Responses Are Associated with Improved Survival

Barth RJ Jr, Fisher DA, Wallace PK, et al (Dartmouth-Hitchcock Med Ctr and Norris Cotton Cancer Ctr, Lebanon, NH)
Clin Cancer Res 16:5548-5556, 2010

Purpose.—To determine whether an autologous dendritic cell (DC) vaccine could induce antitumor immune responses in patients after resection of colorectal cancer metastases and whether these responses could be enhanced by activating DCs with CD40L.

Experimental Design.—Twenty-six patients who had undergone resection of colorectal metastases were treated with intranodal injections of an autologous tumor lysate— and control protein [keyhole limpet hemocyanin (KLH)]—pulsed DC vaccine. Patients were randomized to receive DCs that had been either activated or not activated with CD40L. All patients were followed for a minimum of 5.5 years.

Results.—Immunization induced an autologous tumor-specific T-cell proliferative or IFNγ enzyme-linked immunospot response in 15 of 24 assessable patients (63%) and a tumor-specific DTH response in 61%. Patients with evidence of a vaccine-induced, tumor-specific T-cell proliferative or IFNγ response 1 week after vaccination had a markedly better recurrence-free survival (RFS) at 5 years (63% versus 18%, $P = 0.037$) than nonresponders. In contrast, no association was observed between induction of KLH-specific immune responses and RFS. CD40L maturation induced CD86 and CD83 expression on DCs but had no effect on immune responses or RFS.

Conclusion.—Adjuvant treatment of patients after resection of colorectal metastases with an autologous tumor lysate—pulsed, DC vaccine—induced, tumor-specific immune responses in a high proportion of patients. There was an association between induction of tumor-specific immune responses and RFS. Activation of this DC vaccine with CD40L did not lead to increased immune responses (Figs 1 and 2).

▶ Patients who have resection of colorectal liver metastases have a high risk of recurrent disease. If they are treated with chemotherapy, there is an increase in recurrence-free survival but many patients recur by 3 years after resection. This

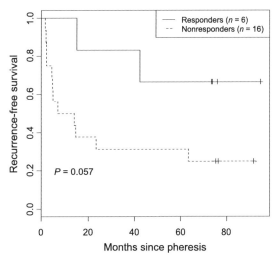

FIGURE 1.—Autologous tumor-specific proliferative response 1 wk after DC immunization is associated with an improved RFS (log-rank $P = 0.057$). (Reprinted with permission from American Association for Cancer Research, Inc. Barth RJ Jr, Fisher DA, Wallace PK, et al. A randomized trial of *ex vivo* CD40L activation of a dendritic cell vaccine in colorectal cancer patients: tumor-specific immune responses are associated with improved survival. *Clin Cancer Res.* 2010;16:5548-5556.)

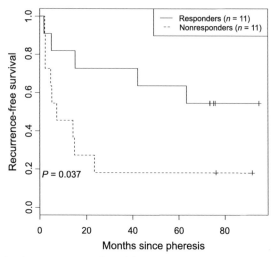

FIGURE 2.—Autologous tumor-specific proliferative or IFNγ ELISPOT response 1 wk after DC immunization is associated with an improved RFS (log-rank $P = 0.037$). (Reprinted with permission from American Association for Cancer Research, Inc. Barth RJ Jr, Fisher DA, Wallace PK, et al. A randomized trial of *ex vivo* CD40L activation of a dendritic cell vaccine in colorectal cancer patients: tumor-specific immune responses are associated with improved survival. *Clin Cancer Res.* 2010;16:5548-5556.)

is a very novel study of 26 patients who had undergone resection of colorectal metastasis. They are treated with an autologous dendritic cell vaccine. In the patients who had immune response, there was an increase in recurrence-free survival (Fig 1, autologous tumor—specific proliferative response and Fig 2, tumor-specific proliferative or interferon gamma response).

While this is a small study, it demonstrates that an immune response can correlate with recurrence-free survival.

What was novel about this study is that the authors chose to perform the treatment in an adjuvant setting with no measurable disease after colorectal metastasis resection. This is the setting that one predicts would have best results because of the patients' immunocompetence and very small tumor burden.

T. J. Eberlein, MD

A Combination of Serum Markers for the Early Detection of Colorectal Cancer

Wild N, Andres H, Rollinger W, et al (Roche Diagnostics GmbH, Penzberg, Germany)
Clin Cancer Res 16:6111-6121, 2010

Purpose.—Fecal occult blood testing is recommended as first-line screening to detect colorectal cancer (CRC). We evaluated markers and marker combinations in serum as an alternative to improve the detection of CRC.

TABLE 3.—Sensitivities (%) of Marker Candidates by Tumor Stages at 95% Specificity

	N/N^a	CEA	Seprase	CYFRA 21-1	OPN	Ferritin	Anti-p53
Colorectal cancer							
Stage 0	6/6	16.7	16.7	16.7	16.7	16.7	33.3
Stage I	53/50	13.2	36.0	13.2	13.2	13.2	16.0
Stage II	68/67	36.8	49.3	26.5	22.1	30.9	17.9
Stage III	76/76	34.2	51.3	23.7	27.6	34.2	15.8
Stage IV	68/66	88.2	31.8	80.9	54.4	13.2	24.2
Stage 0–III[b]	233/229	30.9	45.4	22.3	23.2	27.0	18.8
All stages	301/295	43.9	42.4	35.5	30.2	23.9	20.0
Adenoma							
Advanced adenoma	143/141	7.7	11.3	8.4	9.1	9.8	5.6

[a]Reduced sample number for seprase and anti-p53 due to sample volume.
[b]Thirty additional samples included with staging as given by a pathologist, I–III or II–III.

TABLE 5.—Specificity of the Marker Combination Against Disease Controls and Other Cancer

	N	Specificity (%)[a]
Disease controls	141	60.3 (53.0–67.2)
Chronic bowel diseases[b]	44	47.7 (34.6–61.1)
Colitis	29	62.1 (45.1–77.1)
Diverticulitis	30	63.3 (46.7–77.9)
Inflammatory GI disease[c]	22	68.2 (48.5–84.0)
Other[d]	4	100.0 (47.3–100)
Ulcer	12	66.7 (39.1–87.7)
Other cancer	176	75.0 (69.1–80.3)
Bladder cancer	8	87.5 (52.9–99.4)
Breast cancer	44	77.3 (64.5–87.1)
Endometrium	15	86.7 (63.7–97.6)
Kidney cancer	23	69.6 (50.4–84.8)
Lung cancer	30	46.7 (30.8–63.0)
Ovary cancer	23	69.6 (50.4–84.8)
Prostate cancer	33	97.0 (86.4–99.8)

[a]Apparent specificities when the algorithm was applied using a cutoff derived from the control cohort at 98% specificity, 90% CI.
[b]Colitis ulcerativa, infection-related diarrhea, Morbus Crohn.
[c]Appendicitis, cholangitis, mesenteritis, pancreatitis, proctitis.
[d]Carcinoid, lipoma.

Experimental Design.—Using penalized logistic regression, 6 markers were selected for evaluation in 1,027 samples (301 CRC patients, 143 patients with adenoma, 266 controls, 141 disease controls, and 176 patients with other cancer). The diagnostic performance of each marker and of marker combinations was assessed.

Results.—To detect CRC from serum samples, we tested 22 biomarkers. Six markers were selected for a marker combination, including the known tumor markers CEA (carcinoembryonic antigen) and CYFRA 21-1 as well as novel markers or markers that are less routinely used for the detection of CRC: ferritin, osteopontin (OPN), anti-p53, and seprase. CEA showed the best sensitivity at 95% specificity with 43.9%, followed by seprase (42.4%), CYFRA 21-1 (35.5%), OPN (30.2%), ferritin (23.9%), and anti-p53 (20.0%). A combination of these markers gave 69.6% sensitivity at 95% specificity and 58.7% at 98% specificity. Focusing on International Union against Cancer (UICC) stages 0–III reduced the sensitivity slightly to 68.0% and 53.3%, respectively. In a subcollective, with matched stool samples (75 CRC cases and 234 controls), the sensitivity of the marker combination was comparable with fecal immunochemical testing (FIT) with 82.4% and 68.9% versus 81.8% and 72.7% at 95% and 98% specificity, respectively.

Conclusions.—The performance of the serum marker combination is comparable with FIT. This provides a novel tool for CRC screening to trigger a follow-up colonoscopy for a final diagnosis (Tables 3 and 5).

▶ The authors in this study looked at a range of 22 different biomarkers; 6 were selected for marker combination. Their sensitivities by tumor stage of colorectal cancer at 95% specificity are seen in Table 3. When comparing this panel of markers with other cancers, the results ranged from excellent (97%) in prostate cancer to 46.7% in lung cancer (Table 5).

The authors concluded that a combination of these 6 serum markers would initiate a follow-up colonoscopy for definitive diagnosis of early detection of colorectal cancer. They plan to focus on a true screening population with increased numbers of patients.

T. J. Eberlein, MD

Association of *KRAS* p.G13D Mutation With Outcome in Patients With Chemotherapy-Refractory Metastatic Colorectal Cancer Treated With Cetuximab

De Roock W, Jonker DJ, Di Nicolantonio F, et al (Univ of Leuven, Belgium; Univ of Ottawa, Ontario, Canada; Univ of Turin Med School, Italy; et al)
JAMA 304:1812-1820, 2010

Context.—Patients with metastatic colorectal cancer who have *KRAS* codon 12– or *KRAS* codon 13–mutated tumors are presently excluded from treatment with the anti–epidermal growth factor receptor monoclonal antibody cetuximab.

Objective.—To test the hypothesis that *KRAS* codon 13 mutations are associated with a better outcome after treatment with cetuximab than observed with other *KRAS* mutations.

Design, Setting, and Patients.—We studied the association between *KRAS* mutation status (p.G13D vs other *KRAS* mutations) and response and survival in a pooled data set of 579 patients with chemotherapy-refractory colorectal cancer treated with cetuximab between 2001 and 2008. Patients were included in the CO.17, BOND, MABEL, EMR202600, EVEREST, BABEL, or SALVAGE clinical trials or received off-study treatment. Univariate and multivariate analyses, adjusting for possible prognostic factors and

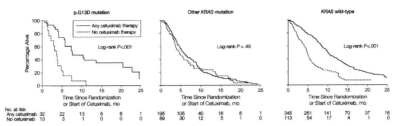

FIGURE 1.—Overall Survival: Predictive Analysis by *KRAS* Status for Patients Receiving Any Cetuximab-Based Therapy vs No Cetuximab. The no cetuximab group for all patients from the pooled data set is the best supportive care group from the CO.17 trial. (Reprinted from De Roock W, Jonker DJ, Di Nicolantonio F, et al. Association of *KRAS* p.G13D mutation with outcome in patients with chemotherapy-refractory metastatic colorectal cancer treated with cetuximab. *JAMA.* 2010;304:1812-1820. Copyright 2010 American Medical Association. All rights reserved.)

data set, were performed. The effect of the different mutations was studied in vitro by constructing isogenic cell lines with wild-type *KRAS*, p.G12V, or p.G13D mutant alleles and treating them with cetuximab.

Main Outcome Measures.—The main efficacy end point was overall survival. Secondary efficacy end points were response rate and progression-free survival.

Results.—In comparison with patients with other *KRAS*-mutated tumors, patients with p.G13D-mutated tumors (n = 32) treated with cetuximab had longer overall survival (median, 7.6 [95% confidence interval {CI}, 5.7-20.5] months vs 5.7 [95% CI, 4.9-6.8] months; adjusted hazard ratio [HR], 0.50; 95% CI, 0.31-0.81; *P* =.005) and longer progression-free survival (median, 4.0 [95% CI, 1.9-6.2] months vs 1.9 [95% CI, 1.8-2.8] months; adjusted HR, 0.51; 95% CI, 0.32-0.81; *P* =.004). There was a significant interaction between *KRAS* mutation status (p.G13D vs other *KRAS* mutations) and overall survival benefit with cetuximab treatment (adjusted HR, 0.30; 95% CI, 0.14-0.67; *P* =.003). In vitro and mouse model analysis showed that although p.G12V mutated colorectal cells were insensitive to cetuximab, p.G13D-mutated cells were sensitive, as were *KRAS* wild-type cells.

Conclusions.—In this analysis, use of cetuximab was associated with longer overall and progression-free survival among patients with chemotherapy-refractory colorectal cancer with p.G13D-mutated tumors than with other *KRAS*-mutated tumors. Evaluation of cetuximab therapy in these tumors in prospective randomized trials may be warranted (Fig 1).

▶ Patients with metastatic colorectal cancer and *KRAS*-mutated tumor do no benefit from antiepidermal growth factor receptor monoclonal antibodies. This study looked at a specific *KRAS* mutation p.G13D and response and survival in patients with chemotherapy-refractory colorectal cancer treated with cetuximab. As seen in Fig 1, the use of cetuximab was associated with longer overall and progression-free survival among patients with this specific mutated tumor.

This implies that specific treatments will be effective depending on genetic pathways mutated in a specific patient's tumor. Further prospective trials will be needed to confirm these results.

T. J. Eberlein, MD

TFAP2E–DKK4 and Chemoresistance in Colorectal Cancer

Ebert MPA, Tänzer M, Balluff B, et al (Ruprecht-Karls-Universität Heidelberg, Mannheim, Germany; Technische Universität, Munich; et al)
N Engl J Med 366:44-53, 2012

Background.—Chemotherapy for advanced colorectal cancer leads to improved survival; however, predictors of response to systemic treatment are not available. Genomic and epigenetic alterations of the gene encoding transcription factor AP-2 epsilon (*TFAP2E*) are common in human cancers. The gene encoding dickkopf homolog 4 protein (*DKK4*) is a potential downstream target of *TFAP2E* and has been implicated in chemotherapy resistance. We aimed to further evaluate the role of *TFAP2E* and *DKK4* as predictors of the response of colorectal cancer to chemotherapy.

Methods.—We analyzed the expression, methylation, and function of *TFAP2E* in colorectal-cancer cell lines in vitro and in patients with colorectal cancer. We examined an initial cohort of 74 patients, followed by four cohorts of patients (total, 220) undergoing chemotherapy or chemoradiation.

Results.—*TFAP2E* was hypermethylated in 38 of 74 patients (51%) in the initial cohort. Hypermethylation was associated with decreased expression of *TFAP2E* in primary and metastatic colorectal-cancer specimens and cell lines. Colorectal-cancer cell lines overexpressing *DKK4* showed increased chemoresistance to fluorouracil but not irinotecan or oxaliplatin. In the four other patient cohorts, *TFAP2E* hypermethylation was significantly associated with nonresponse to chemotherapy (P<0.001). Conversely, the probability of response among patients with hypomethylation was approximately six times that in the entire population (overall estimated risk ratio, 5.74; 95% confidence interval, 3.36 to 9.79). Epigenetic alterations of *TFAP2E* were independent of mutations in key regulatory cancer genes, microsatellite instability, and other genes that affect fluorouracil metabolism.

Conclusions.—*TFAP2E* hypermethylation is associated with clinical nonresponsiveness to chemotherapy in colorectal cancer. Functional assays confirm that *TFAP2E*-dependent resistance is mediated through *DKK4*. In patients who have colorectal cancer with *TFAP2E* hypermethylation, targeting of *DKK4* may be an option to overcome *TFAP2E*-mediated drug resistance. (Funded by Deutsche Forschungsgemeinschaft and others.) (Table 2).

▶ Dickkopf homolog 4 protein (DKK4) is a potential downstream target of TFAP2E and has been implicated in fluorouracil resistance. This is a study looking at cohort of patients followed by 4 other cohorts that underwent chemotherapy or chemoradiation for rectal cancer. The goal of this study was to evaluate the role of TFAP2E and DKK4 as predictors of chemotherapy response in patients with colorectal cancer. As is seen in Table 2, all 4 cohorts showed a negative association of methylation and treatment response; that is, patients with hypermethylation had lower response to chemotherapy. As seen in Fig 3 in the original article, all 4 cohorts of patients demonstrated the same relationship. This is also true whether the patients had metastatic colorectal cancer or underwent chemoradiation for

TABLE 2.—*TFAP2E* Methylation in Four Cohorts of Patients with Colorectal Cancer, According to Response to Treatment*

Cohort No. and Center	No. of Patients	Cancer Type	Response Evaluation	Response	Nonresponse	P Value
I Bochum	74	Metastatic colorectal cancer	RECIST			<0.001
Hypermethylated *TFAP2E*				3	17	
Hypomethylated *TFAP2E*				33	21	
II Dresden	36	Metastatic colorectal cancer	RECIST			<0.001
Hypermethylated *TFAP2E*				1	22	
Hypomethylated *TFAP2E*				13	0	
III Mannheim	42	Primary rectal cancer	Histology			<0.001
Hypermethylated *TFAP2E*				5	14	
Hypomethylated *TFAP2E*				20	3	
IV Munich	68	Primary rectal cancer	Histology			<0.001
Hypermethylated *TFAP2E*				3	28	
Hypomethylated *TFAP2E*				29	8	
I and II (combined RECIST)	110		RECIST			<0.001
Hypermethylated *TFAP2E*				4	39	
Hypomethylated *TFAP2E*				46	21	
III and IV (combined histology)	110		Histology			<0.001
Hypermethylated *TFAP2E*				8	42	
Hypomethylated *TFAP2E*				49	11	
I, II, III, and IV	220		Both			<0.001
Hypermethylated *TFAP2E*				12	81	
Hypomethylated *TFAP2E*				95	32	

Editor's Note: Please refer to original journal article for full references.

*P values were calculated with the use of Fisher's exact test. RECIST denotes Response Evaluation Criteria in Solid Tumors (version 1.1)[7] (see the Supplementary Appendix, available at NEJM.org).

rectal cancer (Fig 3B in the original article). This may serve as a potential genetic and molecular marker that would predict response to fluorouracil chemotherapy. As we develop new genomic information, these kinds of markers will become more common and will be important knowledge for a surgeon to have.

T. J. Eberlein, MD

Association Between Time to Initiation of Adjuvant Chemotherapy and Survival In Colorectal Cancer: A Systematic Review and Meta-Analysis

Biagi JJ, Raphael MJ, Mackillop WJ, et al (Queen's Univ, Kingston, Ontario, Canada)
JAMA 305:2335-2342, 2011

Context.—Adjuvant chemotherapy (AC) improves survival among patients with resected colorectal cancer. However, the optimal timing from surgery to initiation of AC is unknown.

Objective.—To determine the relationship between time to AC and survival outcomes via a systematic review and meta-analysis.

Data Sources.—MEDLINE (1975 through January 2011), EMBASE, the Cochrane Database of Systematic Reviews, and the Cochrane Central Register of Controlled Trials were searched to identify studies that described the relationship between time to AC and survival.

Study Selection.—Studies were only included if the relevant prognostic factors were adequately described and either comparative groups were balanced or results adjusted for these prognostic factors.

Data Extraction.—Hazard ratios (HRs) for overall survival and disease-free survival from each study were converted to a regression coefficient (β) and standard error corresponding to a continuous representation per 4 weeks of time to AC. The adjusted β from individual studies were combined using a fixed-effects model. Inverse variance ($1/SE^2$) was used to weight individual studies. Publication bias was investigated using the trim and fill approach.

Results.—We identified 10 eligible studies involving 15 410 patients (7 published articles, 3 abstracts). Nine of the studies were cohort or population based and 1 was a secondary analysis from a randomized trial of chemotherapy. Six studies reported time to AC as a binary variable and 4 as 3 or more categories. Meta-analysis demonstrated that a 4-week increase in time to AC was associated with a significant decrease in both overall survival (HR, 1.14; 95% confidence interval [CI], 1.10-1.17) and disease-free survival (HR, 1.14; 95% CI, 1.10-1.18). There was no significant heterogeneity among included studies. Results remained significant after adjustment for potential publication bias and when the analysis was repeated to exclude studies of largest weight.

Conclusion.—In a meta-analysis of the available literature on time to AC, longer time to AC was associated with worse survival among patients with resected colorectal cancer.

▶ This is an excellent study that reviews all of the relevant studies that have prognostic factors and comparative groups that were balanced and results adjusted for the various prognostic factors. In carefully evaluating these studies, the authors showed through meta-analysis that a 4-week increase time to adjuvant chemotherapy was associated with a significant decrease in both survival and disease-free survival.

This study emphasizes the importance to all surgeons who do colorectal surgery of expediting referral to colleagues for adjuvant chemotherapy.

There are some potential limitations to this study. There may be an inherent bias caused by the patients' postoperative performance status. It is not known by these authors whether patients actually fully completed the adjuvant chemotherapy. These studies generally did not include oxaliplatin, so whether the conclusion could be extrapolated to studies with oxaliplatin is not known. Finally, this study relies on nonrandomized and retrospective data. Nonetheless, the conclusion is very strong, and it also suggests that chemotherapy should be more strictly controlled as a variable in future adjuvant chemo-therapy trials.

T. J. Eberlein, MD

Cetuximab Plus Irinotecan, Fluorouracil, and Leucovorin as First-Line Treatment for Metastatic Colorectal Cancer: Updated Analysis of Overall Survival According to Tumor *KRAS* and *BRAF* Mutation Status
Van Cutsem E, Köhne C-H, Láng I, et al (Univ Hosp Gasthuisberg, Leuven, Belgium; Klinikum Oldenburg, Germany; Univ Hosp Carl Gustav Carus, Dresden; et al)
J Clin Oncol 29:2011-2019, 2011

Purpose.—The addition of cetuximab to irinotecan, fluorouracil, and leucovorin (FOLFIRI) as first-line treatment for metastatic colorectal cancer (mCRC) was shown to reduce the risk of disease progression and increase the chance of response in patients with *KRAS* wild-type disease. An updated survival analysis, including additional patients analyzed for tumor mutation status, was undertaken.

Patients and Methods.—Patients were randomly assigned to receive FOLFIRI with or without cetuximab. DNA was extracted from additional slide-mounted tumor samples previously used to assess epidermal growth factor receptor expression. Clinical outcome according to the tumor muta-tion status of *KRAS* and *BRAF* was assessed in the expanded patient series.

Results.—The ascertainment rate of patients analyzed for tumor *KRAS* status was increased from 45% to 89%, with mutations detected in 37% of tumors. The addition of cetuximab to FOLFIRI in patients with *KRAS* wild-type disease resulted in significant improvements in overall survival (median, 23.5 v 20.0 months; hazard ratio [HR], 0.796; $P = .0093$), progression-free survival (median, 9.9 v 8.4 months; HR, 0.696; $P = .0012$), and response (rate 57.3% v 39.7%; odds ratio, 2.069; $P < .001$) compared with FOLFIRI alone. Significant interactions between *KRAS* status and treatment effect were noted for all key efficacy end points. *KRAS* mutation status was confirmed as a powerful predictive biomarker for the efficacy of cetuximab plus FOLFIRI. *BRAF* tumor mutation was a strong indicator of poor prognosis.

Conclusion.—The addition of cetuximab to FOLFIRI as first-line therapy improves survival in patients with *KRAS* wild-type mCRC. *BRAF* tumor mutation is an indicator of poor prognosis (Table 3).

▶ Irinotecan, fluorouracil, and leucovorin (FOLFIRI), with the addition of cetux-imab, have been used to treat metastatic colorectal cancer. This is a randomized trial looking at *KRAS* and *BRAF* mutation to predict clinical outcome. As seen in Fig 2A in the original article, addition of cetuximab to FOLFIRI resulted in signif-icant improvement in overall survival. Fig 2B in the original article shows that patients whose tumor had wild-type *KRAS* also benefited from cetuximab plus

TABLE 3.—Efficacy Data for Patients With *KRAS* Wild-Type Tumors According to Tumor *BRAF* Mutation Status

Parameter	*KRAS* Wild-Type/*BRAF* Wild-Type (n = 566)		*KRAS* Wild-Type/*BRAF* Mutant (n = 59)	
	FOLFIRI (n = 289)	Cetuximab + FOLFIRI (n = 277)	FOLFIRI (n = 33)	Cetuximab + FOLFIRI (n = 26)
Overall survival				
No. of events	229	207	33	22
Median, months	21.6	25.1	10.3	14.1
95% CI	20.0 to 24.9	22.5 to 28.7	8.4 to 14.9	8.5 to 18.5
Hazard ratio	0.830		0.908	
95% CI	0.687 to 1.004		0.507 to 1.624	
P (log-rank test)	.0547		.74	
Progression-free survival*				
No. of events	153	123	20	14
Median, months	8.8	10.9	5.6	8.0
95% CI	7.6 to 9.4	9.4 to 11.8	3.5 to 8.1	3.6 to 9.1
Hazard ratio	0.673		0.934	
95% CI	0.528 to 0.858		0.425 to 2.056	
P (log-rank test)	**.0013**		.87	
Best overall response*				
Complete response	0	3	0	0
%		1.1		
Partial response	123	166	5	5
%	42.6	59.9	15.2	19.2
Stable disease	135	80	16	17
%	46.7	28.9	48.5	65.4
Progressive disease	18	14	8	2
%	6.2	5.1	24.2	7.7
Not evaluable	13	14	4	2
%	4.5	5.1	12.1	7.7
Best overall response rate[†], %	42.6	61.0	15.2	19.2
95% CI	36.8 to 48.5	55.0 to 66.8	5.1 to 31.9	6.6 to 39.4
Odds ratio	2.175		1.084	
95% CI	1.551 to 3.051		0.264 to 4.446	
P (CMH test)	**< .001**		.91	

NOTE. P < .05 for bold values.
Abbreviations: FOLFIRI, irinotecan, leucovorin and fluorouracil; CMH, Cochran-Mantel-Haenszel.
Editor's Note: Please refer to original journal article for full references.
*As assessed by an independent review committee for the primary confirmatory analysis.[1]
[†]Best overall response rate = (complete response + partial response).

FOLFIRI. In contrast, patients whose tumors carried mutations in *KRAS* showed no evidence of benefit from the addition of cetuximab to FOLFIRI (Fig 2B in the original article). Patients whose tumors were wild type for both the gene of *KRAS* and the gene of *BRAF* showed benefit from the addition of cetuximab to FOLFIRI (Fig 2C in the original article, Table 3). In this study, there is no evidence of an independent treatment impact by tumor *BRAF* mutation status.

Utilization of these tumor markers may predict patient outcome to cetuximab and FOLFIRI chemotherapy. A subset of responders may then be eligible for aggressive tumor resection.

T. J. Eberlein, MD

Detection of Tumor DNA at the Margins of Colorectal Cancer Liver Metastasis

Holdhoff M, Schmidt K, Diehl F, et al (Ludwig Ctr for Cancer Genetics and Therapeutics and Howard Hughes Med Inst at Johns Hopkins Kimmel Cancer Ctr, Baltimore, MD; Inostics GmbH, Hamburg, Germany; et al)
Clin Cancer Res 17:3551-3557, 2011

Purpose.—Defining an adequate resection margin of colorectal cancer liver metastases is essential for optimizing surgical technique. We have attempted to evaluate the resection margin through a combination of histopathologic and genetic analyses.

Experimental Design.—We evaluated 88 samples of tumor margins from 12 patients with metastatic colon cancer who each underwent partial hepatectomy of one to six liver metastases. Punch biopsies of surrounding liver tissue were obtained at 4, 8, 12, and 16 mm from the tumor border. DNA from these biopsies was analyzed by a sensitive PCR-based technique, called BEAMing, for mutations of *KRAS*, *PIK3CA*, *APC*, or *TP53* identified in the corresponding tumor.

Results.—Mutations were identified in each patient's resected tumor and used to analyze the 88 samples circumscribing the tumor-normal border. Tumor-specific mutant DNA was detectable in surrounding liver tissue in 5 of these 88 samples, all within 4 mm of the tumor border. Biopsies that were 8, 12, and 16 mm from the macroscopic visible margin were devoid of detectable mutant tumor DNA and of microscopically visible cancer cells. Tumors with a significant radiologic response to chemotherapy were not associated with any increase in mutant tumor DNA in beyond 4 mm of the main tumor.

Conclusions.—Mutant tumor-specific DNA can be detected beyond the visible tumor margin, but never beyond 4 mm, even in patients whose tumors were larger prior to chemotherapy. These data provide a rational basis for determining the extent of surgical excision required in patients undergoing resection of liver metastases.

▶ This is a novel study that attempted to objectively define an adequate resection margin of colorectal cancer liver metastasis. Some of the patients had chemotherapy and shrinkage of their tumor. The authors found that mutant tumor-specific DNA was detectable beyond the visible tumor margin. However, it did not seem to extend beyond 4 mm.

Using this very sophisticated technology and perhaps applying it to other solid tumor margins might provide a more rational basis for resection margins. In the meantime, it appears that a normal negative histologic margin would be sufficient when resecting hepatic colorectal metastases.

T. J. Eberlein, MD

Occult Tumor Burden Predicts Disease Recurrence in Lymph Node–Negative Colorectal Cancer

Hyslop T, Weinberg DS, Schulz S, et al (Thomas Jefferson Univ, Philadelphia, PA; Fox Chase Cancer Ctr, Philadelphia, PA; et al)
Clin Cancer Res 17:3293-3303, 2011

Purpose.—Lymph node involvement by histopathology informs colorectal cancer prognosis, whereas recurrence in 25% of node-negative patients suggests the presence of occult metastasis. GUCY2C (guanylyl

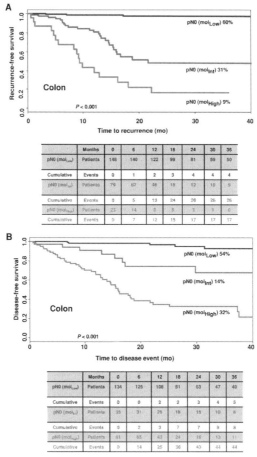

FIGURE 2.—Time to recurrence (A) and disease-free survival (B) in patients with pN0 colon cancer stratified by recursive partitioning. Tables below Kaplan—Meier plots summarize the number of patients at risk as well as cumulative events for each outcome. Censored values in time to recurrence reflect death from another cancer, a noncancer-related death, and death because of the cancer treatment, or loss of follow-up of individual patients (22). Censored patients in disease-free survival reflect loss to follow-up (22). *Editor's Note*: Please refer to original journal article for full references. (Reprinted with permission from American Association for Cancer Research, Inc. Hyslop T, Weinberg DS, Schulz S, et al. Occult tumor burden predicts disease recurrence in lymph node—negative colorectal cancer. *Clin Cancer Res.* 2011;17:3293-3303.)

cyclase C) is a marker of colorectal cancer cells that identifies occult nodal metastases associated with recurrence risk. Here, we defined the association of occult tumor burden, quantified by GUCY2C reverse transcriptase-PCR (RT-PCR), with outcomes in colorectal cancer.

Experimental Design.—Lymph nodes (range: 2−159) from 291 prospectively enrolled node-negative colorectal cancer patients were analyzed by histopathology and GUCY2C quantitative RT-PCR. Participants were followed for a median of 24 months (range: 2−63). Time to recurrence and disease-free survival served as primary and secondary outcomes, respectively. Association of outcomes with prognostic markers, including molecular tumor burden, was estimated by recursive partitioning and Cox models.

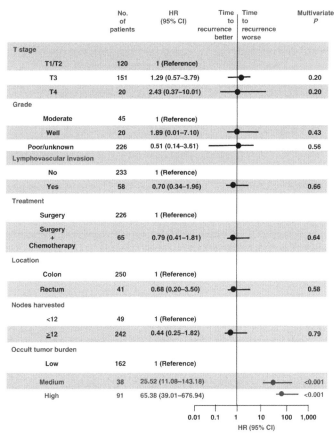

FIGURE 4.—Cox proportional hazards analyses of time to recurrence in patients with pN0 colorectal cancer stratified by recursive partitioning. HRs (circles) with 95% CIs (horizontal lines) and *P* values for multivariable analyses describe interactions between prognostic characteristics and time to recurrence. Parameters that are significantly prognostic (*P* < 0.05) are highlighted in red. For interpretation of the references to color in this figure legend, the reader is referred to web version of this article. (Reprinted with permission from American Association for Cancer Research, Inc. Hyslop T, Weinberg DS, Schulz S, et al. Occult tumor burden predicts disease recurrence in lymph node−negative colorectal cancer. *Clin Cancer Res.* 2011;17:3293-3303.)

Results.—In this cohort, 176 (60%) patients exhibited low tumor burden (Mol$_{Low}$), and all but four remained free of disease [recurrence rate 2.3% (95% CI, 0.1–4.5%)]. Also, 90 (31%) patients exhibited intermediate tumor burden (Mol$_{Int}$) and 30 [33.3% (23.7–44.1)] developed recurrent disease. Furthermore, 25 (9%) patients exhibited high tumor burden (Mol$_{High}$) and 17 [68.0% (46.5–85.1)] developed recurrent disease ($P <$ 0.001). Occult tumor burden was an independent marker of prognosis. Mol$_{Int}$ and Mol$_{High}$ patients exhibited a graded risk of earlier time to recurrence [Mol$_{Int}$, adjusted HR 25.52 (11.08–143.18); $P < 0.001$; Mol$_{High}$, 65.38 (39.01–676.94); $P < 0.001$] and reduced disease-free survival [Mol$_{Int}$, 9.77 (6.26–87.26); $P < 0.001$; Mol$_{High}$, 22.97 (21.59–316.16); $P < 0.001$].

Conclusion.—Molecular tumor burden in lymph nodes is independently associated with time to recurrence and disease-free survival in patients with node-negative colorectal cancer (Figs 2 and 4).

▶ This is a prospective study looking at 291 patients. All these patients had histologically negative nodes. Additionally, these nodes underwent reverse transcriptase polymerase chain reaction quantitative analysis. As seen in Fig 2, recurrence (A) and disease-free survival (B) correlated with molecular disease burden in the lymph nodes. This was also true for stage 1 and stage 2 patients. Using Cox proportional hazards analysis, medium and high molecular disease burden in lymph nodes correlated with significant reduction in disease-free survival. These molecular analyses, along with other potential tumor markers, may help select patients for further more aggressive adjuvant therapies in spite of negative nodal histopathology (Figs 2 and 4).

T. J. Eberlein, MD

Clinical and Economic Comparison of Laparoscopic to Open Liver Resections Using a 2-to-1 Matched Pair Analysis: An Institutional Experience

Bhojani FD, Fox A, Pitzul K, et al (Univ Health Network, Toronto, Ontario, Canada)
J Am Coll Surg 214:184-195, 2012

Background.—Surgical resection of hepatic lesions is associated with intraoperative and postoperative morbidity and mortality. Our center has introduced a laparoscopic liver resection (LLR) program over the past 3 years. Our objective is to describe the initial clinical experience with LLR, including a detailed cost analysis.

Study Design.—We evaluated all LLRs from 2006 to 2010. Each was matched to 2 open cases for number of segments removed, patient age, and background liver histology. Model for End-Stage Liver Disease (MELD) and the Charlson comorbidity index were calculated retrospectively. Nonparametric statistical analysis was used to compare surgical and economic outcomes. Analyses were performed including and excluding converted cases.

Results.—Fifty-seven patients underwent attempted LLR. Demographic characteristics were similar between groups. Estimated blood loss was lower in the LLR vs the open liver resection (OLR) group, at 250 mL and 500 mL, respectively (p < 0.001). Median operating room times were 240 minutes and 270 minutes in the LLR and OLR groups, respectively (p = 0.14). Eight cases were converted to open (14%): 2 for bleeding, 2 for anatomic uncertainty, 1 for tumor size, 1 for margins, 1 for inability to localize the tumor, and 1 for adhesions. Median length of stay was lower for LLR at 5 days vs 6 days for OLR (p < 0.001). There was no difference in frequency of ICU admission, reoperation, 30-day emergency room visit, or 30-day readmission rates. Median overall cost for LLR was lower at $11,376 vs $12,523 for OLR (p = 0.077).

Conclusions.—Our experience suggests that LLR confers the clinical advantages of reduced operating room time, estimated blood loss, and length of stay while decreasing overall cost. LLR, therefore, appears to be a clinically and fiscally advantageous approach in properly selected patients (Fig 2, Table 3).

▶ This article is from Toronto General Hospital and the University of Toronto. The authors compare laparoscopic liver resections to open liver resections using a 2-to-1 matched pair analysis.

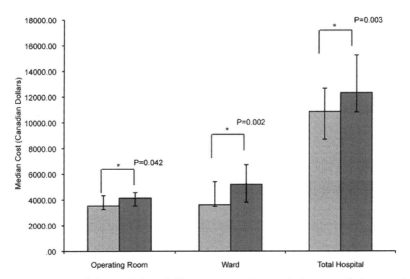

FIGURE 2.—Detailed cost analysis, excluding cases converted to open, by department, for laparoscopic liver resection and open liver resection cohorts expressed in 2010 inflation-adjusted Canadian dollars with interquartile ranges. Light gray bar, laparoscopic liver resection; dark gray bar, open liver resection. (Reprinted from Journal of American College of Surgeons, Bhojani FD, Fox A, Pitzul K, et al. Clinical and economic comparison of laparoscopic to open liver resections using a 2-to-1 matched pair analysis: an institutional experience. *J Am Coll Surg.* 2012;214:184-195. Copyright 2012, with permission from the American College of Surgeons.)

TABLE 3.—Comparison of Intraoperative and Perioperative Outcomes Between Laparoscopic Liver Resection and Open Liver Resection Cohorts

Outcome	Intention-to-Treat Analysis			Converted Cases Excluded		
	Laparoscopic Cohort (n = 57)	Open Cohort (n = 114)	p Value	Laparoscopic Cohort (n = 49)	Open Cohort (n = 98)	p Value
Incision to close time, min, median (range)	160 (65–536)	193 (70–407)	0.079	150 (65–446)	197 (70–407)	0.002*
Total OR time, min, median (range)	240 (128–605)	270 (137–500)	0.141	229 (128–543)	279 (137–500)	0.007*
Estimated blood loss, mL, median (range)	250 (0–6,000)	500 (100–4,000)	<0.001*	200 (0–2,000)	500 (100–4,000)	<0.001*
Intraoperative transfusion, yes, n (%)	7 (12)	12 (11)	0.731	3 (6)	12 (12)	0.387
Length of stay, d, median (range)	5 (2–51)	6 (4–57)	<0.001*	4 (2–38)	6 (4–57)	<0.001*
Postoperative transfusion, yes, n (%)	11 (24)	10 (8)	0.048*	8 (16)	10 (10)	0.286
Complications (with maximum grade), n (%)						
No	35 (61)	86 (75)	0.06	31 (63)	75 (76)	0.091
Yes	22 (39)	28 (25)	1.000	18 (37)	23 (24)	0.679
I	4 (18)	4 (14)	0.407	4 (22)	3 (13)	0.350
II	13 (59)	13 (46)	0.278	11 (61)	10 (43)	0.437
III	2 (9)	6 (21)	1.000	2 (11)	5 (22)	0.363
IV	3 (14)	4 (14)	1.000	1 (6)	4 (17)	1.000
Reoperation, n (%)	1 (2)	3 (3)	1.000	1 (2)	3 (3)	0.269
Transfer to ICU, n (%)	4 (7)	7 (6)	0.329	1 (2)	7 (7)	1.000
Mortality, n (%)	1 (2)	0	0.754	0	0	1.000
30-d ER visit, n (%)	3 (5)	8 (7)	0.552	3 (6)	6 (6)	1.000
30-d Readmission, n (%)	0	3 (3)	1.000	0	2 (2)	0.553
Home on diuretic, n (%)	2 (3)	3 (3)		2 (4)	2 (2)	0.601

ER, emergency room; OR, operating room.
*Statistically significant.

As seen in Table 3, laparoscopic liver resection has some clinical advantage through reduced operating room time, blood loss, and length of stay. It also has reduced cost.

Although this is not a randomized prospective trial, it does show some advantage in selected patients who undergo laparoscopic liver resection.

T. J. Eberlein, MD

Activation of the Phosphoinositide-3-Kinase and Mammalian Target of Rapamycin Signaling Pathways Are Associated With Shortened Survival in Patients With Malignant Peritoneal Mesothelioma
Varghese S, Chen Z, Bartlett DL, et al (The Univ of Maryland School of Medicine, Baltimore; Natl Cancer Inst, Bethesda, MD)
Cancer 117:361-371, 2011

Background.—Malignant peritoneal mesothelioma (MPM) is a rare malignancy of the serosal membranes of the abdominal cavity. This cancer is ultimately fatal in almost all afflicted individuals; however, there is marked variability in its clinical behavior: Some patients die rapidly, and others survive for many years. In the current study, the authors investigated the molecular nature of MPM to obtain insights into the heterogeneity of its clinical behavior and to identify new therapeutic targets for intervention.

Methods.—Fresh pretreatment tumor samples were collected from 41 patients with MPM who underwent surgical cytoreduction and received regional intraoperative chemotherapy perfusion. From those samples, gene expression analyses were performed. The major cellular pathways that were identified in this cancer were inhibited using a pathway-specific inhibitor.

Results.—Unsupervised clustering of genes identified 2 distinct groups of patients with significantly different survivals (Group A: median survival, 24 months; Group B: median survival, 69.5 months; $P = .035$). Phosphoinositide-3-kinase (PI3K) and the closely interacting mammalian target of rapamycin (mTOR) signaling pathways were overexpressed predominantly in the poor survival group; and the genes of these pathways, phosphoinositide-3-kinase, catalytic, α polypeptide (PIK3CA) and rapamycin-insensitive companion of mammalian target of rapamycin (RICTOR), were highly significantly predictive of shortened patient survival in Group A. The role of these pathways in MPM tumor progression was also investigated by treating 2 MPM cell lines with BEZ235, a dual-class PI3K and mTOR inhibitor, and the authors observed significant inhibition of downstream cell signaling and cell proliferation.

Conclusions.—Taken together, the results from this study revealed that, based on gene expression profiles, there were 2 distinct patient groups with significantly different survival and that targeting the PI3K and mTOR

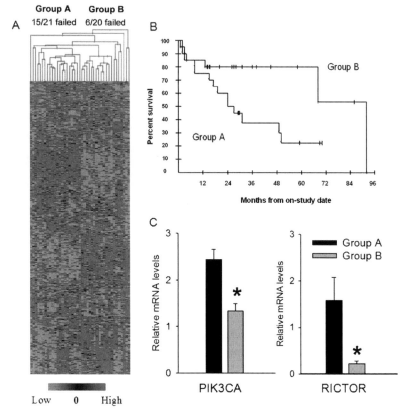

FIGURE 2.—An unsupervised hierarchical cluster analysis of gene expression data from 41 malignant peritoneal mesothelioma (MPM) tumors is shown. (A) This dendrogram of a 2-way cluster analysis of 4748 genes extracted from MPM tumors illustrates the 2 distinct classes of patients with significantly different survival. Data are presented in a matrix format in which the rows represent the individual gene, and the columns represent the tumor from each patient. Red represents high gene expression, and green represents low gene expression, as indicated in the scale bar ($\log_2$-transformed scale). (B) This Kaplan-Meier plot illustrates the actuarial overall survival of patients with MPM in Groups A and B as microarray classes clustered on the basis of gene expression similarities ($P =.035$). (C) Real-time polymerase chain reaction of phosphoinositide-3-kinase, catalytic, α polypeptide (PIK3CA) and rapamycin-insensitive companion of mammalian target of rapamycin (RICTOR) expression in tumors from patients who had poor survival (Group A) versus good survival (Group B) was based on microarray classes; relative messenger RNA (mRNA) levels are reported as the mean ± standard error of the mean. Asterisks indicate $P < .001$. For interpretation of the references to color in this figure legend, the reader is referred to web version of this article. (Reprinted from Varghese S, Chen Z, Bartlett DL, et al. Activation of the phosphoinositide-3-kinase and mammalian target of rapamycin signaling pathways are associated with shortened survival in patients with malignant peritoneal mesothelioma. *Cancer.* 2011;117:361-371. Copyright 2011 American Cancer Society. This material is reproduced with permission of Wiley-Liss, Inc., a subsidiary of John Wiley & Sons, Inc.)

signaling pathways may have significant therapeutic value in patients with MPM (Fig 2).

▶ Malignant peritoneal mesothelioma is a rare malignancy. Surgical resection and intra-abdominal chemotherapy are the mainstays of the treatment. The authors of this study did gene expression analyses of fresh tumor-resected specimens. As seen in Fig 2, the authors identified 2 distinct groups of patients with significantly different survivals. Phosphoinositide-3-kinase and the closely interacting mammalian target of rapamycin signaling pathways were overexpressed in the poor-survival group.

Understanding the biology of individual patients' tumor will help select treatments that are much more personalized. Clearly these poor prognostic genes and pathways should represent targets for new therapies in this disease.

T. J. Eberlein, MD

Hepatocellular

Hepatic Arterial Infusion of Doxorubicin-Loaded Microsphere for Treatment of Hepatocellular Cancer: A Multi-Institutional Registry

Martin RCG II, Rustein L, Enguix DP, et al (Univ of Louisville, KY; Maine Med Ctr, Portland, ME; Le Fe Hosp, Spain; et al)
J Am Coll Surg 213:493-500, 2011

Background.—Hepatic intra-arterial therapy for unresectable hepatocellular cancer (HCC) has been shown to improve overall survival, but can have significant toxicity. A recent prospective randomized controlled trial demonstrated superior response rates and significantly less morbidity and doxorubicin-related adverse events with drug-eluting beads with doxorubicin (DEBDOX) compared with conventional chemoembolization. The aim of this study was to confirm the efficacy of DEBDOX for the treatment of unresectable HCC.

Study Design.—This open-label, multicenter, multinational single-arm study included 118 intermediate-staged HCC patients who were not candidates for transplantation or resection. Patients received DEBDOX at each treatment. Complications and response rates to treatment were analyzed.

Results.—There were 118 patients who received a total of 186 DEBDOX treatments with a median total treatment dose of 75 mg (range 38 to 150 mg), and median overall total hepatic exposure of 150 mg (range 150 to 600 mg). Five lesions were targeted, with a median size of 5.3 cm (range 1.0 to 16.9 cm). Severe adverse events related to liver dysfunction were seen after 4% of treatments. Overall survival was a median of 14.2 months (range 5 to 30 months), with progression-free survival of 13 months and hepatic-specific progression-free survival of 16 months. Okuda class less than 1 at time of treatment, reduction of alpha-fetoprotein of 1,000 ng/mL at the first post-treatment evaluation, delivery of more than 200 mg doxorubicin, and less than 25% liver involvement were all predictors of favorable overall survival assessed by multivariable analyses.

Conclusions.—Hepatic intra-arterial injection of DEBDOX is safe and effective in the treatment of HCC, as demonstrated by a minimal complication rate and robust and durable tumor response (Tables 3-5).

▶ Unresectable hepatocellular cancer is associated with very poor survival. Transarterial chemoembolization has been associated with a number of problems

TABLE 3.—Bead Infusion-Related Morbidity

Side Effect	All Grades		Severe Grade*	
	n	%	n	%
Nausea	6	14	1	2
Vomiting	6	14	1	2
Hypertension	1	2	1	2
Liver dysfunction/failure	4	9	2	5
Anorexia	2	5	1	2
Pain	3	7	0	0
Pancreatitis	3	7	1	2
Hematological	3	7	2	5
Bleeding	5	11	4	9
Other	11	25	0	0

Side effects: n = 44 DEBDOX treatments.
DEBDOX, drug-eluting beads with doxorubicin.
*Defined as Grade 3 or higher.

TABLE 4.—Response Rates for all 118 Patients Evaluated

Response	3 mo (n=118)	6 mo (n=114)	12 mo (n=112)	18 mo (n=106)*
Complete response, n (%)	15 (13)	12 (11)	8 (7)	3
Partial response, n (%)	48 (41)	54 (47)	32 (29)	10
Stable disease, n (%)	44 (37)	45 (39)	22 (20)	12
Progression of disease, n (%)	1 (1)	1 (1)	4 (4)	3
Not reached time point, n	0	0	40	76
Dead of disease, n	3	1	4	2
Dead of complication, n	1	1	2	0

*Percentages not included for 18-month data due to the number of patients not available for follow-up at that time point.

TABLE 5.—Multivariable Predictors of Overall Survival

Parameter	Hazard Ratio	95% CI	p Value
CLIP	1.3	0.89−2.1	0.06
Okuda class <1	1.85	1.08−4.0	0.0001*
Bilobar disease	0.87	0.56−3.4	0.13
No. of lesions	0.78	0.65−3.9	0.1
Child-Pugh (A vs B)	0.68	0.54−4.2	0.3
Reduction in AFP >1,000 ng/mL	1.96	1.2−4.2	0.0006*
No. of bead treatments	3.03	1.02−4.5	0.05*
>200 mg delivered	2.8	1.1−3.4	0.04*
Extent of liver involved (<25%)	1.5	1.08−1.9	0.003*

AFP, alpha-fetoprotein; CLIP, Cancer of the Liver Italian Program.
*Statistically significant.

because of the variations in chemotherapeutic agents used and variability in the treatments given. This study was performed to evaluate safety and efficacy of drug-eluting beads loaded with doxorubicin. As seen in Table 3, this treatment was actually associated with relatively few side effects. As seen in Table 4, more than half of the patients had complete or partial response by 6 months of treatment and more than one-third had similar responses at 1 year. As seen in Table 5, Okuda class < 1 at the time of treatment, reduction of AFP by 1000 ng/mL at the time of first posttreatment evaluation, being able to deliver 200 mg of doxorubicin, and having liver involvement less than 25% were all predictors of favorable overall survival using this treatment.

Future studies may try to get more drugs to the tumor through repeated treatments, rather than using additional embolic material. In this small study, a few of the patients were able to go to transplantation using this regimen as a bridge.

T. J. Eberlein, MD

Hepatocellular Carcinoma
El-Serag HB (Michael E. DeBakey Veterans Affairs Med Ctr, Houston, TX)
N Engl J Med 365:1118-1127, 2011

Background.—Hepatocellular cancer is diagnosed in over half a million persons worldwide each year. Liver cancer is the fifth most common cancer in men and the seventh in women, with 85% of cases occurring in developing countries, especially where infection with hepatitis B (HBV) is endemic—Southeast Asia and sub-Saharan Africa. Rarely does hepatocellular manifest before age 40 years and cases peak at about age 70 years. Infection with hepatitis C virus (HCV) is the fastest-rising cause of cancer-related death in the United States. The 5-year survival of HCV-related cancer is less than 12%. The greatest proportional increase in cases is seen in Hispanics and white persons age 45 to 60 years. Risk factors, diagnosis, treatment, and prevention of hepatocellular carcinoma were investigated.

Risk Factors.—The major risk factors for hepatocellular carcinoma are infection with HBV or HCV, alcoholic liver disease, and nonalcoholic fatty liver disease. Less common risk factors are hereditary hemochromatosis, alpha$_1$-antitrypsin deficiency, autoimmune hepatitis, some porphyrias, and Wilson's disease. The distribution of risk factors varies by geographic area and race or ethnic group. Usually the risk factors produce cirrhosis, found in 80% to 90% of patients with hepatocellular carcinoma.

Worldwide, chronic HBV infection is seen in about half of all cases and virtually all pediatric cases. Where HBV infection is transmitted from mother to newborn, up to 90% of infected persons have chronic disease, with HBV often incorporated into host DNA. The risk of hepatocellular carcinoma in persons who are positive for hepatitis B surface antigen (HBsAg) is further increased if the individual is male, elderly, infected for a long time, has a family history of hepatocellular carcinoma, was exposed to aflatoxin, uses alcohol or tobacco, is coinfected with HBV or hepatitis delta virus, has high levels of HBV hepatocellular replication, or is infected with HBV genotype C.

Hepatocellular carcinoma occurs 15 to 20 times more often in persons infected with HCV than those who are not infected. Most of the excess risk is found in those with advanced hepatic fibrosis or cirrhosis. Risk factors for hepatocellular carcinoma in persons infected with HCV include older age at the time of infection, male gender, coinfection with human immunodeficiency virus (HIV) or HBV, and probably diabetes or obesity. Prolonged heavy alcohol use is another strong indicator of higher risk. Coffee drinking may reduce the risk in some areas, such as Japan and southern Europe. It is also related to reduced insulin levels and a lower risk for type 2 diabetes.

Diagnosis.—Noninvasive imaging tests, especially at specialized centers, can be used to diagnose hepatocellular carcinoma in persons with cirrhosis and a focal hepatic mass exceeding 2 cm in diameter. Typical imaging shows areas of early arterial enhancement and delayed washout in the venous or delayed phase of four-phase multidetector computed tomography (CT) or in dynamic contrast-enhanced magnetic resonance imaging (MRI). These changes are related to increased vascularity in the carcinoma. Concordant findings on CT and MRI are recommended if the lesions measure 1 to 2 cm in diameter. An alpha-fetoprotein level of 400 ng/mL or higher is also highly predictive of hepatocellular carcinoma. An image-guided biopsy is considered if the focal hepatic mass has atypical features, the CT and MRI findings do not match, or no cirrhosis is present. A negative biopsy result does not rule out malignant disease; the nodule should be reassessed every 3 to 6 months until it disappears, enlarges, or displays diagnostic characteristics. Risk of tumor seeding along the needle track after biopsy is low. It can be hard to measure liver nodules smaller than 1 cm; it is best to monitor them via ultrasonography (US) every 3 to 6 months for 1 to 2 years.

Treatment.—Choice of treatment is related to cancer stage, resources available, and level of practitioner expertise. Recommendations for staging-guided treatment use systems such as the Barcelona Clinic Liver Cancer staging and the Child-Pugh system. Genomic analysis is used to identify possible prognostic biomarkers, but requires validation. High serum and tissue levels of vascular endothelial growth factor are significantly associated with poor survival, but the clinical usefulness of this is unclear.

Very early stage disease is difficult to diagnosis, but surgical resection at this stage produces an overall survival of 90%. Choice of therapy is dictated by severity of liver dysfunction, extent of portal hypertension, and presence of coexisting conditions. Patients with solitary tumors and no portal hypertension can undergo surgical resection. Patients with early-stage hepatocellular carcinoma are best managed with liver transplantation or, if transplantation is not possible, local ablation. For patients with intermediate-stage cancer the best choice is transarterial chemoembolization (TACE), which improves 2-year survival by 20% to 25% compared to conservative treatment. Radioembolization with yttrium-90 microspheres has been used as palliative treatment for patients with Child-Pugh class A cirrhosis and intermediate-stage disease. Radical therapy is not appropriate for patients with advanced-stage disease. Carefully selected patients may have an increased survival with TACE, but the primary treatment option for these patients is oral sorafenib. Other small molecules being studied for use in these patients include bevacizumab and cetuximab. In the terminal stage of disease, which includes cancer symptoms related to liver failure, vascular involvement, or extrahepatic spread, 1-year survival is less than 10%. None of the treatments mentioned is of benefit.

The clinical effectiveness of antiviral therapy for infection with HBV or HCV and for surveillance and treatment is low. Transplantation, resection, and TACE are not widely used. It is difficult to implement surveillance that requires repeated assessments over relatively short time periods and strategies to ensure prompt recall. The diagnostic evaluation is complicated, and curative treatments are often unavailable or quite costly.

Prevention.—All newborns and persons without immunity at high risk for HBV infection should be given HBV vaccine, which is both safe and effective. Antiviral therapy that controls HBV infection in HBsAg-positive patients and that eradicates HCV in patients with viremia may substantially reduce, but does not eliminate the risk of hepatocellular carcinoma in patients with viral hepatitis. Risk may be reduced by administering either interferon or lamivudine. Persons infected with HCV who do not have cirrhosis and receive interferon-based treatment with a sustained viral response have up to 75% reduction in risk of hepatocellular carcinoma. Maintenance interferon therapy for patients with HCV infection and cirrhosis with no sustained viral response does not reduce the cancer risk. Surveillance is recommended for high risk patients. One approach is US of the liver and measurement of serum alpha-fetoprotein levels every 6 to 12 months for patients with cirrhosis or advanced hepatic fibrosis regardless of its cause. HBV carriers with or without cirrhosis who are Africans over age 20 years or Asians over age 40 years or who have a family history of hepatocellular carcinoma can also benefit from this approach. Surveillance is not recommended for HCV-infected persons

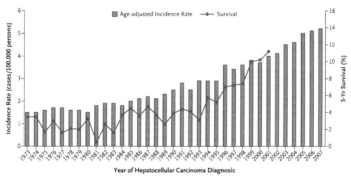

FIGURE 2.—Age-Adjusted Incidence and 5-Year Survival Rates for Patients with Hepatocellular Carcinoma in the United States, 1973–2007. (Reprinted from El-Serag HB. Hepatocellular carcinoma. *N Engl J Med.* 2011;365:1118-1127. © 2011 Massachusetts Medical Society.)

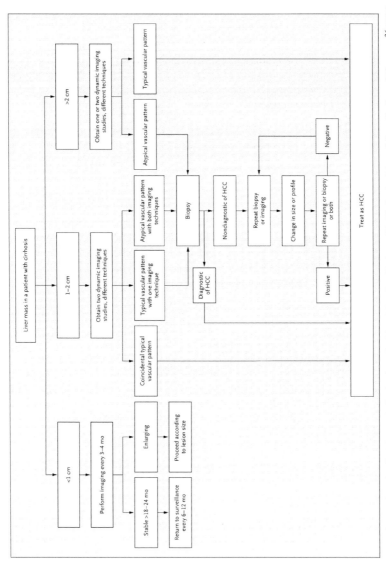

FIGURE 3.—Proposed Procedure for the Diagnostic Evaluation of a Liver Mass in a Patient with Cirrhosis. Adapted from Bruix and Sherman.[26] HCC denotes hepato-cellular carcinoma. *Editor's Note*: Please refer to original journal article for full references. (Reprinted from El-Serag HB. Hepatocellular carcinoma. *N Engl J Med*. 2011;365:1118-1127. © 2011 Massachusetts Medical Society.)

with mild or no hepatic fibrosis. Alpha-fetoprotein levels in serum are inadequate as the only means of surveillance. US has a sensitivity of about 65% and a specificity of over 90% for early detection. CT and MRI are not generally recommended for surveillance because their sensitivity, specificity, and negative and positive predictive values are unknown and because they are expensive and carry risks for radiation exposure, allergic reaction to contrast medium, nephrotoxicity with CT, and nephrogenic fibrosing dermatopathy when gadolinium is used for MRI in patients with renal insufficiency (Figs 2 and 3).

▶ This is an outstanding review article on hepatocellular carcinoma. It reviews not only the epidemiology of the disease but the current data with regard to prevention, diagnosis, and treatment. The references are up to date, and the discussion of clinical trials is focused, succinct, yet comprehensive. Certainly, for anyone doing liver/transplant surgery, I recommend this article (Figs 2 and 3).

T. J. Eberlein, MD

Pancreatic

Efficacy of stapler versus hand-sewn closure after distal pancreatectomy (DISPACT): a randomised, controlled multicentre trial
Diener MK, Seiler CM, Rossion I, et al (Univ of Heidelberg, Germany; et al)
Lancet 377:1514-1522, 2011

Background.—The ideal closure technique of the pancreas after distal pancreatectomy is unknown. We postulated that standardised closure with a stapler device would prevent pancreatic fistula more effectively than would a hand-sewn closure of the remnant.

Methods.—This multicentre, randomised, controlled, parallel group-sequential superiority trial was done in 21 European hospitals. Patients with diseases of the pancreatic body and tail undergoing distal pancreatectomy were eligible and were randomly assigned by central randomisation before operation to either stapler or hand-sewn closure of the pancreatic remnant. Surgical performance was assessed with intraoperative photo documentation. The primary endpoint was the combination of pancreatic fistula and death until postoperative day 7. Patients and outcome assessors were masked to group assignment. Interim and final analysis were by intention to treat in all patients in whom a left resection was done. This trial is registered, ISRCTN18452029.

Findings.—Between Nov 16, 2006, and July 3, 2009, 450 patients were randomly assigned to treatment groups (221 stapler; 229 hand-sewn closure), of whom 352 patients (177 stapler, 175 hand-sewn closure) were analysed. Pancreatic fistula rate or mortality did not differ between stapler (56 [32%] of 177) and hand-sewn closure (49 [28%] of 175; OR $0 \cdot 84$, 95% CI $0 \cdot 53-1 \cdot 33$; p=$0 \cdot 56$). One patient died within the first 7 days after surgery in the hand-sewn group; no deaths occurred in the stapler group. Serious adverse events did not differ between groups.

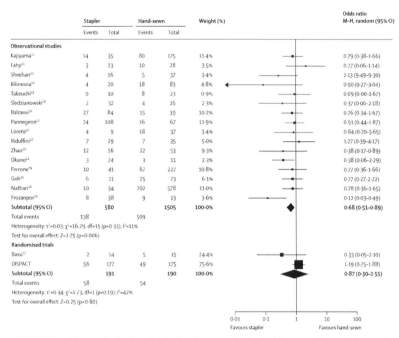

FIGURE 2.—Meta-analysis of randomised and non-randomised trials comparing scalpel resection of the pancreatic tail followed by hand-sewn closure of the pancreatic remnant with stapler resection and closure for distal pancreatectomy. Separate analysis of status of evidence before and after the DISPACT trial. M-H=Mantel-Haenszel. (Reprinted from The Lancet, Diener MK, Seiler CM, Rossion I, et al. Efficacy of stapler versus hand-sewn closure after distal pancreatectomy (DISPACT): a randomised, controlled multicentre trial. *Lancet.* 2011;377:1514-1522. © 2011, with permission from Elsevier.)

Interpretation.—Stapler closure did not reduce the rate of pancreatic fistula compared with hand-sewn closure for distal pancreatectomy. New strategies, including innovative surgical techniques, need to be identified to reduce this adverse outcome (Fig 2, Tables 2 and 3).

▶ This is a randomized, multicenter, controlled trial that consisted of 21 centers, all with extensive experience for the surgical treatment of pancreatic disease. There was no difference in patient characteristics between the 2 arms of this study. Most patients who had distal pancreatectomies also had splenectomy and lymph node dissection. As seen in Table 2, there is no difference in pancreatic fistula rate or mortality. Other serious events did not differ between the groups (Table 3). This study contributes to a meta-analysis, which is seen in Fig 2 and discussed in the discussion portion of the manuscript (Fig 2). Further studies using different techniques, such as laparoscopic surgical intervention or the use of biologic glue, are ongoing.

T. J. Eberlein, MD

TABLE 2.—Primary and Secondary Endpoints

	Stapler n=177	Hand-Sewn n=175	Total	OR (95% CI)	p Value
Primary endpoint					
Pancreatic fistula (day 3–7) and death (until day 7)	56 (32%)	49 (28%)	105 (30%)	0.84 (0.53–1.33)	0.56*
Clinical grading					
Grade A	32 (57%)	33 (67%)	65 (62%)	1.05 (0.61–1.82)	0.27†
Grade B	17 (30%)	12 (25%)	29 (28%)	0.69 (0.32–1.49)	‥
Grade C	7 (13%)	4 (8%)	11 (11%)	0.55 (0.16–1.90)	‥
Mortality (until day 7)	0 (0%)	1 (<1%)	1 (<1%)	‥	0.31‡
Secondary endpoints					
Pancreatic fistula (30 days)	63 (36%)	64 (37%)	127 (36%)	1.04 (0.68–1.61)	0.84‡
Clinical grading					
Grade A	27 (43%)	28 (44%)	55 (43%)	1.06 (0.60–1.88)	0.92†
Grade B	20 (32%)	20 (31%)	40 (32%)	1.01 (0.52–1.96)	‥
Grade C	16 (25%)	16 (25%)	32 (25%)	1.01 (0.49–2.09)	‥
Mortality (30 days)	1 (<1%)	2 (1%)	3 (1%)	2.04 (0.18–22.7)	0.55‡
Total operating time (min)	187.7 (78.9)	192.4 (82.2)	190.0 (80.5)	1.00 (1.00–1.00)	0.70§
Resection time for distal pancreatectomy (min)	68.4 (46.0)	70.8 (45.6)	69.6 (45.7)	1.00 (1.00–1.01)	0.43§
Wound dehiscence	1 (<1%)	2 (1%)	3 (1%)	2.04 (0.18–22.7)	0.55§
Wound infection	11 (6%)	9 (5%)	20 (6%)	0.82 (0.33–2.03)	0.66‡
Intra-abdominal fluid collection or abscess	34 (19%)	34 (19%)	68 (19%)	1.01 (0.60–1.72)	0.95‡
Concomitant occurrence of pancreatic fistula and fluid collection or abscess	16 (9%)	14 (8%)	30 (9%)	1.14 (0.54–2.42)	0.73‡
New onset of diabetes mellitus	16 (9%)	23 (13%)	39 (11%)	1.52 (0.78–2.99)	0.22‡
Length of hospital stay (days)	15.1 (13.5)	15.7 (15.9)	15.4 (14.7)	1.00 (0.99–1.02)	0.86§
Safety					
Mortality (90 days)	6 (3%)	6 (3%)	12 (3%)	‥	0.98‡
Mortality (12 months)	16 (9%)	18 (10%)	34 (10%)	‥	0.69‡
Patients with at least one serious adverse event	87 (49%)	70 (40%)	157 (45%)	‥	0.08‡

Data are number (% of group total), mean (SD), odds ratio (OR; 95% CI), or p value.
*p value for primary analysis (logistic regression with surgical skills as covariate, two-sided).
†Mantel-Haenszel test.
‡X2 test.
§Wilcoxon U test.

TABLE 3.—Serious Adverse Events Reported

	Stapler n=124	Hand-Sewn n=123	Total n=247	p Value
Maximum intensity				0·16
Mild	18 (15%)	9 (7%)	27 (11%)	··
Moderate	54 (44%)	56 (46%)	110 (45%)	··
Severe	50 (41%)	58 (47%)	108 (44%)	··
Missing	2	0	2	··
Causality to intervention				0·18
Unrelated	53 (43%)	50 (41%)	103 (42%)	··
Possibly related	23 (18%)	29 (24%)	52 (21%)	··
Probably related	9 (7%)	2 (1%)	11 (4%)	··
Definitely related	38 (31%)	39 (32%)	77 (31%)	··
Not assessable	1 (<1%)	3 (2%)	4 (2%)	··
Category of SAE				0·25
Pancreatic fistula	25 (20%)	28 (22%)	53 (21%)	··
Delayed gastric emptying	3 (2%)	0 (0%)	3 (1%)	··
Bleeding	8 (7%)	11 (9%)	19 (8%)	··
Abscess or fluid collection	20 (16%)	11 (9%)	31 (13%)	··
Cholangitis	3 (2%)	1 (1%)	4 (2%)	··
Wound infection	2 (2%)	8 (7%)	10 (4%)	··
Other surgical morbidity	21 (17%)	22 (18%)	43 (17%)	··
Cardiocirculatory	8 (7%)	6 (5%)	14 (6%)	··
Pulmonary	4 (3%)	8 (7%)	12 (5%)	··
Pancreatic cancer or metastasis	16 (13%)	10 (8%)	26 (10%)	··
Renal	2 (2%)	4 (3%)	6 (2%)	··
Other general variables	9 (7%)	10 (8%)	19 (8%)	··
Not assessable	3 (2%)	4 (3%)	7 (3%)	··
SAE results in death				0·69
No	108 (87%)	105 (85%)	213 (86%)	··
Yes	16 (13%)	18 (15%)	34 (14%)	··

SAE=serious adverse event.

Tissue Biomarkers for Prognosis in Pancreatic Ductal Adenocarcinoma: A Systematic Review and Meta-analysis

Jamieson NB, Carter CR, McKay CJ, et al (Glasgow Royal Infirmary, UK)
Clin Cancer Res 17:3316-3331, 2011

Purpose.—The management of pancreatic ductal adenocarcinoma (PDAC) continues to present a great challenge particularly with regard to prediction of outcome following pancreaticoduodenectomy. Molecular markers have been extensively investigated by numerous groups with the aim of enhancing prognostication; however, despite hundreds of studies that have sought to assess the potential prognostic value of molecular markers in predicting the clinical course following resection of PDAC, at this time, no molecular marker assay forms part of recommended clinical practice.

Experimental Design.—We conducted a systematic review and meta-analysis of the published literature for immunohistochemistry-based biomarkers of PDAC outcome. A dual search strategy was applied to the PubMed database on January 6, 2010, to identify cohort studies that reported associations between immunohistochemical biomarker expression and survival outcomes in PDAC, and conformed to the REMARK (REporting recommendations for tumor MARKer prognostic studies) criteria.

Results.—A total of 103 distinct proteins met all inclusion criteria. Promising markers that emerged for the prediction of overall survival included BAX (HR = 0.31, 95% CI: 0.71—0.56), Bcl-2 (HR = 0.41, 95% CI: 0.27—0.63), survivin (HR = 0.46, 95% CI: 0.29—0.73), Ki-67: (HR = 2.42, 95% CI: 1.87—3.14), COX-2 (HR = 1.39, 95% CI: 1.13—1.71), E-cadherin (HR = 1.80, 95% CI: 1.33—2.42), and S100 calcium-binding proteins, in particular S100A2 (HR = 3.23, 95% CI: 1.58—6.62).

Conclusions.—We noted that that there was incomplete adherence to the REMARK guidelines with inadequate methodology reporting as well as failure to perform multivariate analysis. Addressing the persistent incomplete adoption of these criteria may eventually result in the incorporation of molecular marker assessment within PDAC management algorithms.

▶ This is a systematic review and meta-analysis of the published literature for biomarkers of pancreatic ductal adenocarcinoma outcome. These authors identified a number of markers as potential predictors of overall survival. These include BAX, Bcl-2, Survivin, Ki-67, COX-2, E-cadherin, and S100A2. Certainly surgeons who care for patients with pancreatic cancer should make every effort to assess these biomarkers prospectively in their cancer patients.

T. J. Eberlein, MD

Miscellaneous

Clinical Significance of *miR-146a* in Gastric Cancer Cases

Kogo R, Mimori K, Tanaka F, et al (Kyushu Univ, Beppu, Japan; et al)
Clin Cancer Res 17:4277-4284, 2011

Purpose.—The profiles of microRNAs change significantly in gastric cancer. *MiR-146a* is reported to be a tumor suppressor in pancreatic cancer, breast cancer, and prostate cancer. We investigated the clinical significance of *miR-146a* in gastric cancer, in particular focusing on hypothetical *miR-146a* target genes, such as epidermal growth factor receptor (*EGFR*) and interleukin-1 receptor-associated kinase (*IRAK1*).

Experimental Design.—We examined *miR-146a* levels in 90 gastric cancer samples by q-real-time (qRT)—PCR and analyzed the association between *miR-146a* levels and clinicopathologic factors and prognosis. The regulation of *EGFR* and *IRAK1* by *miR-146a* was examined with *miR-146a*—transfected gastric cancer cells. Moreover, we analyzed the association between *miR-146a* levels and the G/C single nucleotide polymorphism (SNP) within *pre-miR-146a* seed sequences in 76 gastric cancer samples, using direct sequencing of genomic DNA.

Results.—In 90 clinical samples of gastric cancer, *miR-146a* levels in cancer tissues were significantly lower than those in the corresponding

TABLE 2.—Univariate and Multivariate Analysis for Overall Survival (Cox Proportional Hazards Regression Model)

Factors	Univariate Analysis			Multivariate Analysis		
	RR	95% CI	P value	RR	95% CI	P Value
Age (<64/65<)	0.95	0.68–1.34	0.76			
Sex (Male/Female)	0.77	0.51–1.10	0.153			
Histologic grade[a] (Poor & Signet/Well & Moderate)	1.24	0.88–1.79	0.214			
T factor (T2–T4/T1)	3.72	1.73–15.7	<0.001[b]	2.22	0.79–10.2	0.14
Lymph node metastasis (Positive/Negative)	3.57	1.96–8.88	<0.001[b]	2.76	1.45–7.01	<0.001[b]
Lymphatic invasion (Positive/Negative)	2.13	1.27–4.34	0.002[b]	0.79	0.41–1.85	0.555
Venous invasion (Positive/Negative)	1.86	1.31–2.64	<0.001[b]	1.48	1.03–2.15	0.036[b]
MiR-146a level (Low/High)	1.67	1.28–2.43	0.003[b]	1.53	1.06–2.26	0.022[b]

Abbreviations: RR, Relative risk; CI, Confidence interval.
[a]Well differentiated adenocarcinoma (Well), Moderately differentiated adenocarcinoma (Moderate), Poorly differentiated adenocarcinoma (Poor), Signet ring cell carcinoma (Signet).
[b]$P < 0.05$.

noncancerous tissue ($P < 0.001$). Lower levels of *miR-146a* were associated with lymph node metastasis and venous invasion ($P < 0.05$). Moreover, a lower level of *miR-146a* was an independent prognostic factor for overall survival ($P = 0.003$). Ectopic expression of *miR-146a* inhibited migration and invasion and downregulated *EGFR* and *IRAK1* expression in gastric cancer cells. In addition, G/C SNP within the pre-*miR-146a* seed sequence significantly reduced *miR-146a* levels in the GG genotype compared with the CC genotype.

Conclusions.—*MiR-146a* contains an SNP, which is associated with mature *miR-146a* expression. *MiR-146a* targeting of *EGFR* and *IRAK1* is an independent prognostic factor in gastric cancer cases (Table 2).

▶ *MiR-146a* is reported as a tumor suppressor in pancreatic cancer, breast cancer, and prostate cancer. The authors analyzed 90 patients with gastric cancer to determine the role of *miR-146a* in overall survival. As seen in Table 2, lower levels of *miR-146a* were associated with lymph node metastasis and venous invasion. Additionally, it was an independent prognostic factor for overall survival.

From this analysis, it appears to be an independent prognostic factor in gastric cancer cases. While this study may show prognostic significance of this biomarker, further research will be needed to utilize this information as a therapeutic tool. In the meantime, it may well be a marker for more aggressive adjuvant therapy.

T. J. Eberlein, MD

Durable Complete Responses in Heavily Pretreated Patients with metastatic Melanoma Using T-Cell Transfer Immunotherapy

Rosenberg SA, Yang JC, Sherry RM, et al (Natl Cancer Inst, Bethesda, MD)
Clin Cancer Res 17:4550-4557, 2011

Purpose.—Most treatments for patients with metastatic melanoma have a low rate of complete regression and thus overall survival in these patients is poor. We investigated the ability of adoptive cell transfer utilizing autologous tumor-infiltrating lymphocytes (TIL) to mediate durable complete regressions in heavily pretreated patients with metastatic melanoma.

Experimental Design.—Ninety-three patients with measurable metastatic melanoma were treated with the adoptive transfer of autologous TILs administered in conjunction with interleukin-2 following a lymphodepleting preparative regimen on three sequential clinical trials. Ninety-five percent of these patients had progressive disease following a prior systemic treatment. Median potential follow-up was 62 months.

Results.—Objective response rates by Response Evaluation Criteria in Solid Tumors (RECIST) in the 3 trials using lymphodepleting preparative regimens (chemotherapy alone or with 2 or 12 Gy irradiation) were 49%, 52%, and 72%, respectively. Twenty of the 93 patients (22%) achieved a complete tumor regression, and 19 have ongoing complete regressions beyond 3 years. The actuarial 3- and 5-year survival rates for the entire group were 36% and 29%, respectively, but for the 20 complete responders were 100% and 93%. The likelihood of achieving a complete response was similar regardless of prior therapy. Factors associated with objective response included longer telomeres of the infused cells, the number of $CD8^+CD27^+$ cells infused, and the persistence of the infused cells in the circulation at 1 month (all $P_2 < 0.001$).

Conclusions.—Cell transfer therapy with autologous TILs can mediate durable complete responses in patients with metastatic melanoma and has similar efficacy irrespective of prior treatment.

▶ This is a study using a combination of tumor-infiltrating lymphocytes (TILs) administered with high-dose interleukin-2 following a lymphodepleting regimen in patients who have been heavily treated previously and still have metastatic progressive disease. This regimen led to a significant proportion (up to 40%) of patients with metastatic melanoma. Of the 20 patients in the study who have complete regression, 19 are still ongoing 3 to 7 years after treatment. As seen in Fig 3 in the original article, mean telomere length, the number of $CD27^+$ and $CD8^+$ lymphocytes, and the percentage persistence of the infused cells in peripheral blood at 1 month predicted complete response.

It should be emphasized that not all patients with metastatic melanoma are eligible for this approach. First, the patients need at least a 2-cm-diameter area of metastatic tumor that is suitable for resection and can generate tumor-infiltrating lymphocytes.

This type of therapy will be used more frequently if further research develops a simpler, faster, and less costly method to grow TILs; immunotherapy expertise is also needed.

T. J. Eberlein, MD

Sentinel-Lymph-Node Biopsy for Cutaneous Melanoma
Gershenwald JE, Ross MI (Univ of Texas M.D. Anderson Cancer Ctr, Houston)
N Engl J Med 364:1738-1745, 2011

A 38-year-old woman presented to her dermatologist with a 2-month history of changes in a mole on her right upper back. The mole had been present for a few years, but recently the patient had noticed episodes of itching and observed blood on her blouse. On skin examination, this pigmented lesion was 8 mm in diameter and had irregular borders and variegated color. An excisional biopsy was performed; pathological examination revealed a superficial spreading melanoma, 2.8 mm thick (i.e., in depth), with ulceration and six mitotic figures per square millimeter. Subsequent examination of the patient revealed a healing biopsy site over the right upper back. There was no clinical adenopathy and no evidence of in-transit or satellite metastases. The patient had no specific symptoms indicative of metastatic disease. A surgical oncologist was consulted, who recommended that the patient undergo wide excision of the primary tumor and sentinel-lymph-node biopsy in the same operative setting.

▶ This is an excellent summary about sentinel lymph node biopsy for patients with melanoma. It begins with a case but then details many of the major clinical studies and reviews guidelines as well as recommendations. Certainly, any surgical oncologist who is performing sentinel lymph node biopsy will benefit from reading this well-written review.

T. J. Eberlein, MD

---

gp100 Peptide Vaccine and Interleukin-2 in Patients with Advanced Melanoma
Schwartzentruber DJ, Lawson DH, Richards JM, et al (Indiana Univ Health Goshen Ctr for Cancer Care, Goshen; Emory Univ, Atlanta; Oncology Specialists, Park Ridge, IL; et al)
N Engl J Med 364:2119-2127, 2011

Background.—Stimulating an immune response against cancer with the use of vaccines remains a challenge. We hypothesized that combining a melanoma vaccine with interleukin-2, an immune activating agent, could improve outcomes. In a previous phase 2 study, patients with metastatic melanoma receiving high-dose interleukin-2 plus the gp100:209-217(210M) peptide

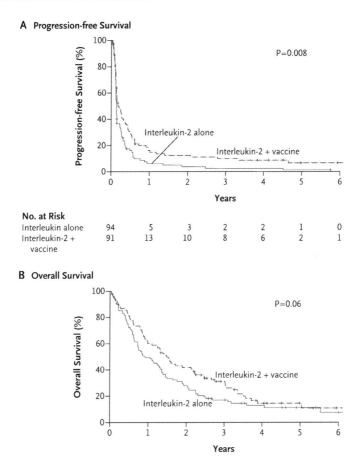

A Progression-free Survival

P=0.008

Interleukin-2 alone

Interleukin-2 + vaccine

No. at Risk

Interleukin alone	94	5	3	2	2	1	0
Interleukin-2 + vaccine	91	13	10	8	6	2	1

B Overall Survival

P=0.06

Interleukin-2 + vaccine

Interleukin-2 alone

No. at Risk

Interleukin alone	94	46	26	14	8	4	1
Interleukin-2 + vaccine	91	54	37	20	8	4	1

FIGURE 1.—Progression-free and overall survival. Progression-free survival (Panel A) was longer among patients receiving vaccine and interleukin-2 than among those receiving interleukin-2 alone. The median progression-free survival among patients who received the vaccine was 2.2 months (95% confidence interval [CI], 1.7 to 3.9), as compared with 1.6 months (95% CI, 1.5 to 1.8) among patients who did not receive the vaccine. There was a trend toward longer overall survival (Panel B) among patients receiving vaccine and interleukin-2 than among those receiving interleukin-2 alone. The median survival among patients who received the vaccine was 17.8 months (95% CI, 11.9 to 25.8), as compared with 11.1 months (95% CI, 8.7 to 16.3) among patients who did not receive the vaccine. (Reprinted from Schwartzentruber DJ, Lawson DH, Richards JM, et al. gp100 peptide vaccine and interleukin-2 in patients with advanced melanoma. *N Engl J Med.* 2011;364:2119-2127. © 2011 Massachusetts Medical Society.)

vaccine had a higher rate of response than the rate that is expected among patients who are treated with interleukin-2 alone.

Methods.—We conducted a randomized, phase 3 trial involving 185 patients at 21 centers. Eligibility criteria included stage IV or locally advanced stage III cutaneous melanoma, expression of HLA*A0201, an absence of brain metastases, and suitability for high-dose interleukin-2 therapy. Patients were randomly assigned to receive interleukin-2 alone (720,000 IU per kilogram of body weight per dose) or gp100:209-217(210M) plus incomplete Freund's adjuvant (Montanide ISA-51) once per cycle, followed by interleukin-2. The primary end point was clinical response. Secondary end points included toxic effects and progression-free survival.

Results.—The treatment groups were well balanced with respect to baseline characteristics and received a similar amount of interleukin-2 per cycle. The toxic effects were consistent with those expected with interleukin-2 therapy. The vaccine–interleukin-2 group, as compared with the interleukin-2–only group, had a significant improvement in centrally verified overall clinical response (16% vs. 6%, P=0.03), as well as longer progression-free survival (2.2 months; 95% confidence interval [CI], 1.7 to 3.9 vs. 1.6 months; 95% CI, 1.5 to 1.8; P=0.008). The median overall survival was also longer in the vaccine–interleukin-2 group than in the interleukin-2–only group (17.8 months; 95% CI, 11.9 to 25.8 vs. 11.1 months; 95% CI, 8.7 to 16.3; P=0.06).

Conclusions.—In patients with advanced melanoma, the response rate was higher and progression-free survival longer with vaccine and interleukin-2 than with interleukin-2 alone. (Funded by the National Cancer Institute and others; ClinicalTrials.gov number, NCT00019682.) (Fig 1).

▶ This is a randomized, phase 3 trial involving 185 patients from 21 different institutions. As seen in Table 2 in the original article, vaccine plus high-dose interleukin-2 tended to have a more favorable response, especially complete responses, when compared with high-dose interleukin-2 alone. However, patients with vaccine and high-dose interleukin-2 tended to have significantly more arrhythmias and metabolic abnormalities associated with their treatment protocol.

If one evaluates Fig 1, they would see that vaccine plus interleukin-2 seemed to have a survival appearance particularly from 6 months through 3 years of follow-up. After that, the advantage to vaccine and interleukin seemed to dissipate.

Metastatic melanoma remains a difficult disease to treat. However, this randomized trial shows that a combination of vaccine and interleukin-2 can activate the immune response and create significant improvement in progression-free survival but not overall survival. Finally, this treatment is very expensive and will require further modification to enhance efficacy and reduce cost.

T. J. Eberlein, MD

Improved Survival with Vemurafenib in Melanoma with BRAF V600E Mutation

Chapman PB, for the BRIM-3 Study Group (Memorial Sloan-Kettering Cancer Ctr, NY; et al)
N Engl J Med 364:2507-2516, 2011

Background.—Phase 1 and 2 clinical trials of the BRAF kinase inhibitor vemurafenib (PLX4032) have shown response rates of more than 50% in patients with metastatic melanoma with the BRAF V600E mutation.

Methods.—We conducted a phase 3 randomized clinical trial comparing vemurafenib with dacarbazine in 675 patients with previously untreated, metastatic melanoma with the BRAF V600E mutation. Patients were randomly assigned to receive either vemurafenib (960 mg orally twice daily) or dacarbazine (1000 mg per square meter of body-surface area intravenously every 3 weeks). Coprimary end points were rates of overall and progression-free survival. Secondary end points included the response rate, response duration, and safety. A final analysis was planned after 196 deaths and an interim analysis after 98 deaths.

Results.—At 6 months, overall survival was 84% (95% confidence interval [CI], 78 to 89) in the vemurafenib group and 64% (95% CI, 56 to 73) in the dacarbazine group. In the interim analysis for overall survival and final analysis for progression-free survival, vemurafenib was associated with a relative reduction of 63% in the risk of death and of 74% in the risk of either death or disease progression, as compared with dacarbazine ($P<0.001$ for both comparisons). After review of the interim analysis by an independent data and safety monitoring board, crossover from dacarbazine to vemurafenib was recommended. Response rates were 48% for vemurafenib and 5% for dacarbazine. Common adverse events associated with vemurafenib were arthralgia, rash, fatigue, alopecia, keratoacanthoma or squamous-cell carcinoma, photosensitivity, nausea, and diarrhea; 38% of patients required dose modification because of toxic effects.

Conclusions.—Vemurafenib produced improved rates of overall and progression-free survival in patients with previously untreated melanoma with the BRAF V600E mutation. (Funded by Hoffmann—La Roche; BRIM-3 ClinicalTrials.gov number, NCT01006980.) (Figs 1 and 2).

▶ This is a phase 3, randomized, prospective clinical trial comparing vemurafenib with dacarbazine in 675 patients with previously untreated metastatic melanoma but all who had *BRAF V600E* mutation. As seen in both Figs 1 and 2, vemurafenib resulted in significant improvement in overall survival and progression-free survival in these patients. While almost 40% of the patients had to have dose modification because of toxicity, the toxicity was relatively manageable and consisted of diarrhea, hyporkeratosis, pruritus, alopecia, and other rashes.

Almost half the patients in the study treated with vemurafenib had response

It is noted that about 18% of the patients treated with vemurafenib had at least 1 squamous cell cancer of the skin or a keratoacanthoma. The mechanism for this

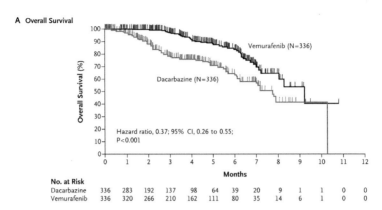

A Overall Survival

No. at Risk

Dacarbazine	336	283	192	137	98	64	39	20	9	1	1	0	0
Vemurafenib	336	320	266	210	162	111	80	35	14	6	1	0	0

B Subgroup Analyses of Overall Survival

Subgroup	No. of Patients	Hazard Ratio (95% CI)
All patients	672	0.37 (0.26–0.55)
Age		
<65 yr	512	0.40 (0.25–0.62)
≥65 yr	160	0.33 (0.16–0.67)
Age group		
≤40 yr	117	0.53 (0.23–1.23)
41–54 yr	225	0.25 (0.12–0.55)
55–64 yr	170	0.47 (0.22–0.99)
65–74 yr	110	0.12 (0.03–0.47)
≥75 yr	50	0.60 (0.23–1.55)
Sex		
Female	293	0.49 (0.28–0.86)
Male	379	0.30 (0.18–0.51)
Region		
North America	172	0.44 (0.20–0.93)
Western Europe	405	0.33 (0.20–0.53)
Australia or New Zealand	77	0.59 (0.20–1.78)
Other	18	0.00 (0.00–NR)
ECOG status		
0	457	0.31 (0.18–0.54)
1	215	0.42 (0.25–0.72)
Disease stage		
IIIC	33	0.53 (0.07–3.76)
M1a	74	0.31 (0.07–1.47)
M1b	126	0.91 (0.33–2.52)
M1c	439	0.32 (0.21–0.50)
IIIC, M1a, or M1b	233	0.64 (0.29–1.38)
Lactate dehydrogenase level		
Normal	390	0.37 (0.19–0.69)
Elevated	282	0.36 (0.22–0.57)

Vemurafenib Better ← → Dacarbazine Better

FIGURE 1.—Overall survival. Panel A shows Kaplan–Meier estimates of survival in patients in the intention-to-treat population. Patients could be evaluated for overall survival if they had undergone randomization at least 2 weeks before the clinical cutoff date. An inadequate number of patients were evaluated after 7 months of follow-up in either study group to provide reliable Kaplan–Meier estimates of the survival curves. The vertical lines indicate that patients' data were censored. Panel B shows hazard ratios and 95% confidence intervals (CI) for rates of overall survival in prespecified subgroups of patients, according to various baseline characteristics. In both panels, data are shown for patients who received no study treatment (48 patients in the dacarbazine group and 2 patients in the vemurafenib group) and for 1 patient who was assigned to the dacarbazine group but who received vemurafenib. NR denotes not reached. (Reprinted from Chapman PB, for the BRIM-3 Study Group. Improved survival with vemurafenib in melanoma with BRAF V600E mutation. *N Engl J Med.* 2011;364:2507-2516. © 2011 Massachusetts Medical Society.)

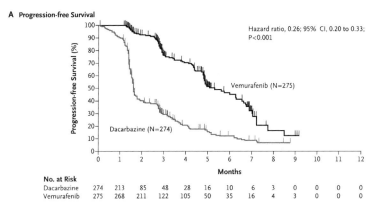

FIGURE 2.—Progression-free survival. Panel A shows Kaplan–Meier estimates of progression-free survival in patients in the intention-to-treat population. Patients could be evaluated for progression-free survival if they had undergone randomization at least 9 weeks before clinical cutoff date. The median progression-free survival was 5.3 months for vemurafenib and 1.6 months for dacarbazine. The vertical lines indicate that patients' data were censored. Panel B shows hazard ratios and 95% confidence intervals (CI) for progression-free survival in prespecified subgroups of patients, according to baseline characteristics. In both panels, data are shown for patients who received no study treatment (48 patients in the dacarbazine group and 2 patients in the vemurafenib group) and for 1 patient who was assigned to the dacarbazine group and who received vemurafenib. NR denotes not reached. (Reprinted from Chapman PB, for the BRIM-3 Study Group. Improved survival with vemurafenib in melanoma with BRAF V600E mutation. *N Engl J Med.* 2011;364:2507-2516. © 2011 Massachusetts Medical Society.)

development of cutaneous melanoma still requires investigation. Another important issue associated with patients treated with vemurafenib is the mechanism of how patients become resistant to this drug. This drug may well form the basis of future combination therapies in patients who have melanoma and risk of recurrence or metastatic disease.

T. J. Eberlein, MD

11 Vascular Surgery

Introduction

There were several seminal vascular-related publications during the past year that have been highlighted in the current edition of the YEAR BOOK OF SURGERY. The CAESAR trial complemented last year's PIVOTAL trial and again demonstrated that there is no difference in all-cause mortality for endovascular repair of small abdominal aortic aneurysms (diameter 4.1 − 5.4 cm) when compared with expectant management. The ACE trial confirmed the findings of the other randomized, controlled trials (DREAM, EVAR-1, OVER) comparing open and endovascular repair for abdominal aortic aneurysms by failing to show a difference in outcome among low- to moderate-risk patients. The Carotid Occlusion Surgery Study Randomized Trial failed to demonstrate a benefit in terms of ipsilateral stroke prevention for extraintracranial bypass despite a significant risk in the medical arm, finally overcoming the highly criticized EC/IC Bypass Study. Lastly, the PARTNERS trial demonstrated that the 30-day and 1-year outcomes were comparable between transcatheter and open aortic valve replacement among high-risk patients. Although percutaneous valves are likely outside the scope of practice for most vascular surgeons, we will likely be involved in the management of the access-related complications.

The articles selected contribute to our overall understanding of aortic pathologies, particularly with regards to the management of aneurysms. A report using the M2S database (M2S, Inc., West Lebanon, NH) suggests that a large percentage of endovascular abdominal aortic aneurysm repairs across the country are being performed at a size threshold below 55 mm and outside the manufacturers' instructions for use. Not surprisingly, the repairs performed outside the manufacturers' guidelines were associated with a higher incidence of endoleaks. A report from the Eurostar Registry has attempted to define the natural history of aneurysm growth after endovascular repair in the absence of an identifiable endoleak. The authors found that the aneurysm rupture risk within the first 4 years was quite small with the predictors of rupture being a growth rate > 8 mm and a Vanguard graft (Boston Scientific, Natick, MA). Fortunately, an additional report documented that the late conversion from an endovascular repair to an open repair is relatively safe and several technical tips were provided. A classification scheme for blunt aortic injuries, along with treatment recommendations, has been developed based upon the external contour of the aorta. The authors have suggested that intimal injuries are relatively benign while frank ruptures are lethal. Somewhat surprisingly, the 5-year survival rates are better for the open repair of descending thoracic aneurysm when compared with endovascular repair among good risk Medicare patients, suggesting some type of device-related phenomenon as a contributing factor.

The management of cerebrovascular occlusive disease continues to evolve with the emphasis on endovascular therapies. A report from the Medicare population comparing carotid angioplasty and stenting with endarterectomy failed to demonstrate a difference in periprocedural outcomes although the endovascular approach was associated with a higher mortality and myocardial infarction rate at 1 year. The endovascular approach has also been extended to the management of carotid artery dissections with reasonable midterm outcomes, potentially overcoming the inherent limitations of the open approach for this unusual problem. Early carotid endarterectomy (<6 hrs) may be associated with improved neurologic outcome for symptomatic patients and does not appear to cause new intracranial lesions. Finally, a small but elegant randomized controlled trial demonstrated that prior or simultaneous carotid endarterectomy and coronary artery bypass grafting may improve outcome in patients with asymptomatic carotid stenoses, providing further fuel to the ongoing debate about the role of the combined procedures.

The optimal management of both claudication and limb-threatening ischemia remains unresolved despite the widespread proliferation of the endovascular approach. A meta-analysis suggested that a supervised exercise program is comparable to endovascular treatment and better than medical management alone. However, the underlying data are quite limited given the magnitude of the problem. A small randomized controlled trial demonstrated that heparin bonded ePTFE grafts may be associated with improved patency rates when used for femorofemoral or femoropopliteal bypass grafts, providing another alternative to patients without adequate autogenous conduit. A report examining the role of duplex surveillance after femoropopliteal endovascular interventions suggests that the natural history of the index lesions is clearly different from infrainguinal vein bypass grafts, thereby questioning the role of a dedicated surveillance protocol. A sobering report demonstrated that there is a significant decrement in functional outcome after both open and endovascular treatment of critical limb ischemia, emphasizing the "terminal" nature of the disease process. Lastly, a report from the NISQIP database suggested that the mortality rates for major lower extremity amputations exceeded those for revascularizations. Despite the authors' best attempts, the study is clearly limited by a selection bias, but it does serve to question the prevalent belief that amputation is safer than bypass for critically ill patients.

The balance of the articles selected advance our understanding of dialysis access, venous disease, and visceral occlusive disease. A retrospective study suggests that the 2-stage brachiobasilic autogenous hemodialysis access is superior to the 1-stage alternative and begs for a larger randomized controlled trial. A small series hypothesizes that many of the venous outflow stenoses at the costoclavicular junction of hemodialysis access are related to extrinsic compression, similar to venous thoracic outlet, and that this can be effectively remediated with surgical decompression. The importance of venous outflow lesions in the iliac system and their appropriate diagnosis and treatment with intravascular ultrasound and stenting, respectively, are emphasized in two separate reports. Importantly, venous outflow lesions are likely contributory in the settings of acute deep venous thrombosis, chronic venous insufficiency and combined lymphatic/venous insufficiency. An interesting report documented a significant incidence of pulmonary emboli after repair of popliteal vein injuries in the civilian population. Notably, most of these patients were systemically anticoagulated, suggesting that the optimal treatment may also include an inferior vena cava filter. Finally, a report has documented the outcome after endovascular reinterventions for visceral artery occlusive lesions. Although the outcomes were reasonable, a few patients presented with acute mesenteric ischemia, thereby emphasizing the importance of routine surveillance.

Thomas S. Huber, MD, PhD
Associate Editor

Aneurysm

Comparison of Surveillance Versus Aortic Endografting for Small Aneurysm Repair (CAESAR): Results from a Randomised Trial

Cao P, for the CAESAR Trial Group (Hospital S. Camillo — Forlanini, Rome, Italy; et al)
Eur J Vasc Endovasc Surg 41:13-25, 2011

Background.—Randomised trials have failed to demonstrate benefit from early surgical repair of small abdominal aortic aneurysm (AAA) compared with surveillance. This study aimed to compare results after endovascular aortic aneurysm repair (EVAR) or surveillance in AAA <5.5 cm.

Methods.—Patients (50—79 years) with AAA of 4.1—5.4 cm were randomly assigned, in a 1:1 ratio, to receive immediate EVAR or surveillance by ultrasound and computed tomography (CT) and repair only after a defined threshold (diameter ≥5.5 cm, enlargement >1 cm/year, symptoms) was achieved. The main end point was all-cause mortality. Recruitment is closed; results at a median follow-up of 32.4 months are here reported.

Results.—Between 2004 and 2008, 360 patients (early EVAR = 182; surveillance = 178) were enrolled. One perioperative death after EVAR and two late ruptures (both in the surveillance group) occurred. At 54 months, there was no significant difference in the main end-point rate [hazard ratio (HR) 0.76; 95% confidence interval (CI) 0.30—1.93; $p = 0.6$] with Kaplan—Meier estimates of all-cause mortality of 14.5% in the EVAR and 10.1% in the surveillance group. Aneurysm-related mortality, aneurysm rupture and major morbidity rates were similar. Kaplan—Meier estimates of aneurysms growth ≥5 mm at 36 months were 8.4% in the EVAR group and 67.5% in the surveillance group (HR 10.49; 95% CI 6.88—15.96;

$p < 0.01$). For aneurysms under surveillance, the probability of delayed repair was 59.7% at 36 months (84.5% at 54 months). The probability of receiving open repair at 36 months for EVAR feasibility loss was 16.4%.

Conclusion.—Mortality and rupture rates in AAA <5.5 cm are low and no clear advantage was shown between early or delayed EVAR strategy. However, within 36 months, three out of every five small aneurysms under surveillance might grow to require repair and one out of every six might lose feasibility for EVAR.

Surveillance is safe for small AAA if close supervision is applied. Long-term data are needed to confirm these results.

Clinical Trial Registration Information.—This study is registered, NCT Identifier: NCT00118573.

▶ The results of the Comparison of surveillance versus Aortic Endografting for Small Aneurysm Repair (CAESAR) trial complement the PIVOTAL Trial[1] and provide additional level 1 evidence that there is no survival advantage for repairing small (4.1–5.4 cm) abdominal aortic aneurysms (AAA) with the endovascular approach (EVAR) when compared with expectant management or surveillance. Notably, there were no differences in all-cause mortality (the primary end point of the study) or aneurysm-related mortality. However, the incidence of adverse events was greater in the patients assigned to early EVAR (21% vs 15% at 54 months, $P > .001$). There was an aneurysm-related death in both treatment groups (EVAR, perioperative pancreatitis; surveillance, ruptured aneurysm) and a total of 2 ruptured aneurysms in the surveillance group. Notably, the ruptured aneurysms occurred in patients who had been followed up with for some time and had been scheduled for operative repair because their aneurysms had exceeded the size threshold (ie, > 5.5 cm). The study confirmed several of the observations from the earlier randomized trials examining the treatment of both open and EVAR for AAAs. Notably, the annual rupture risk (< 1%) and growth rate (1.5–2 mm) for AAAs < 5.5 cm are both quite small. Furthermore, the overwhelming majority of patients with small AAAs in the size range of the trial will ultimately exceed the repair threshold and require operative treatment (ie, 60% at 36 months, 85% at 54 months), particularly those with the larger small aneurysms. Lastly, EVAR repair of these small aneurysms appears to be safe and well tolerated despite the fact that early repair does not appear to provide a survival benefit. It is interesting to note that 16% of the patients in the surveillance group were ultimately not deemed candidates for EVAR (ie, lost feasibility for EVAR) primarily because of changes in the infrarenal neck. However, it is worth emphasizing that there is a large volume of quality evidence that fails to demonstrate a survival benefit for EVAR when compared with the open approach. There are several limitations to the study that merit consideration. Notably, the study did not reach its original enrollment targets and was stopped prematurely based on a futility analysis; it is conceivable that a benefit may have been seen for EVAR had the original target been reached. The participating centers were very experienced with EVAR and had to fulfill several inclusion criteria. Accordingly, the study findings may not apply outside of these centers of excellence. The overwhelming majority of the patients in the study were men (96%); thus, the findings may not be applicable to women. The AAA rupture risk for women may exceed that for men for a specific diameter measurement with a 5.0-cm threshold being more appropriate for women. The safety of expectant management or surveillance is contingent upon close, conscientious follow-up as detailed in the study, and patients that are deemed noncompliant may benefit from earlier, definitive repair.

T. S. Huber, MD, PhD

Reference

1. Ouriel K, Clair DG, Kent KC, Zarins CK; Positive impact of Endovascular Options for treating Aneurysms Early (PIVOTAL) Investigators. Endovascular repair compared with surveillance for patients with small abdominal aortic aneurysms. *J Vasc Surg.* 2010;51:1081-1087.

A randomized controlled trial of endovascular aneurysm repair versus open surgery for abdominal aortic aneurysms in low- to moderate-risk patients
Becquemin J-P, for the ACE trialists (Univ Paris XII, France)
J Vasc Surg 53:1167-1173, 2011

Background.—Several studies, including three randomized controlled trials (RCTs), have shown that endovascular repair (EVAR) of abdominal aortic aneurysms (AAA) offered better early results than open surgical repair (OSR) but a similar medium-term to long-term mortality and a higher incidence of reinterventions. Thus, the role of EVAR, most notably in low-risk patients, remains debated.

Methods.—The ACE (Anevrysme de l'aorte abdominale: Chirurgie versus Endoprothese) trial compared mortality and major adverse events after EVAR and OSR in patients with AAA anatomically suitable for EVAR and at low-risk or intermediate-risk for open surgery. A total of 316 patients with >5 cm aneurysms were randomized in institutions with proven expertise for both treatments: 299 patients were available for analysis, and 149 were assigned to OSR and 150 to EVAR. Patients were monitored for 5 years after treatment. Statistical analysis was by intention to treat.

Results.—With a median follow-up of 3 years (range, 0-4.8 years), there was no difference in the cumulative survival free of death or major events rates between OSR and EVAR: 95.9% ± 1.6% vs 93.2% ± 2.1% at 1 year and 85.1% ± 4.5% vs 82.4% ± 3.7% at 3 years, respectively ($P = .09$). In-hospital mortality (0.6% vs 1.3%; $P = 1.0$), survival, and the percentage of minor complications were not statistically different. In the EVAR group, however, the crude percentage of reintervention was higher (2.4% vs 16%, $P < .0001$), with a trend toward a higher aneurysm-related mortality (0.7% vs 4%; $P = .12$).

Conclusions.—In patients with low to intermediate risk factors, open repair of AAA is as safe as EVAR and remains a more durable option.

▶ The Anevrysme de l'aorte abdominale: Chirurgie versus Endoprothese (ACE) Trial joins the 3 other randomized, controlled trials (EVAR-1, DREAM, OVER) comparing open (OSR) versus endovascular (EVAR) aneurysm repair. Not surprisingly, the long-term survival and freedom from major complications were comparable between the groups. However, the authors did not find an early mortality benefit for EVAR, as seen in the other trials, largely because of the low perioperative rate in the OSR group (EVAR, 1.3%, OSR, 0.6%). The endovascular approach was associated with the predictable perioperative outcome benefits (eg, shorter length of stay, shorter mechanical ventilation, fewer transfusions) and a higher rate of reintervention (2.4% vs 16%). Somewhat surprisingly, there was a trend toward a higher aneurysm-related mortality rate in the EVAR group although this is somewhat irrelevant in the absence of an overall survival difference. The ACE Trial was restricted to low- to moderate-risk patients as defined by the Society for Vascular Surgery/American Association for Vascular Surgery comorbidity severity scoring scale although it is not completely clear that the patients had a significantly lower risk than in the other randomized trials. The study begs the question as to how the data should be used in terms of everyday practice. It certainly further strengthens the findings from the 3 earlier trials, and I look forward to a formal meta-analysis. However, I am not certain that it will impact the number of open repairs, despite the small reported advantage, given the overwhelming patient preference for the endovascular approach. It is nice to know that OSR remains as safe as EVAR, and this can be very reassuring for the small percentage of patients that are not candidates for EVAR with the commercially available devices.

T. S. Huber, MD, PhD

Predictors of Abdominal Aortic Aneurysm Sac Enlargement After Endovascular Repair

Schanzer A, Greenberg RK, Hevelone N, et al (Univ of Massachusetts Med School, Worcester; Cleveland Clinic Foundation, OH; Harvard School of Public Health, Boston, MA)
Circulation 123:2848-2855, 2011

Background.—The majority of infrarenal abdominal aortic aneurysm (AAA) repairs in the United States are performed with endovascular methods. Baseline aortoiliac arterial anatomic characteristics are fundamental criteria for appropriate patient selection for endovascular aortic repair (EVAR) and key determinants of long-term success. We evaluated compliance with anatomic guidelines for EVAR and the relationship between baseline aortoiliac arterial anatomy and post-EVAR AAA sac enlargement.

Methods and Results.—Patients with pre-EVAR and at least 1 post-EVAR computed tomography scan were identified from the M2S, Inc. imaging database (1999 to 2008). Preoperative baseline aortoiliac anatomic characteristics were reviewed for each patient. Data relating to the specific AAA endovascular device implanted were not available. Therefore, morphological measurements were compared with the most liberal and the most conservative published anatomic guidelines as stated in each manufacturer's instructions for use. The primary study outcome was post-EVAR

AAA sac enlargement (>5-mm diameter increase). In 10 228 patients undergoing EVAR, 59% had a maximum AAA diameter below the 55-mm threshold at which intervention is recommended over surveillance. Only 42% of patients had anatomy that met the most conservative definition of device instructions for use; 69% met the most liberal definition of device instructions for use. The 5-year post-EVAR rate of AAA sac enlargement was 41%. Independent predictors of AAA sac enlargement included endoleak, age ≥80 years, aortic neck diameter ≥28 mm, aortic neck angle >60°, and common iliac artery diameter >20 mm.

Conclusion.—In this multicenter observational study, compliance with EVAR device guidelines was low and post-EVAR aneurysm sac enlargement was high, raising concern for long-term risk of aneurysm rupture.

▶ The authors have used the M2S, Inc (West Lebanon, New Hampshire), image repository to document aortic sac enlargement after endovascular aneurysm repair (EVAR) in an attempt to identify predictors of enlargement, primarily focusing on aortoiliac anatomy and the device manufacturers' indications for use (IFU). Somewhat disconcertingly, they found that most repairs were performed for aneurysms < 55 mm in maximal diameter, a large percentage of repairs (31%—58%) were performed outside of the manufacturers' IFU, and a significant percentage (41%) of the aneurysms sacs increased in size > 5 mm by 5 years after repair. Furthermore, they identified the presence of an endoleak, advanced age, and several anatomic features as predictors of sac enlargement, establishing a relationship between use outside of the IFU, endoleak, and sac growth. These findings suggest that the current application of EVAR across the country is less than ideal. However, several points merit further comment to further frame and potentially refute this contention. The ADAM and UK small aneurysm trials clearly defined 55 mm as an appropriate diameter threshold for aneurysm repair, but this threshold may not be appropriate for women, given their higher diameter-specific rupture risk. Furthermore, the consistent message from the small aneurysm trials was that it wasn't necessarily if the aneurysm needed to be repaired, but when, particularly for those aneurysms approaching 55 mm. Although endoleak and sac enlargement after EVAR are associated with the need for further remedial procedures and rupture, they are really surrogate markers for more important adverse outcomes. It is unclear from the data whether these outcomes were (or are) associated with either death or aneurysm-related death. It is impossible to determine from the M2S data whether the endoleaks and sac enlargement were addressed, and it is important to remember that the majority can be remediated with a catheter-based procedure. The study paralleled the widespread dissemination and clinical maturation of the EVAR technology, and thus it is not particularly surprising that the compliance with the IFU decreased as the surgical community gained experience. Despite the authors' contention to the contrary, it is likely that the cases submitted to M2S were more complicated from an anatomic standpoint and may not be very representative of all patients undergoing EVAR in our country. This important publication underscores the fact that compliance with the manufacturers' IFUs is likely associated with better outcome while challenging us all to constantly reassess our operative indications for EVAR, particularly given the randomized trials demonstrating no difference with open repair.

T. S. Huber, MD, PhD

Annual rupture risk of abdominal aortic aneurysm enlargement without detectable endoleak after endovascular abdominal aortic repair
Koole D, for the European Collaborators on Stent-Graft Techniques for Aortic Aneurysm Repair (EUROSTAR) (Univ Med Ctr Utrecht, The Netherlands; et al)
J Vasc Surg 54:1614-1622, 2011

Objectives.—Whether abdominal aortic aneurysm (AAA) enlargement after endovascular aneurysm repair (EVAR), without an identifiable endoleak, is a risk factor for AAA rupture remains controversial. To our knowledge, studies including large patient numbers investigating this topic have not been done. Therefore, a considerable number of conversions to open AAA repair have been performed in this patient group. This study evaluated AAA rupture risk in patients without detectable endoleaks but with AAA enlargement after EVAR treatment.

Methods.—Baseline characteristics and follow-up data were collected prospectively by case record forms. Follow-up visits were scheduled at 1, 3, 6, 12, 18, and 24 months, and annually thereafter. The follow-up assessment included clinical examination and imaging studies. Patients were divided into three groups according to the degree of shrinkage or enlargement of the aneurysm. Group A included patients with >8 mm aneurysm shrinkage, group B consisted of patients with ≤8 mm shrinkage to ≤8 mm enlargement, and group C patients had an aneurysm enlargement of >8 mm.

Results.—The basis for this analysis was 6337 patients who were enrolled prospectively in the European Collaborators on Stent-Graft Techniques for Aortic Aneurysm Repair (EUROSTAR) database between 1996 and 2006. Group A included 691 patients; group B, 5307 patients; and group C, 339 patients. Ruptures occurred in 3 patients in group A, in 14 patients in group B, and in 9 patients in group C. The annual rate of rupture in group C was <1% in the first 4 years but accelerated to 7.5% up to 13.6% in the years thereafter. The mortality rate of elective conversion to open AAA repair was 6.0%.

Conclusions.—The risk of rupture in patients with an AAA enlargement of 8 mm after EVAR, without detectable endoleaks, is <1% in the first 4 years. No ruptures were seen in patients with AAA enlargement without detectable endoleaks who were not treated with Vanguard stent grafts (Boston Scientific Corp, Natick, Mass) and had AAA diameters <70 mm. For this group, conversion to open repair might not be mandatory, and regular follow-up can be advised instead. After 4 years of follow-up, this study observed an increased annual rupture risk, which might indicate the need for conversion; however, groups are small, and follow-up bias could play a role.

▶ This study helps define the optimal management of patients with continued aneurysm growth after endovascular aneurysm repair (EVAR) without an identifiable endoleak. Using the EUROSTAR Registry, the authors reported that the annual rupture risk for aneurysms that had enlarged more than 8 mm was less than 1% during the first 4 years, but greater than 7.5% thereafter. They identified aneurysm enlargement greater than 8 mm (hazard ratio 5.89) and Vanguard stent grafts (hazard ratio 4.52) as the strongest predictors of rupture in their multivariate model. Although it is worth noting that only the aneurysms that had been originally repaired with a Vanguard graft ruptured with a maximal diameter less than 70 mm. These data confirm the consistent theme that aneurysms can rupture after EVAR but suggest that the risk is quite modest (certainly within the first 4 years) and may not merit early conversion. Similar to the treatment of all aneurysms, the operative decision for open conversion reflects a balance between the operative risk and the risk of rupture. It is also worth noting that the mortality rate for open conversion in the current study was 6%, whereas the mortality rate for rupture was 62%. The data seem to support the authors' recommendations for a conservative approach (ie, expectant management) within the first 4 years for most grafts with aneurysms less than 70 mm provided that an endoleak has been aggressively excluded. The optimal treatment after 4 years remains to be determined, but open conversion may be justified. These recommendations do not apply to the Vanguard and early Excluder grafts (ie, high porosity) given their propensity for rupture and sac enlargement, respectively. These recommendations must be interpreted with some caution given the registry nature of the data, the limited long-term follow-up, and the accuracy of the diameter measurements but clearly suggest that continued sac enlargement in the absence of an endoleak may not be an ominous sign.

T. S. Huber, MD, PhD

Late open conversion and explantation of abdominal aortic stent grafts

Brinster CJ, Fairman RM, Woo EY, et al (Hosp of the Univ of Pennsylvania, Philadelphia)

J Vasc Surg 54:42-47, 2011

Objectives.—To evaluate indications for, operative strategy during, and outcomes following late open surgical conversion following endovascular aneurysm repair (EVAR).

Methods.—Between 2002 and 2009, patients undergoing open abdominal aortic aneurysm repair at a university hospital were entered prospectively into a database which was examined to identify patients undergoing open conversion >30 days after EVAR.

Results.—Over 7 years, 21 patients required late open conversion of EVAR. The average patient age was 75 years (range, 59-88), and there were 16 male (76%) patients. The mean interval to conversion was 33.4 months (range, 2-73). Eight patients (38%) presented with proximal type I endoleak; 4 patients (19%) presented with type II endoleak and aneurysm expansion; 5 patients (24%) presented with graft migration and aneurysm expansion; and 5 patients (24%) presented with de novo visceral aneurysms. Rupture (1) and infection (1) were also observed. There were five (24%) emergent cases. Most patients (12/21, 57%) had more than one reason for conversion. There were no perioperative deaths; three patients (14%) had major complications. Grafts requiring conversion were AneuRx (6; Medtronic AVE, Santa Rosa, Calif), Zenith (6; Cook Inc, Bloomington, Ind), Talent (3; Medtronic), Excluder (2; W. L. Gore, Flagstaff, Ariz), Anaconda (1; TERUMO Corp, Ann Arbor, Mich), Ancure (1; Guidant, Menlo Park, Calif), Quantum LP (1; Cordis Corp, Miami Lakes, Fla), and Powerlink (1; Endologix, Irvine, Calif). The surgical approach was retroperitoneal in 16 (76%) and transperitoneal in four (19%) patients. Initial proximal aortic control was supraceliac (9/21), suprarenal (7/21), or infrarenal (5/21), with stepwise distal clamping to reduce ischemic time. Complete endograft removal was performed in 17/21 patients; in 4/21 the distal anastomosis was performed to the endograft after proximal segment explantation. Reconstruction was completed with tube (19/21) or aortoiliac (2/21) grafts; in one case, homograft was used. Mean intraoperative blood loss was 1.9 L (range, 0.4-6.5 L), mean intensive care unit (ICU) stay was 3 days (range, 2-6), and the mean hospital stay was 10 days (range, 4-39).

Conclusions.—While technically challenging, delayed open conversion of EVAR can be accomplished with low morbidity and mortality in both the elective and emergent settings. These results reinforce the justification for long-term surveillance of endografts following EVAR.

▶ The authors have documented their experience with open conversion after endovascular aneurysm repair (EVAR). Although the series is relatively small, they reported no deaths and fairly low morbidity rates. Indeed, the outcomes are among the best reported and reflect a favorable trend spanning the last decade. The indications encompassed a variety of failure modes, including endoleak, aneurysm expansion, and graft migration, and it is noteworthy that the patients averaged 2 failure modes each (eg, graft migration and type 1 endoleak). Notably, a variety of different devices were used for the index repair, suggesting that failure or need for conversion is not limited to a specific device. Despite the favorable outcome rates, open conversion is a major surgical procedure associated with significant blood loss (mean estimated blood loss, 1.9 L), prolonged hospital stay, and resource utilization. Although not stated in the article, these procedures should likely be concentrated in centers of excellence given their relative infrequency and overall complexity. The authors highlight several technical points that merit emphasis. The left retroperitoneal approach facilitates the proximal aortic dissection and placement of the cross clamp at the level of the renal arteries, the superior mesenteric artery (SMA), or the celiac axis as dictated by the extent of the device. It is often necessary to place the clamp on the supra-SMA or supraceliac aorta initially, but it can usually be repositioned further distally after removal of the aortic device. Exposing the right iliac vessels can be difficult through the retroperitoneal approach in large patients, but can be facilitated by ligating the inferior mesenteric artery, allowing the viscera to be reflected further to the patient's right. The aortoiliac segment is usually inflamed, thereby complicating the dissection and the anastomoses. The authors were able to remove all device components in the majority of cases although they emphasized that this is not always possible for devices with suprarenal fixation (eg, Zenith, Cook Inc, Bloomington, Indiana) and those in which the iliac limbs were well incorporated. The suprarenal component may be cut using wire cutters with the residual segment of the device incorporated into the proximal anastomosis. The iliac device limbs can be used for the distal anastomosis, precluding their removal, although this usually mandates long-term surveillance, similar to that for the index EVAR.

Lastly, the report underscores the importance of long-term surveillance after EVAR. Although most EVAR failures can be remediated with catheter-based interventions, open conversion is occasionally required (eg, 1%) and will likely become more common with the widespread application of EVAR, the longer duration of follow-up and the use of EVAR for patients with challenging anatomy.

T. S. Huber, MD, PhD

A new classification scheme for treating blunt aortic injury
Starnes BW, Lundgren RS, Gunn M, et al (Univ of Washington, Seattle)
J Vasc Surg 55:47-54, 2012

Background.—There are numerous questions about the treatment of blunt aortic injury (BAI), including the management of small intimal tears, what injury characteristics are predictive of death from rupture, and which patients actually need intervention. We used our experience in treating BAI during the past decade to create a classification scheme based on radiographic and clinical data and to provide clear treatment guidelines.

Methods.—The records of patients admitted with BAI from 1999 to 2008 were retrospectively reviewed. Patients with a radiographically or operatively confirmed diagnosis (echocardiogram, computed tomography, or angiography) of BAI were included. We created a classification system based on the presence or absence of an aortic external contour abnormality, defined as an alteration in the symmetric, round shape of the aorta: (1) intimal tear (IT)—absence of aortic external contour abnormality and intimal defect and/or thrombus of <10 mm in length or width; (2) large intimal flap (LIF)—absence of aortic external contour abnormality and intimal defect and/or thrombus of ≥10 mm in length or width; (3) pseudoaneurysm—presence of aortic external contour abnormality and contained rupture; (4) rupture—presence of aortic external contour abnormality and free contrast extravasation or hemothorax at thoracotomy.

Results.—We identified 140 patients with BAI. Most injuries were pseudoaneurysm (71%) at the isthmus (70%), 16.4% had an IT, 5.7% had a LIF, and 6.4% had a rupture. Survival rates by classification were IT, 87%; LIF, 100%; pseudoaneurysm, 76%; and rupture, 11% (one patient). Of the ITs, LIFs, and pseudoaneurysms treated nonoperatively, none worsened, and 65% completely healed. No patient with an IT or LIF died. Most patients with ruptures lost vital signs before presentation or in the emergency department and did not survive. Hypotension before or at hospital presentation and size of the periaortic hematoma at the level of the aortic arch predicted likelihood of death from BAI.

Conclusions.—As a result of this new classification scheme, no patient without an external aortic contour abnormality died of their BAI. ITs can be managed nonoperatively. BAI patients with rupture will die, and resources could be prioritized elsewhere. Those with LIFs do well, and currently, most at our institution are treated with a stent graft. If a pseudoaneurysm is going to rupture, it does so early. Hematoma at the arch on computed tomography scan and hypotension before or at arrival help to predict which pseudoaneurysms need urgent repair (Table 6).

▶ The authors have defined a new classification scheme for blunt aortic injuries and have attempted to define their natural history. The classification scheme was based on the presence or absence of an abnormality in the external contour of the aorta on CT scan. The 4 classes were defined as intimal tear, large intimal flap, pseudoaneurysm, and rupture with abnormalities in the external contour occurring in the latter 2 groups. Notably, most injuries (71%) involved pseudoaneurysms at the isthmus of the aorta. None of the patients with isolated intimal injuries (ie, tears or large flaps) and an intact external contour went on to rupture their aorta, suggesting that these are relatively benign lesions. However, there was a tremendous amount of selection bias as demonstrated by the fact that most (ie, 6/8) of the patients with large intimal flaps underwent operative repair. The serial imaging studies in these patients with intimal injuries

---

TABLE 6.—University of Washington Clinical Treatment Guidelines for Blunt Aortic Injury

1. All patients with radiographic evidence of blunt aortic injury (BAI) should undergo anti-impulse therapy with β-blockade, if tolerated, coupled with antiplatelet therapy (81 mg aspirin).
2. Observation alone with interval follow-up computed tomography angiography (CTA) within 30 days is appropriate for all intimal tears <10 mm.
3. Selective management of large intimal flaps (>10 mm) is appropriate with repeat imaging within 7 days to assess for progression. Evidence of progression should be managed, when possible, with endovascular repair.
4. All patients with an aortic external contour abnormality should be considered for semielective (≤1 week) endovascular repair if there is a high likelihood of survival from other associated injuries. These patients should be monitored with CT imaging as follows: 1 month, 6 months, 1 year, and every other year thereafter. Patients with hypotension on presentation and aortic arch hematoma >15 mm should be repaired with endovascular methods on a more *urgent* basis.
5. Intentional left subclavian artery coverage *without* revascularization is well tolerated in a majority of patients with BAI.
6. Patients with traumatic brain injury and an aortic external contour abnormality should be considered for earlier repair if a deliberate increase in mean arterial pressure is deemed beneficial for the patient.

further supported their benign nature because essentially all of them remained stable or healed, with almost half healing at 1 month. Among the patients with pseudoaneurysms, the overall mortality rate was 24%, with 9 out of 24 deaths resulting from the blunt aortic injury. Similar to the case of large intimal injuries, most patients with pseudoaneurysms underwent repair or attempted repair. Importantly, none of the patients treated nonoperatively ruptured their pseudoaneurysms or developed any progression on serial CT scans. Essentially, all the patients with ruptured aneurysms died, with most deaths resulting from the aortic injury. Multivariate analysis demonstrated that hypotension (systolic blood pressure < 90 mm Hg) and the size of the periaortic hematoma for patients with pseudoaneurysms were associated with death from blunt aortic injury. The report echoes the consistent findings in the literature that aortic ruptures from blunt injuries are lethal and that patients who survive the initial few hours in the hospital are likely a self-selected group unlikely to rupture or die from their aortic injury. The authors' treatment guidelines (see Table 6) are very reasonable and merit consideration. However, it is worth emphasizing that all patients require serial CT follow-up with the duration dictated by the nature and extent of their injury, particularly given the potential for device-related complications such as collapse.

T. S. Huber, MD, PhD

Survival After Open Versus Endovascular Thoracic Aortic Aneurysm Repair in an Observational Study of the Medicare Population

Goodney PP, Travis L, Lucas FL, et al (Dartmouth-Hitchcock Med Ctr, Lebanon, NH; Maine Med Ctr, Portland; et al)
Circulation 124:2661-2669, 2011

Background.—The goal of this study was to describe short- and long-term survival of patients with descending thoracic aortic aneurysms (TAAs) after open and endovascular repair (TEVAR).

Methods and Results.—Using Medicare claims from 1998 to 2007, we analyzed patients who underwent repair of intact and ruptured TAA, identified from a combination of procedural and diagnostic *International Classification of Disease*, ninth revision, codes. Our main outcome measure was mortality, defined as perioperative mortality (death occurring before hospital discharge or within 30 days), and 5-year survival, from life-table analysis. We examined outcomes across repair type (open repair or TEVAR) in crude, adjusted (for age, sex, race, procedure year, and Charlson comorbidity score), and propensity-matched cohorts. Overall, we studied 12573 Medicare patients who underwent open repair and 2732 patients who underwent TEVAR. Perioperative mortality was lower in patients undergoing TEVAR compared with open repair for both intact (6.1% versus 7.1%; *P*=0.07) and ruptured (28% versus 46%; *P*<0.0001) TAA. However, patients with intact TAA selected for TEVAR had significantly worse survival than open patients at 1 year (87% for open, 82% for TEVAR; *P*=0.001) and 5 years (72% for open; 62% for TEVAR; *P*=0.001).

Furthermore, in adjusted and propensity-matched cohorts, patients selected for TEVAR had worse 5-year survival than patients selected for open repair.

Conclusions.—Although perioperative mortality is lower with TEVAR, Medicare patients selected for TEVAR have worse long-term survival than patients selected for open repair. The results of this observational study suggest that higher-risk patients are being offered TEVAR and that some do not benefit on the basis of long-term survival. Future work is needed to identify TEVAR candidates unlikely to benefit from repair.

▶ The authors have examined the perioperative and 5-year mortality rates in Medicare patients undergoing open and endovascular repair (TEVAR) for both intact and ruptured descending thoracic aneurysms. The perioperative mortality rates were comparable for the intact aneurysms (6.1% vs 7.1%, $P = .07$) but favored TEVAR for the ruptures (28% vs 46%, $P < .0001$). Somewhat surprisingly, the 5-year survival rates favored the open approach for the intact aneurysms (unadjusted, 72% vs 62%, $P = .001$) for all of the analyses performed (ie, unadjusted, adjusted, propensity matched) and were comparable or better for the ruptures (unadjusted 26% vs 23%, $P = .37$). These findings contradict many of the single-institution and industry-sponsored studies that have reported favorable perioperative outcomes and comparable long-term survival after TEVAR. The explanation for the mortality differences at 5 years is not clear from the data, but the observed differences in the propensity-matched group (ie, similar low-risk cohorts differing only by the treatment) suggest some type of device-related complications. The current findings differ significantly from those reported for the endovascular repair of intact infrarenal aneurysms that have consistently failed to demonstrate a survival difference after 2 years. The current data also suggest that there has been a rapid adoption of the endovascular approach after the commercial release of the initial device and that the application has been extended to higher risk patients. The data raise some important issues about the current application of TEVAR for descending thoracic aneurysms. First, the survival benefit for open repair suggests that it may be a better approach for good-risk patients with intact aneurysms, negating the perceived, short-term advantage for the less invasive endovascular approach. Second, the increased mortality rate in the TEVAR group suggests that expectant or nonoperative management may be a better treatment option for certain high-risk patients. Needless to say, there are several shortcomings of the current study that limit the strength of the observations, including the administrative database and the lack of anatomic criteria. However, the findings clearly mandate a reassessment of the widespread application of TEVAR and justify an appropriate randomized trial.

T. S. Huber, MD, PhD

Carotid

Extracranial-Intracranial Bypass Surgery for Stroke Prevention in Hemodynamic Cerebral Ischemia: The Carotid Occlusion Surgery Study Randomized Trial
Powers WJ, for the COSS Investigators (Univ of North Carolina School of Medicine, Chapel Hill; et al)
JAMA 306:1983-1992, 2011

Context.—Patients with symptomatic atherosclerotic internal carotid artery occlusion (AICAO) and hemodynamic cerebral ischemia are at high risk for subsequent stroke when treated medically.

Objective.—To test the hypothesis that extracranial-intracranial (EC-IC) bypass surgery, added to best medical therapy, reduces subsequent ipsilateral ischemic stroke in patients with recently symptomatic AICAO and hemodynamic cerebral ischemia.

Design.—Parallel-group, randomized, open-label, blinded-adjudication clinical treatment trial conducted from 2002 to 2010.

Setting.—Forty-nine clinical centers and 18 positron emission tomography (PET) centers in the United States and Canada. The majority were academic medical centers.

Participants.—Patients with arteriographically confirmed AICAO causing hemispheric symptoms within 120 days and hemodynamic cerebral ischemia identified by ipsilateral increased oxygen extraction fraction measured by PET. Of 195 patients who were randomized, 97 were randomized to receive surgery and 98 to no surgery. Follow-up for the primary end point until occurrence, 2 years, or termination of trial was 99% complete. No participant withdrew because of adverse events.

Interventions.—Anastomosis of superficial temporal artery branch to a middle cerebral artery cortical branch for the surgical group. Antithrombotic therapy and risk factor intervention were recommended for all participants.

Main Outcome Measure.—For all participants who were assigned to surgery and received surgery, the combination of (1) all stroke and death from surgery through 30 days after surgery and (2) ipsilateral ischemic stroke within 2 years of randomization. For the nonsurgical group and participants assigned to surgery who did not receive surgery, the combination of (1) all stroke and death from randomization to randomization plus 30 days and (2) ipsilateral ischemic stroke within 2 years of randomization.

Results.—The trial was terminated early for futility. Two-year rates for the primary end point were 21.0% (95% CI, 12.8% to 29.2%; 20 events) for the surgical group and 22.7% (95% CI, 13.9% to 31.6%; 20 events) for the nonsurgical group ($P = .78$, Z test), a difference of 1.7% (95% CI, −10.4% to 13.8%). Thirty-day rates for ipsilateral ischemic stroke were 14.4% (14/97) in the surgical group and 2.0% (2/98) in the nonsurgical group, a difference of 12.4% (95% CI, 4.9% to 19.9%).

Conclusion.—Among participants with recently symptomatic AICAO and hemodynamic cerebral ischemia, EC-IC bypass surgery plus medical therapy compared with medical therapy alone did not reduce the risk of recurrent ipsilateral ischemic stroke at 2 years.

Trial Registration.—clinicaltrials.gov Identifier: NCT00029146.

▶ This elegant randomized, controlled trial asks the lingering question of whether an extracranial-intracranial (EC/IC) bypass (ie, superficial temporal to middle cerebral artery) is effective in reducing stroke in symptomatic (event < 120 days) patients with an internal carotid artery occlusion. This is a relevant question because internal carotid artery occlusions are associated with a significant incidence of transient ischemic attacks or strokes at both the time of the initial event and thereafter. Similar to the maligned EC/IC Bypass Study,[1] the bypass did not provide any benefit in terms of ipsilateral stroke prevention at 2 years (surgery, 21.0% vs medical, 22.7%) despite excellent bypass patency rates (96% at last follow-up) and improved cerebral perfusion as documented by positron emission tomography scans. The study overcomes many of the criticisms of the original EC/IC Bypass Study including the multiple crossovers between treatment groups and the inability to identify the subgroup of patients with cerebral ischemia that may benefit from the procedure. It is noteworthy that the adverse event rates for the bypasses, both perioperative and longer term, were similar between the 2 trials. One of the surprising findings of the study was that the stroke risk associated with medical management was significantly lower than the 40% rate used in the power calculations. This underscores the importance of aggressive medical treatment that should include antithrombotic agents, blood pressure control, lipid/triglyceride lower agents, and glucose control. This publication should finally lay to rest the EC/IC bypass as a stroke prevention operation in the setting of an acute internal carotid artery occlusion. However, it shows that this subset of patients is at 23% risk of development of a further ipsilateral stroke within 2 years despite optimal medical management, a neurological event rate comparable to the medical arm in NASCET.[2]

T. S. Huber, MD, PhD

References

1. Failure of extracranial-intracranial arterial bypass to reduce the risk of ischemic stroke. Results of an international randomized trial. The EC/IC Bypass Study Group. *N Engl J Med.* 1985;313:1191-1200.
2. Beneficial effect of carotid endarterectomy in symptomatic patients with high-grade carotid stenosis. North American Symptomatic Carotid Endarterectomy Trial Collaborators. *N Engl J Med.* 1991;325:445-453.

Outcomes After Carotid Artery Stenting and Endarterectomy in the Medicare Population

Wang FW, Esterbrooks D, Kuo Y-F, et al (Creighton Univ, Omaha, NE; Univ of Texas Med Branch, Galveston; et al)
Stroke 42:2019-2025, 2011

Background and Purpose.—Carotid artery stenting (CAS) is an alternative to carotid endarterectomy (CEA) for stroke prevention. The value of this therapy relative to CEA remains uncertain.

Methods.—In 10 958 Medicare patients aged 66 years or older between 2004 and 2006, we analyzed in-hospital, 1-year stroke, myocardial infarction, and death rate outcomes and the effects of potential confounding variables.

Results.—CAS patients (87% were asymptomatic) had a higher baseline risk profile, including having a higher percentage of coronary and peripheral arterial disease, heart failure, and renal failure. In-hospital stroke rate (1.9% CAS versus 1.4% CEA; $P=0.14$) and mortality (CAS 0.9% versus 0.6% CEA; $P=0.20$) were similar. By 1 year, CAS patients had similar stroke rates (5.3% CAS versus 4.1% CEA; $P=0.12$) but higher all-cause mortality rates (9.9% CAS versus 6.1% CEA; $P<0.001$). Using Cox multivariable models, there was a similar stroke risk (hazard ratio, 1.28; 95% CI, 0.90−1.79) but CAS patients had a significantly higher mortality (HR, 1.32; 95% CI, 1.02−1.71). Sensitivity analyses suggested that unmeasured confounders could be responsible for the mortality difference. In multivariable analysis, stroke risk was highest in the patients symptomatic at the time of revascularization.

Conclusions.—CAS patients had a similar stroke risk but an increased mortality rate at 1 year compared with CEA patients, possibly related to the higher baseline risk profile in the CAS patient group.

▶ The report documents the outcome after carotid angioplasty/stenting (CAS) and carotid endarterectomy (CEA) among Medicare patients between 2004 and 2006 in an attempt to provide "real world" data for the 2 procedures. There were no differences in the periprocedural stroke and mortality rates despite a higher burden of comorbidities among those undergoing CAS, although there was a trend toward worse outcomes among symptomatic patients. CAS was associated with greater mortality and a higher incidence of myocardial infarction at 1 year despite no difference in stroke, although the risk of stroke was higher for the symptomatic patients at this time point. Multivariate analysis demonstrated that CAS was associated with death and myocardial infarction, although sensitivity analyses suggested that the confounder could have contributed to the observed mortality differences. Despite the authors' objectives, it is unclear whether those provide real world data, since 87% of the patients were asymptomatic, and reimbursement was limited to patients enrolled in postapproval investigational studies and those deemed to be higher surgical risk for CEA. Given these restrictions, it is not surprising that the incidence of comorbidities was greater among CAS patients. It is important to emphasize that the symptomatic status of the patients is one of the strongest predictors of outcome. The inclusion of such a large percentage of asymptomatic patients likely accounted for the negative findings in terms of the stroke outcomes but also likely obscured additional relevant differences in outcome between CAS and CEA for symptomatic patients as suggested by the randomized trials. The data must also be interpreted with some caution given the administrative database and the lack of important clinical, anatomic, and procedural factors. Importantly, stroke was not documented by a formal neurological examination, as dictated by all of the carotid revascularization trials. Overall, the data are encouraging and suggest that CAS is probably a safe alternative to CEA as suggested by the carotid revascularization endarterectomy versus stenting trial. One of the remaining challenges is to help define the patient populations best served by these 2 complementary therapies or medical management alone.

T. S. Huber, MD, PhD

Endovascular stent therapy for extracranial and intracranial carotid artery dissection: single-center experience
Ohta H, Natarajan SK, Hauck EF, et al (Univ at Buffalo, NY)
J Neurosurg 115:91-100, 2011

Object.—The objective of this study was to evaluate endovascular stent therapy for carotid artery dissections (CADs).

Methods.—Retrospective review of data at Millard Fillmore Gates Hospital identified 43 patients with 44 CADs (intracranial and/or extracranial) treated with carotid artery (CA) stent placement between January 2000 and June 2009.

Results.—Thirty-two CADs were spontaneous and 12 were traumatic; 35 were symptomatic. Lesion locations included the extracranial internal CA (ICA; 24 cases), extracranial ICA with common CA involvement (4 cases), and extracranial ICA—intracranial ICA (16 cases). Carotid artery occlusion was 100% in 15 cases (34.1%), 99% in 6 cases (13.6%), 70%—98% in 13 cases (29.5%), and <70% in 10 cases (22.7%). Five patients suffered pseudoaneurysms. Stent deployment was successful in 43 (97.7%) of 44 cases. The mean pretreatment score on the National Institutes of Health Stroke Scale was 6.2 ± 6.2. Recanalization (Thrombolysis in Myocardial Infarction Grade 2 or 3) was accomplished for 42 lesions (95.5%). Four patients demonstrated residual parent vessel stenosis (10%-50% in severity). Procedure-related complications occurred in 7 patients and included middle cerebral artery embolism (1 patient), intracranial hemorrhage (2 patients), worsening of dissection (1 patient), stent malpositioning (1 patient), embolic protection filter overload (1 patient), and filter retrieval device fracture (1 patient). Only 2 of these complications caused permanent deficits: the embolism caused a minor but permanent neurological deficit, and 1 intracranial hemorrhage was fatal. At discharge, 36 patients (83.7%) had modified Rankin Scale scores of 0—2 (favorable outcome). During the follow-up interval (mean 19.2 months, range 4—92 months), no patient suffered a new stroke and 1 patient died secondary to preexisting chronic renal failure. In 20 patients with angiographic follow-up, permanent resolution of the dissection was noted in 90.5%; 2 lesions (9.5%) required retreatment.

Conclusions.—Endovascular stent-assisted repair of extra- and intracranial CAD was safe and effective in this experience and can be recommended for selected patients. In particular, patients with symptomatic CADs that are not responsive to medical therapy should be considered for interventional treatment.

▶ The authors report the largest experience with endovascular stent treatment for extracranial and intracranial carotid artery dissections. Notably, one-third of the lesions involved both the extra- and intracranial carotid artery, while the carotid artery was also occluded in one-third of the patients. The overall technical results were excellent, and the perioperative complication rate was acceptable. Similarly, the midterm outcome in terms of both clinical status and vessel patency was good, with the majority of the dissections resolving. The authors provided a nice treatment algorithm and summarized the treatment indications in the Introduction, which included recurrence of neurologic symptoms despite adequate medical treatment, significant brain ischemia, contraindications to anticoagulation, expanding pseudoaneurysms with neurologic symptoms, and traumatic dissections with the latter justified based on a higher mortality rate. It is interesting to note that 20% of the patients were asymptomatic since these patients have been traditionally treated with anticoagulation alone regardless of whether the lesion was presumed to be traumatic or the dissection failed to heal. The impressive results justify the authors' approach while demonstrating a safe, effective treatment for a difficult problem that does not have a good, open surgical solution. Notably, the dissections usually extend to the base of the skull (or extend into the intracranial segment), thereby complicating the open surgical exposure and compromising the potential distal bypass target. The authors provided several technical tips worth noting. Because the dissection vessels are largely filled with thrombus, they recommend the use of embolic protection devices. However, they said that distal protection devices are difficult to navigate through a tortuous, thrombus-filled lumen and that a proximal protection device may be more useful in this setting. Additionally, they favored a closed-cell stent design to avoid the cheese-grating of the thrombus and emphasized the importance of covering the entire extent of the dissection.

T. S. Huber, MD, PhD

Urgent carotid endarterectomy to prevent recurrence and improve neurologic outcome in mild-to-moderate acute neurologic events
Capoccia L, Sbarigia E, Speziale F, et al (Univ of Rome, Italy)
J Vasc Surg 53:622-628, 2011

Objectives.—This study evaluated the safety and benefit of urgent carotid endarterectomy (CEA) in patients with carotid disease and an acute stable neurologic event.

Methods.—The study involved patients with acute neurologic impairment, defined as ≥4 points on the National Institutes of Health Stroke Scale (NIHSS) evaluation related to a carotid stenosis ≥50% who underwent urgent CEA. Preoperative workup included neurologic assessment with the NIHSS on admission or immediately before surgery and at discharge, carotid duplex scanning, transcranial Doppler ultrasound imaging, and head computed tomography or magnetic resonance imaging. End points were perioperative (30-day) neurologic mortality, significant NIHSS score improvement or worsening (defined as a variation ≥4), and hemorrhagic or ischemic neurologic recurrence. Patients were evaluated according to their NIHSS score on admission (4–7 or ≥8), clinical and demographic characteristics, timing of surgery (before or after 6 hours), and presence of brain infarction on neuroimaging.

Results.—Between January 2005 and December 2009, 62 CEAs were performed at a mean of 34.2 ± 50.2 hours (range, 2–280 hours) after the onset of symptoms. No neurologic mortality nor significant NIHSS score worsening was detected. The NIHSS score decreased in all but four patients, with no new ischemic lesions detected. The mean NIHSS score was 7.05 ± 3.41 on admission and 3.11 ± 3.62 at discharge in the entire group ($P < .01$). Patients with an NIHSS score of ≥8 on admission had a bigger score reduction than those with a lower NIHSS score (NIHSS 4–7; mean 4.95 ± 1.03 preoperatively vs 1.31 ± 1.7 postoperatively, NIHSS ≥8 10.32 ± 1.94 vs 4.03 ± 3.67; $P < .001$).

Conclusions.—In patients with acute neurologic event, a high NIHSS score does not contraindicate early surgery. To date, guidelines recommend treatment of symptomatic carotid stenosis ≤2 weeks from onset of symptoms to minimize the neurologic recurrence. Our results suggest that minimizing the time for intervention not only reduces the risk of recurrence but can also improve neurologic outcome.

▶ The authors have examined the impact of urgent carotid endarterectomy (CEA) on patients presenting to their stroke unit with mild to moderate acute neurological events (National Institute of Health Stroke Scale [NIHSS] score < 22) related to a carotid stenosis ≥50%. Notably, the mean time from onset of symptoms to CEA was 34 ± 50 hours, with 35% operated on within 6 hours of the event. The authors found that urgent CEA was safe and not associated with any neurological death or significant worsening of the NIHSS score at the time of discharge. Furthermore, no new significant lesions were found on postoperative CT or MRI imaging. Somewhat surprisingly, the patients with the most severe initial injury (NIHSS score ≥8) were found to have the most significant benefit in terms of improvement of their NIHSS score. These important findings support the national guidelines that recommend CEA within 2 weeks of an acute event and serve to ally most surgeons' concerns about the risk of converting an ischemic injury to a hemorrhagic one with early CEA. Indeed, it has been the practice of many surgeons to delay CEA after an acute event for 4 to 6 weeks or at least until the patient's neurologic improvement had stabilized or plateaued despite the fact that the risk of a recurrence is greatest after the index event. It is unfortunate that a control group was not included to help determine whether the observed neurological improvement was affected (either positively or negatively) by the early CEA. The inclusion/exclusion criteria and the perioperative algorithm (including medical management and imaging) should be reviewed before implementation to determine whether the findings are applicable to a given clinical situation or scenario. Notably, the authors were very aggressive with their medical management, including perioperative anticoagulation, and a surprisingly large number of CEAs were performed without a patch angioplasty (ie, primary repair). I am not certain that the results of this small study (N = 62) will be sufficient to change everyone's practice but concede that the approach is reasonable and safe and merits consideration because it justifies the guidelines advocating early CEA for symptomatic patients.

T. S. Huber, MD, PhD

Short-term results of a randomized trial examining timing of carotid endarterectomy in patients with severe asymptomatic unilateral carotid stenosis undergoing coronary artery bypass grafting
Illuminati G, Ricco J-B, Caliò F, et al (Univ of Rome "La Sapienza," Italy; Univ of Poitiers, France)
J Vasc Surg 54:993-999, 2011

Objective.—This study evaluated the timing of carotid endarterectomy (CEA) in the prevention of stroke in patients with asymptomatic carotid stenosis >70% receiving a coronary artery bypass graft (CABG).

Methods.—From January 2004 to December 2009, 185 patients with unilateral asymptomatic carotid artery stenosis >70%, candidates for CABG, were randomized into two groups. In group A, 94 patients received a CABG with previous or simultaneous CEA. In group B, 91 patients underwent CABG, followed by CEA. All patients underwent preoperative helical computed tomography scans, excluding significant atheroma of the ascending aorta or aortic arch. Baseline characteristics of the patients, type of coronary artery lesion, and preoperative myocardial function were comparable in the two groups. In group A, all patients underwent CEA under general anesthesia with the systematic use of a carotid shunt, and 79 patients had a combined procedure and 15 underwent CEA a few days before CABG. In group B, all patients underwent CEA, 1 to 3 months after CABG, also under general anesthesia and with systematic carotid shunting.

Results.—Two patients (one in each group) died of cardiac failure in the postoperative period. Operative mortality was 1.0% in group A and 1.1% in group B (*P* = .98). No strokes occurred in group A vs seven ipsilateral ischemic strokes in group B, including three immediate postoperative strokes and four late strokes, at 39, 50, 58, and 66 days, after CABG. These late strokes occurred in patients for whom CEA was further delayed due to an incomplete sternal wound healing or because of completion of a cardiac rehabilitation program. The 90-day stroke and death rate was

1.0% (one of 94) in group A and 8.8% (eight of 91) in group B (odds ratio [OR], 0.11; 95% confidence interval [CI], 0.01-0.91; $P = .02$). Logistic regression analysis showed that only delayed CEA (OR, 14.2; 95% CI, 1.32-152.0; $P = .03$) and duration of cardiopulmonary bypass (OR, 1.06; 95% CI, 1.02-1.11; $P = .004$) reliably predicted stroke or death at 90 days.

Conclusions.—This study suggests that previous or simultaneous CEA in patients with unilateral severe asymptomatic carotid stenosis undergoing CABG could prevent stroke better than delayed CEA, without increasing the overall surgical risk.

▶ The authors have examined the long-standing question regarding the optimal treatment of asymptomatic carotid stenosis in patients requiring coronary artery bypass surgery (CABG). In their elegant, randomized, controlled trial, patients were randomly assigned to either carotid endarterectomy (CEA) prior or simultaneous to CABG or CEA after CABG. Somewhat surprisingly, they reported that the 90-day stroke and mortality rates were significantly higher in the group undergoing delayed CEA (1.0 vs 8.8%, $P = .02$) with "delayed CEA" having the largest odds ratio (OR, 14.2; 95% confidence interval, 1.3–152.0) among the predictors in their logistic regression analysis. These findings are particularly noteworthy because patients with significant aortic arch atherosclerotic occlusive disease were excluded from the study in an attempt to eliminate this potential confounding contribution to postoperative stroke, and all patients were on a statin agent. The historic controversy surrounding the 2 combined procedures has focused on the actual need for CEA in asymptomatic patients and the timing of the procedures. The Asymptomatic Carotid Atherosclerosis Study (ACAS)[1] reported that natural history of asymptomatic carotid stenosis greater than 60% was relatively benign (2% stroke risk/year); therefore, it would intuit that the perioperative carotid-based stroke risk at the time of CABG in patients with a significant carotid lesion would be fairly small. However, the observed ipsilateral ischemic stroke rate of 7.7% in the delayed CEA group suggests that CABG may change the natural history of these asymptomatic lesions. The underlying mechanism remains unclear, but it may be related to the induction of a prothrombotic state in the perioperative period. The opponents of the combined procedures (either staged or simultaneous) have also pointed to the reported increased morbidity and mortality rates, suggesting that patients who have a CEA before CABG have a higher myocardial infarction rate, those that have a CABG before CEA have a higher stroke rate, and those with the simultaneous procedures have higher mortality rates. These objections were partially overcome by the low perioperative myocardial infarction and mortality rates in the current study. However, it is worth emphasizing that the overall outcomes in the current study were excellent and significantly better than reported from most other national series. It is unclear whether the results of this single-center study with 185 patients is sufficient to resolve several decades of debate about the utility of combined CEA and CABG for asymptomatic stenoses, but prior or simultaneous CEA certainly merit serious consideration in the scenario defined in the study.

T. S. Huber, MD, PhD

Reference

1. Endarterectomy for asymptomatic carotid artery stenosis. Executive committee for the asymptomatic carotid atherosclerosis study. *JAMA*. 1995;273:1421-1428.

Peripheral Arterial Occlusive Disease

A meta-analysis of the outcome of endovascular and noninvasive therapies in the treatment of intermittent claudication

Ahimastos AA, Pappas EP, Buttner PG, et al (Baker IDI Heart and Diabetes Inst, Melbourne, Australia; James Cook Univ, Townsville, Australia; et al)
J Vasc Surg 54:1511-1521, 2011

Purpose.—Intermittent claudication is a common symptom of peripheral arterial disease. Currently, there is a lack of consensus on the most effective therapies for this problem. We conducted a meta-analysis of randomized trials assessing the efficacy of endovascular therapy (EVT) compared with noninvasive therapies for the treatment of intermittent claudication.

Methods.—Randomized trials comparing the efficacy of EVT and noninvasive therapies, such as medical therapy (MT) and supervised exercise (SVE) in patients with intermittent claudication were identified by a systematic search. Data were pooled, and combined overall effect sizes (standardized differences of mean values) were calculated for a random effect model in terms of ankle-brachial index (ABI) and treadmill walking for initial claudication distance (ICD) and maximum walking distance (MWD). Nine eligible trials (873 participants) were included: two compared EVT and MT alone, four compared EVT and SVE, and three trials compared EVT plus SVE vs SVE alone.

Results.—Heterogeneity between studies was marked. Quantitative data analysis suggested that EVT improved outcomes over MT alone at early follow-up evaluations. Outcomes of EVT plus SVE were better than those of SVE alone in terms of both ABI and treadmill walking at immediate, early, and intermediate follow-up. No substantial differences in outcomes of EVT alone compared with SVE alone were found.

Conclusion.—In patients with intermittent claudication, current evidence supports improved ABI and treadmill walking when EVT is added to MT or SVE during early and intermediate follow-up. There is no evidence that EVT alone provides improved outcome over SVE alone. There is low confidence in these findings for a number of reasons, including the small number of trials, the small size of these studies, the heterogeneity in study design, and the limited use of quality of life tools in assessing outcomes. More consistent data from larger, more homogenous studies, including longer follow-up, are required.

▶ This meta-analysis addresses one of the most important issues facing the large group of providers that care for patients with intermittent claudication. Specifically, what is the optimal treatment algorithm with respect to medical management (MT), supervised exercise therapy (SVE), and endovascular therapy (EVT)? The results of the meta-analysis suggest that EVT is better than MT but comparable to SVE, while the combination of EVT and SVE is better than EVT alone. These findings are somewhat sobering given the widespread application of the EVT for claudicants, particularly among nonvascular surgeons and suggest that SVE should clearly be the initial treatment option. Indeed, it is almost paradoxical that the treatment goal (ie, improved walking) and the treatment (ie, walking) are essentially the same; if patients want to walk further, they just need to walk. It is important to emphasize that the exercise programs analyzed in the meta-analysis were supervised, not patient-directed programs. The results of these supervised programs have been consistently better than those reported from patient-directed programs, although both require a motivated patient. Unfortunately, supervised exercise programs for claudication are not currently reimbursed in our health care system in stark contrast to the lucrative reimbursement for the EVT, particularly in the outpatient setting. The strength of the conclusions from the current study is limited by the relatively limited number of studies and small sample sizes. That is particularly disconcerting given the prevalence of peripheral vascular disease in our country. Furthermore, the meta-analysis focused only ankle-brachial indices and walking distances, whereas quality of life and health care economics are likely equally important. We clearly need additional high-quality evidence to guide our treatment for intermittent claudication because the current approach is likely both suboptimal and nonsustainable from an economic standpoint.

T. S. Huber, MD, PhD

The Scandinavian Propaten® Trial — 1-Year Patency of PTFE Vascular Prostheses with Heparin-Bonded Luminal Surfaces Compared to Ordinary Pure PTFE Vascular Prostheses — A Randomised Clinical Controlled Multi-Centre Trial

Lindholt JS, Gottschalksen B, Johannesen N, et al (Viborg Hosp, Denmark; Slagelse Hosp, Denmark; Univ Hosp of Aarhus, Skejby, Denmark; et al)
Eur J Vasc Endovasc Surg 41:668-673, 2011

Objective.—To compare 1-year potencies' of heparin-bonded PTFE [(Hb-PTFE) (Propaten®)] grafts with those of ordinary polytetraflouroethylene (PTFE) grafts in a blinded, randomised, clinically controlled, multicentre study.

Materials and Methods.—Eleven Scandinavian centres enrolled 569 patients with chronic functional or critical lower limb ischaemia who were scheduled to undergo femoro—femoral bypass or femoro—poplitaeal bypass. The patients were randomised 1:1 stratified by centre. Patency was assessed by duplex ultrasound scanning. A total of 546 patients (96%) completed the study with adequate follow-up.

Results.—Perioperative bleeding was, on average, 370 ml with PTFE grafts and 399 ml with Heparin-bonded PTFE grafts ($p = 0.32$).

Overall, primary patency after 1 year was 86.4% for Hb-PTFE grafts and 79.9% for PTFE grafts (OR = 0.627, 95% CI: 0.398; 0.989, $p = 0.043$). Secondary patency was 88% in Hb-PTFE grafts and 81% in PTFE grafts (OR = 0.569 (0.353; 0.917, $p = 0.020$)).

Subgroup analyses revealed that significant reduction in risk (50%) was observed when Hb-PTFE was used for femoro—popliteal bypass (OR = 0.515 (0.281; 0.944, $p = 0.030$)), and a significant reduction in risk (50%) was observed with Hb-PTFE in cases with critical ischaemia (OR = 0.490 (0.249; 0.962, $p = 0.036$)).

Conclusion.—The Hb-PTFE graft significantly reduced the overall risk of primary graft failure by 37%. Risk reduction was 50% in femoro—popliteal bypass cases and in cases with critical ischaemia.

▶ The authors report the results of a multicenter, randomized, blinded trial comparing standard PTFE and heparin-bonded PTFE (hb-PTFE) grafts for patients undergoing femoro-femoral or femoro-popliteal bypass (both above and below the knee). They reported that both the primary (86% vs 80%, NNT = 15) and secondary (88% vs 81%, NNT = 29) patency rates were significantly better, although the overall clinical significance of these findings are somewhat questionable given the large numbers needed to treat. The subgroup analyses provided some additional useful information, although it is important to emphasize that the primary objective of the study was to compare 1-year patency rates between the graft types. Notably, the subgroup analyses demonstrated a significant difference in patency between the grafts when used in the femoro-popliteal (81% vs 69%) but not the femoro-femoral configuration. Among the femoro-popliteal grafts, there was a significant difference for patients with critical limb ischemia (80% vs 58%) but not for those with intermittent claudication. It is not completely clear how the results of this elegant trial should be translated into clinical practice. Conceding the limitations of the subgroup analyses, the choice of graft probably doesn't make much difference in the femoro-femoral position. Indeed, this is not particularly surprising given the relatively large size of the femoral vessels and the quantity of blood flow through a femoro-femoral graft. The hb-PTFE does appear to provide a worthwhile advantage in the femoro-popliteal configuration, particularly among patients with critical limb ischemia. I believe that everyone would agree that the saphenous vein is the ideal conduit for a femoro-popliteal graft, although it is reassuring that the patency rates for the hg-PTFE in this configuration are reasonable, at least at 1 year. There has been an ongoing concern about the potential for the heparin-bonded grafts to cause heparin-induced thrombocytopenia with thrombosis, although this seems to be more theoretical than a real clinical concern.

T. S. Huber, MD, PhD

Functional Ability in Patients with Critical Limb Ischaemia is Unaffected by Successful Revascularisation

Cieri E, Lenti M, De Rango P, et al (Univ of Perugia, Italy; et al)
Eur J Vasc Endovasc Surg 41:256-263, 2011

Objective.—Patient- and society-oriented measures of outcome have a critical role in determining the effectiveness of any treatment in patients with critical limb ischaemia (CLI). In particular, the impact of an intervention on patient's dependency and functional performance is relevant but is largely unknown.

The aim of the study was to investigate whether the limitations encountered in the activities of daily living (ADLs) measured with the Katz Index (KI) in patients with CLI were changed by the treatment.

Methods.—During the period 2006—2008, 248 consecutive patients undergoing repair for CLI were investigated with an ADL questionnaire for assessing KI before and after a mean of 16.19 months from treatment. Changes in KI were stratified by type of treatment and outcome.

Results.—There were 165 males and 83 females, mean age 73.3 ± 8.3 years; 125 patients showed tissue loss and 123 rest pain alone, 98 received surgical bypass and 150 endovascular repair. Pre-operative KI mean was 10.42. At the post-operative assessment, there was significant worsening in patients' functional outcome (mean KI decreased to 9.78) despite relief of pain (81.5%), tissue healing (72%), good vessel patency (83.8%) and low amputation rate (9.7%). Deterioration of KI was not significantly higher in patients undergoing endovascular repair. Patients receiving major amputation started with worse pre-operative functional score (KI mean 9.42) and did further deteriorate (KI mean 7.71) after demolition surgery. However, patients who received successful revascularisation showed deterioration in the dependence index.

Conclusions.—Successful vascular treatment is not associated with improved functional ability in patients with CLI, especially when already highly dependent in their activities. Large nationwide preventive and educational programmes should be implemented to prevent irreversible and severe health deterioration in populations with CLI.

▶ The authors prospectively examined the changes in functional activity after lower extremity revascularization for critical limb ischemia (ie, rest pain or tissue loss). They reported that revascularization, both surgical bypass and endovascular repair, was associated with a significant decrease in functional activity, despite reasonable outcomes in terms of the traditional measures of surgical success, including resolution of rest pain, wound healing, and vessel patency. They used the Katz Index for functional activity that encompasses 6 activities of daily living (ie, bathing, dressing, toileting, transferring, continence, feeding) scored from 0 to 2 (0, unable to perform task; 1, able to perform with assistance; 2, completely independent). Although likely not familiar to most surgeons, the Katz Index has allegedly been well validated and widely used in the geriatric population. Multivariate analysis identified nonhealing ulcer at baseline, need for amputation, and persistent rest pain after repair as independent predictors of a functional decrement, likely reflecting the severity of the underlying occlusive disease. It is interesting to note that the endovascular treatment was associated with a comparable (if not greater) decrement of function, potentially undermining the role for the less invasive treatment for this patient population. These sobering findings underscore the terminal nature of critical limb ischemia and re-emphasize that the best results from a surgical or technical standpoint may still not be very good from a patient's perspective. It has become obvious that claudication and critical limb ischemia are clearly different disease processes and that the optimal treatment strategies may be different. In our own practice, I think that we have historically been too aggressive with critical limb ischemia and probably too conservative with claudication. I would echo the authors' sentiments that the best treatment strategy for critical limb ischemia is likely patient education and prevention.

T. S. Huber, MD, PhD

Infrainguinal bypass is associated with lower perioperative mortality than major amputation in high-risk surgical candidates
Barshes NR, Menard MT, Nguyen LL, et al (Brigham and Women's Hosp, Boston, MA)
J Vasc Surg 53:1251-1259, 2011

Background.—Major amputation is often selected over infrainguinal bypass in patients with severe systemic comorbidities because it is assumed to have lower perioperative risks, yet this assumption is unproven and largely unexamined.

Methods.—The 2005 to 2008 National Surgical Quality Improvement Project (NSQIP) database was used to identify all patients undergoing either infrainguinal bypass or major amputation using procedural codes. Patients with systemic or local infections were excluded. A subset of high-risk patients were then defined as American Society of Anesthesiologists (ASA) class 4 or 5, or ASA class 3 with renal failure, dyspnea at rest, ventilator dependence, recent congestive heart failure, or recent myocardial infarct. Propensity score matching was used to obtain two high-risk patient groups matched for preoperative characteristics.

Results.—No significant differences in demographic, preoperative, or anesthetic variables were found between the matched, high-risk amputation or bypass groups (792 and 780 patients, respectively). Bypass was associated with a lower 30-day postoperative mortality than amputation (6.54% vs 9.97%; $P = .0147$). Amputation was associated with higher rates of pulmonary embolism (0.9% vs 0% for amputation vs bypass groups, respectively; $P = .009$) and urinary tract infection (5.2% vs 2.7%; $P = .01$), while bypass was associated with higher rates of return to the operating room (14.1% vs 27.6%; $P < .001$) and a trend toward higher postoperative transfusion requirements (0.9% vs 2.1%; $P = .054$). The postoperative time to discharge did not differ between the two groups.

Conclusion.—The decision to perform an infrainguinal bypass or amputation should depend on well-established predictors of graft patency and functional success rather than presumptions about different perioperative risks between the two procedures.

▶ The study attempts to answer whether the perioperative morbidity and mortality rates are lower for high-risk patients undergoing major amputation or infrainguinal bypass in an attempt to dispel the notation that high-risk patients should preferentially undergo a major amputation. The authors have used the National Surgical Quality Improvement Project database and propensity matching to develop groups with similar preoperative characteristics, differing only in the treatment option. The authors found that the postoperative mortality rates were higher for patients undergoing amputation (9.97% vs 6.54%) and that these patients had a significantly higher incidence of pulmonary embolus and urinary tract infections. When the analysis was limited to patients with critical limb ischemia, a similar survival trend was seen, although the differences did not achieve significance ($P = .0557$). Somewhat surprisingly, a significantly higher percentage of the patients undergoing bypass had to return to the operating room (14.1% vs 27.6%). These findings seem to confirm my bias that major amputations are not necessarily safer than infrainguinal bypass procedures, although they need to be interpreted with some caution. Clearly, there is a tremendous amount of selection bias between the 2 treatment groups, despite the authors' elegant analyses. However, conducting the appropriate randomized, controlled trial would likely be unethical. A successful infrainguinal bypass requires an inflow source, a distal target, a suitable conduit, a lesion to bypass, and a patient that will derive a benefit from the procedure. It is not clear from this study whether these components were present in the patients undergoing major amputation (or revascularization for that matter). One could clearly imagine that many of the patients undergoing major amputation lacked suitable conduits or adequate distal targets, thereby making revascularization impossible. Furthermore, it is important to emphasize that the focus of the study was only the perioperative outcome, and accordingly, many longer-term outcome measures such as wound healing, functional outcome, maintenance of ambulatory status, and quality of life were not considered. Despite the limitations, the data seem to dispel the myth that major amputation is safer than revascularization for high-risk patients and mandate that revascularization should be at least considered as a reasonable option in the treatment algorithm.

T. S. Huber, MD, PhD

Clinical outcomes and implications of failed infrainguinal endovascular stents
Gur I, Lee W, Akopian G, et al (Huntington Memorial Hosp, Pasadena, CA; Univ of Southern California, Los Angeles, CA)
J Vasc Surg 53:658-667, 2011

Objective.—While the influence of initial TransAtlantic InterSociety Consensus (TASC) II classification has been clearly shown to influence the primary patency of infrainguinal stenting procedures, its effect on outcomes once stent failure has occurred is less well documented. It is the objective of this paper to determine whether clinical outcomes and implications of anatomic stent failure vary according to initial TASC II classification.

Methods.—Results were analyzed by TASC II classification. Kaplan-Meier survival curves were plotted and differences between groups tested by log-rank method. A Cox proportional hazards regression model was used to perform the multivariate analysis.

Results.—During a 5-year period, 239 angioplasties and stents were performed in 192 patients. Primary patency was lost in 69 stented arteries. Failure was due to one or more hemodynamically significant stenoses in 43 patients, and occlusion in 26 patients. After primary stenting, limbs initially classified as TASC C and D were more likely to fail with occlusion ($P < .0001$), require open operation ($P = .032$), or lose run-off vessels ($P = .0034$) than those classified as TASC A or B. In two patients initially classified as TASC C, stent failure changed the level of open operation to a more distal site. Percutaneous reintervention was performed on 35 limbs. Successful reintervention improved the patency of TASC A and B lesions to 92%, 85%, and 64% and TASC C and D lesions to 78%, 72%, and 50% at 12, 24, and 36 months, respectively. Initial TASC classification was highly predictive of first anatomic failure ($P < .0001$), but it did not predict the durability of subsequent catheter based reintervention ($P = .32$). Ten patients with stent failure required operation, and five underwent amputation; all had failed with occlusion. Overall limb salvage was 89% and periprocedural mortality was 0.4%.

Conclusions.—Following primary stenting of the superficial femoral artery (SFA) and popliteal artery, lesions classified as TASC C or D are more likely to fail with occlusion, lose run-off vessels, and alter the site of subsequent open operation than their TASC A and B counterparts. Although these complications are infrequent, they may negatively impact later attempts at revascularization, and this must be considered when deciding upon the proper treatment strategy for patients with infrainguinal occlusive disease.

▶ The authors have attempted to determine the clinical outcome of angioplasty/stent failure for patients undergoing treatment for their infrainguinal occlusive disease (SFA/pop: 77%). They have reported that the primary patency rates for the TASC A and B lesions (12 mos: 84%; 24 mos: 70%; 36 mos: 55%) were reasonable and better than those for the C and D lesions (12 mos: 60%; 24 mos: 37%; 36 mos; 22%). Interestingly, the patency rates after the endovascular reinterventions were quite good and did not appear to be affected by the initial TASC classification. Not surprisingly, the TASC C and D lesions were more likely to fail, require open operation, and lose run-off vessels than the A and B lesions were. However, the runoff was worsened after angioplasty/stent failure in only 15/192 patients, and the remedial open operation was ultimately changed in only 2 patients. The study attempts to address the important questions as to whether a failed angioplasty/stent causes significant harm to patients by exacerbating their presenting symptoms and/or complicating the ultimate open revascularization. However, the study is framed within the context of the larger question as to whether an endovascular-first approach is appropriate for all patients with infrainguinal occlusive disease. The data would suggest that the adverse events associated with angioplasty/stenting are relatively uncommon but occur more frequently in patients with more advanced disease as reflected by their TASC classification. Somewhat paradoxically, the data can be used to support or refute an endovascular-first approach for the more complicated TASC C and D lesions depending upon surgeon bias. However, a reasonable interpretation of the data, consistent with the findings of the BASIL study, are that patients with advanced infrainguinal occlusive disease and reasonable life expectancy may benefit from open revascularization while those treated with an initial endovascular approach merit close surveillance and remedial intervention for failing lesions.[1]

T. S. Huber, MD, PhD

Reference

1. Adam DJ, Beard JD, Cleveland T, et al. Bypass versus angioplasty in severe ischemia of the leg. (BASIL): multicenter, randomised controlled trial. *Lancet.* 2005;366:1925-1934.

Access

A comparison between one- and two-stage brachiobasilic arteriovenous fistulas
Reynolds TS, Zayed M, Kim KM, et al (Harbor-UCLA Med Ctr, Torrance; Stanford Univ Med Ctr, CA)
J Vasc Surg 53:1632-1639, 2011

Objectives.—Brachiobasilic arteriovenous fistulas (BBAVF) can be performed in one or two stages. We compared primary failure rates as well as primary and secondary patency rates of one- and two-stage BBAVF at two institutions.

Methods.—Patients undergoing one- and two-stage BBAVF at two institutions were compared retrospectively with respect to age, sex, body mass index, use of preoperative venous duplex ultrasound, diabetes, hypertension, and cause of end-stage renal disease. Categorical variables were compared using chi-square and Fisher's exact test, whereas the Wilcoxon rank-sum test was used to compare continuous variables. Patency rates were assessed using the Kaplan-Meier survival analysis and the Cox proportional hazards model with propensity analysis to determine hazard ratios.

Results.—Ninety patients (60 one-stage and 30 two-stage) were identified. Mean follow-up was 14.2 months and the mean time interval between the first and second stage was 11.2 weeks. Although no significant difference in early failure existed (one-stage, 22.9% vs two-stage, 9.1%; $P = .20$), the two-stage BBAVF showed significantly improved primary functional patency at 1 year at 88% vs 61% (*P* = .047) (hazard ratio, 0.2 (95% confidence interval [CI], .04-.80; *P* = .03). Patency for one-stage BBAVF markedly decreased to 34% at 2 years compared with 88% for the two-stage procedure (*P* = .047). Median primary functional patency for one-stage BBAVF was 31 weeks (interquartile range [IQR], 11-54) vs 79 weeks (IQR, 29-131 weeks) for the two-stage procedure, respectively (*P* = .0015). Two-year secondary functional patency for one- and two-stage procedures were 41% and 94%, respectively (*P* = .015).

Conclusions.—Primary and secondary patency at 1 and 2 years as well as functional patency is improved with the two-stage BBAVF when compared with the one-stage procedure. Lower primary failure rates prior to dialysis with the two-stage procedure approached, but did not reach statistical significance. While reasons for these finding are unclear, certain technical aspects of the procedure may play a role (Fig 2).

▶ The authors have retrospectively compared the 1- and 2-stage brachiobasilic autogenous hemodialysis access (BBAVF) in their practice and reported that the patency rates for the 2-stage procedures were superior and the primary failure rate approached significance. Notably, the secondary functional patency rate, perhaps the most important of the outcome measures, was markedly superior for the 2-stage procedure (94% vs 41%, *P* .015) as shown in Fig 2. These findings are particularly relevant given the tremendous emphasis on autogenous access nationwide from the Kidney Disease Outcome Quality Initiative (KDOQI), the Fistula First Breakthrough Initiative, and the Society for Vascular Surgery Clinical

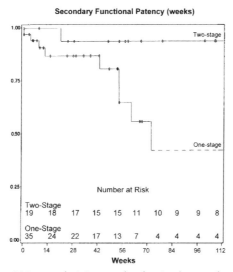

FIGURE 2.—Kaplan—Meier curve depicting secondary functional patency for one-stage and two-stage brachiobasilic arteriovenous fistulas *(BBAVF) (Dashed line indicates standard error >10%)*. (Reprinted from the Journal of Vascular Surgery, Reynolds TS, Zayed M, Kim KM, et al. A comparison between one- and two-stage brachiobasilic arteriovenous fistulas. *J Vasc Surg.* 2011;53:1632-1639. Copyright 2011, with permission from the Society for Vascular Surgery.)

Practice Guidelines. The role of the 1-stage and 2-stage BBAVF have been debated in the literature for some time, with the supporting evidence somewhat weak and comprising only a single, small randomized controlled trial.[1] The theoretical advantage of the 1-stage procedure includes the shorter maturation period (and less catheter dependence) in addition to the obvious that it only includes 1 operative procedure. In contrast, the 2-stage approach avoids an extensive arm incision and corresponding vein dissection until (or unless) the vein has matured sufficiently for use. Indeed, this is particularly relevant for an increasing number of obese patients who are presenting for permanent access. The arterialized vein comprising the BBAVF may be easier to handle during the 2-stage procedure, but this is partially offset by the increased venous hypertension. Notably, the second-stage procedure was performed a mean of 11.2 weeks after the initial procedure with the median time for first cannulation 12.3 weeks vs 19.3 weeks for the 1- and 2-stage procedures, respectively. There are a few technical points regarding the second-stage procedure that merit further comment. As noted by the authors, the median antebrachial cutaneous nerve overlies the basilic vein near the antecubital fossa. This nerve (or a branch thereof) needs to be transected if the BBAVF is simply elevated during the second-stage procedure. Alternatively, the BBAVF can be transected and tunneled over the nerve, although this obviously requires creating another anastomosis. Transecting the BBAVF also affords the opportunity to reroute the vein more lateral on the upper arm through a subcutaneous plane, thereby avoiding having it sitting immediately below the skin incision where it is at risk if the wound were to break down. Furthermore, this more lateral course is ultimately more comfortable for the patient and easier to access for the dialysis technologists. It has been my impression that the BBAVF not only dilates but also elongates during the maturation process, facilitating rerouting of the vein during the second procedure. Unlike the authors, I have routinely obtained an ultrasound of the BBAVF prior to the second procedure to confirm that the diameter is sufficient to justify the morbidity of the procedure. Despite the compelling results, the study must be interpreted with some caution given the relatively small sample size and the retrospective design with all the inherent bias. I suspect that the authors' findings will be supported by further reports and believe that the 2-stage procedure offers an advantage, particularly in obese patients.

T. S. Huber, MD, PhD

Reference

1. El Mallah S. Staged basilic vein transposition for dialysis angioaccess. *Int Angiol.* 1998;17:65-68.

Costoclavicular Venous Decompression in Patients With Threatened Arteriovenous Hemodialysis Access

Glass C, Dugan M, Gillespie D, et al (Univ of Rochester Med Ctr, NY)
Ann Vasc Surg 25:640-645, 2011

Background.—Autologous arteriovenous fistulas are frequently threatened by central venous obstruction. Although this is frequently ascribed to indwelling catheters and neointimal venous remodeling, we believe that extrinsic compression of the subclavian vein as it passes through the costoclavicular junction (CCJ) may play a significant role in a subset of dialysis patients.

Methods.—We reviewed our experience with CCJ decompression for arteriovenous fistula dysfunction at our institution. Decompression followed principles for venous thoracic outlet syndrome: bony decompression with thorough venolysis, followed by central venography through the fistula and endoluminal treatment, if necessary. Patients underwent transaxillary first rib resection, or claviculectomy in the supine position in cases when reconstruction was anticipated. In all cases, the minimum exposure included 360° mobilization of the subclavian vein with resection of surrounding cicatrix to the jugular/innominate junction.

Results.—A total of 10 patients requiring decompression between November 2008 and February 2010 were included. All had severe arm swelling, four had dialysis dysfunction (postcannulation bleeding or maturation failure), two had severe arm pain, and one had a pseudoaneurysm. All patients had subclavian vein stenosis at the CCJ by venography or intravascular ultrasound. The majority of patients had balloon dilation (mean: 2.3 attempts) without success. Six patients underwent transaxillary first rib resection and four had medial claviculectomy. No patients required surgical venous reconstruction. In all, 80% of fistulas remained functionally patent, and all but one patient (who underwent ligation) had complete relief of upper arm edema. Median hospital length of stay was 2 days and mean follow-up was 7 months (range, 1-13). There was no mortality or significant morbidity. Five patients later required central venoplasty (four subclavian, mean: 1.8 attempts and one innominate) and three had stents placed (two subclavian, one innominate).

Conclusion.—A significant number of patients with threatened AV access owing to central venous obstruction have lesions attributable to compression at the CCJ. Surgical decompression by means of first rib or clavicular resection and thorough external venoloysis allowed symptom-free functional salvage in 80% of these patients, all of whom would have lost their access otherwise. Because surgical reconstruction is seldom needed, the transaxillary approach may be preferable to claviculectomy. This lesion should be specifically looked for, and principles of venous thoracic outlet syndrome treatment seem to apply and be effective.

▶ The authors make the novel observation that venous outflow stenoses at the costoclavicular junction in patients with an ipsilateral hemodialysis access is likely secondary to extrinsic compression and should be treated similarly to patients with a venous thoracic outlet obstruction. Although their collective experience with thoracic decompression and venous reconstruction in this setting was quite small, the outcomes were good and, most importantly, salvaged the access or preserved the ipsilateral extremity for future access procedures. Central venous stenoses or occlusions are rapidly becoming the Achilles heel of hemodialysis access and the responsible etiology of most complex or tertiary care access problems in our practice. Many of these lesions can be treated with balloon angioplasty or intraluminal stents, although the long-term success rates for these therapies are limited, particularly for lesions at the costoclavicular junction. Indeed, the placement of an intraluminal stent in this location can be detrimental with the stent prone to fracture secondary to the extrinsic forces. It is not surprising that decompression of the anatomic structures at this location (ie, anterior scalene muscle, first rib, clavicle) may relieve the compression and facilitate successful, remedial endovascular treatment. However, it is not clear from the data where the decompression should fit into the treatment algorithm. I would envision using the technique to salvage a durable, functional autogenous access after failed endovascular attempts or to possibly facilitate an additional access option in a patient with severe central venous occlusive disease and very limited access options. The authors describe using a transaxillary approach when venous reconstruction is not required and a claviculectomy when it is required. It has been our preference to use a supraclavicular approach for patients with thoracic outlet syndrome (both arterial and venous) with the addition of an infraclavicular incision if venous reconstruction is necessary. We also favor immediate, postdecompression venogram (or fistulagram) with endovascular treatment but try to avoid the use of intraluminal stents. The complete mobilization of the subclavian vein and the dissection of the surrounding scar tissue, as described by the authors, is likely an important component of the procedure. Lastly, it is important to emphasize that a significant percentage of the patients will require further endovascular treatment (postdecompression) for recurrent venous stenoses or occlusions.

T. S. Huber, MD, PhD

Venous

Diagnosis and treatment of venous lymphedema
Raju S, Furrh JB IV, Neglén P (The Rane Ctr, Flowood, MS)
J Vasc Surg 55:141-149, 2012

Background.—Chronic venous disease (CVD) is a common cause of secondary lymphedema. Venous lymphedema is sometimes misdiagnosed as primary lymphedema and does not receive optimal treatment. We have routinely used intravascular ultrasound (IVUS) imaging in all cases of limb swelling. The aim of this study is to show that (1) routine use of IVUS can detect venous obstruction missed by traditional venous testing, and (2) iliac-caval venous stenting can yield satisfactory clinical relief and can sometimes reverse abnormal lymphangiographic findings.

Methods.—The study comprised CVD patients who underwent iliac vein stenting. Lymphangiography was abnormal in 72 of 443 CEAP C_3 limbs, with leg swelling as the primary complaint (abnormal lymphangiography group). Clinical features and stent outcome were compared with a control group of 205 of 443 with normal lymphangiography (normal lymphangiographic group).

Results.—Clinical features were a poor guide to the diagnosis of lymphedema. Isotope lymphangiography was not helpful in differentiating primary from secondary lymphedema. Venography had 61% sensitivity to the diagnosis of venous obstruction. IVUS had a sensitivity of 88% for significant ($\geq 50\%$ area stenosis) venous obstruction. At 40 months, cumulative secondary stent patency was similar for the abnormal (100%) and normal lymphangiographic (95%) groups. Swelling improved significantly after stent placement in the abnormal lymphangiographic group (mean [standard deviation] swelling grade improvement 0.8 ± 1.1) but was less ($P < .004$) than in the control group (1.4 ± 1.3). Complete swelling relief was 16% and 44% ($P < .001$) and partial improvement (≥ 1 grade of swelling) was 45% and 66% ($P < .01$) in the abnormal and normal lymphangiographic groups, respectively. Associated pain was present in 50% and 36% of the swollen limbs in the abnormal and normal lymphangiographic groups. Pain relief (≥ 3 visual analog scale) at 40 months was 87% and 83%, respectively ($P = .3$), with 65% and 71%, experiencing complete pain relief. Quality of life criteria improved after stent placement in both groups but to a better extent in the normal lymphangiographic group. Abnormal lymphangiography improved or normalized in 9 of 36 (25%) of those tested after stent correction.

Conclusions.—Prevailing practice patterns and diagnostic deficiencies probably result in the misdiagnosis of many cases of venous lymphedema as "primary" lymphedema. IVUS is recommended to rule out venous obstruction as the associated or initiating cause of lymphedema. Iliac venous stenting to correct the obstruction has excellent long-term patency and good clinical outcome, although results are not as good as in those with normal lymphatic function.

▶ This report focuses attention on the presence of combined venous and lymphatic disease and underscores the importance of treating any venous outflow disease in patients being evaluated for lymphedema. The authors emphasize that approximately 20% to 30% of patients with chronic venous disease have concurrent lymphatic dysfunction, while conversely, a significant proportion of patients with lymphedema (both primary and secondary) likely have a component of venous insufficiency. In this study, the authors reported that patient with limb swelling (CEAP C3) and an abnormal isotope lymphangiogram had significant improvement in their leg swelling and pain with a trend toward a significant improvement in their quality of life after iliac venous stenting. Admittedly, the results were not as good in the patients with the abnormal lymphangiogram when compared with the normal control group, but traditional treatment for lymphedema with compression has been fairly unsatisfactory for both patients and providers, with the overall compliance rates quite poor. The authors emphasize the importance of intravascular ultrasound scan as the definitive diagnostic study for the venous outflow stenoses while highlighting the limitations of the more traditional venous imaging studies, including duplex ultrasound scan and contrast venography. Although the patients were analyzed based on the presence of an abnormal isotope lymphangiogram, the exact role of this test in the diagnostic/treatment algorithm is unclear from the study, and it has not been an important component of our own practice. I would contend that the lymphangiogram results may be more "academic" than practical, as the take home message from the study seems to be that patients with clinically relevant edema (whether from venous our lymphatic disease) should undergo imaging of the iliac system with intravascular ultrasound scan.

T. S. Huber, MD, PhD

Iliofemoral stenting for venous occlusive disease
Titus JM, Moise MA, Bena J, et al (Cleveland Clinic Foundation, OH)
J Vasc Surg 53:706-712, 2011

Background.—Venous hypertension is a significant cause of patient morbidity and decreased quality of life. Common etiologies of venous hypertension include deep venous thrombosis (DVT) or congenital abnormalities resulting in chronic outflow obstruction. We have implemented an aggressive endovascular approach for the treatment of iliac venous occlusion with angioplasty and stenting. The purpose of this study was to determine the patency rates with this approach at a large tertiary care center.

Materials/Methods.—All patients undergoing iliofemoral venous angioplasty and stenting over a 4-year period were identified from a vascular surgical registry. Charts were reviewed retrospectively for patient demographics, the extent of venous system involvement, the time course of the venous pathology, and any underlying cause. Technical aspects of the procedure including previous angioplasty or stenting attempts and presence of collaterals on completion venogram were then recorded. Patency upon follow-up was determined using primarily ultrasound scans; other imaging methods were used if patency was not clear using an ultrasound scan.

Results.—A total of 36 patients (40 limbs) were stented from January 2005 through December 2008. Of these patients, 27 were women (75%). Both lower extremities were involved in 4 patients. Thrombolysis was performed in 19 patients (52.8%). Thrombosis was considered acute (<30 days) in 13 patients (38%). The majority of patients who had a recognized underlying etiology were diagnosed with May-Thurner syndrome (15 patients; 42%). In 9 patients, an etiology was not determined (25%). The mean follow-up time period in the study population was 10.5 months. One stent in the study occluded acutely and required restenting. Primary patency rates at 6, 12, and 24 months were 88% (75.2-100), 78.3% (61.1-95.4), and 78.3% (61.1-95.4), respectively. Secondary patency rates for the same time frames were 100% (100.0, 100.0), 95% (85.4, 100.0), and

95% (85.4, 100.0). Better outcomes were seen in stenting for May-Thurner syndrome and idiopathic causes, whereas external compression and thrombophilia seemed to portend less favorable outcomes ($P < .001$). Symptomatic improvement was reported in 24 of 29 patients (83%) contacted by telephone follow-up.

Conclusion.—Iliofemoral venous stenting provides a safe and effective option for the treatment of iliac venous occlusive disease. Acceptable patency rates can be expected through short-term follow-up, especially in the case of May-Thurner syndrome. Further experience with this approach and longer-term follow-up is necessary. Thrombophilia workup should be pursued aggressively in this population, and further studies should be undertaken to determine the optimal length of anticoagulation therapy after stent placement.

▶ This report highlights the importance of venous outflow obstruction as a potential etiology of both deep venous thrombosis and chronic venous insufficiency while emphasizing the benefit of iliofemoral stents. The significance of these venous outflow lesions has been appreciated more recently as reflected by a variety of publications, including this one. The study documents excellent outcomes in terms of patency rates, symptomatic relief, and complications but highlights the fact that responses for patients with thrombophilia and extrinsic compression (not secondary to May-Thurner) are inferior. Outflow obstructions in the iliofemoral veins are common in the setting of acute deep venous thrombosis and are often the underlying etiology. They can (and should) be corrected at the time of any chemical or mechanical lysis. The significance of these venous outflow lesions in the setting of chronic venous insufficiency is less clear, but they probably play a more significant role than previously appreciated. Unfortunately, there are no good hemodynamic assessments or measurements for the venous circulation to incriminate the significance of an outflow lesion. In our own algorithm for patients with chronic venous insufficiency, we have corrected the superficial and perforator incompetence prior to investigating and/or correcting the iliofemoral outflow stenoses, but it may be more appropriate to address the outflow component earlier. The technical conduct of treating iliofemoral venous lesions is different from the corresponding arterial lesions as noted in the Methods section. Specifically, primary stenting is likely superior to angioplasty alone. The self-expanding stents should be sized to the native vessel, and this requires large stents (median diameter 14 mm, range 9-28) with the appropriate choice facilitated using intravascular ultrasound. The stents can extend into the inferior vena cava and the common femoral vein, and it is not necessary to using "kissing stents" at the confluence of the common iliac veins. Percutaneous access can be obtained from the popliteal, femoral, or internal jugular veins with the choice dictated by the distribution of the thrombus and surgeon preference. Inferior vena caval filters should be used for patients at high risk for emboli, and the temporary filters may have an important role in this setting for patients with an identifiable, temporary cause for their thromboembolic event.

T. S. Huber, MD, PhD

Incidence and Outcome of Pulmonary Embolism following Popliteal Venous Repair in Trauma Cases

Tofigh AM, Karvandi M (Shahid Beheshti Univ of Med Sciences, Tehran, Iran)
Eur J Vasc Endovasc Surg 41:406-411, 2011

Objectives and Design.—Popliteal vein repair and ligation are the two-main approaches to the treatment of the venous component of major, complex, knee injuries with vascular involvement. We have studied the incidence of pulmonary embolism following popliteal vein repair in trauma cases using computed tomography (CT) angiography and report the outcome.

Material and Methods.—From June 2006 to December 2009, 45 patients with popliteal vein injury were operated on in our vascular unit using lateral venorrhaphy, end-to-end anastomosis, a saphenous vein interposition graft and venous patch repair. All the patients were operated on using a medial approach to the knee. On the third postoperative day, all patients underwent a colour Doppler scan of the repaired popliteal vein to study patency, and pulmonary artery CT angiography using a 64-slice multidetector CT scan unit to establish the incidence of pulmonary embolism.

Results.—The number of patients treated by each method were: lateral venorrhaphy 20 (44%), end-to-end anastomosis 13 (29%), saphenous vein interposition graft 9 (20%) and venous patch repair three (7%). Two patients (4%) died because of sudden cardio-respiratory arrest the day after surgery with massive bilateral pulmonary artery embolism at autopsy. Popliteal colour duplex ultrasound imaging showed seven (16%) cases of complete vein thrombosis and seven (16%) cases of partial vein thrombosis. CT angiography showed pulmonary embolism in 11 (26%) patients. From seven patients with complete thrombosis three patients, and from seven patients with incomplete thrombosis five patients showed pulmonary embolism on CT angiography. Other than two cases of early mortality, five (12%) patients developed clinical manifestations of pulmonary embolism and 11 (26%) patients had pulmonary embolism detected by CT angiography. Seven (16%) of our patients had mild-to-severe pulmonary embolism and 13 patients (29%) had proven pulmonary embolism. The total mortality rate was 7%.

Conclusion.—A surprisingly high incidence of pulmonary embolism was observed after popliteal vein repair in civil trauma patients. Additional prophylactic methods such as using higher doses of heparin and using inferior vena cava (IVC) filters might be needed to prevent this potentially fatal complication.

▶ The authors investigated the incidence of pulmonary embolus after popliteal vein repair following civilian trauma, diagnosed by CT angiography on postinjury day 3, and found a staggering 29% rate. Notably, 16% of the patients had symptomatic pulmonary emboli, and there were 2 deaths from massive emboli. These findings are particularly noteworthy because the authors provided the textbook standard of care for the injuries, including a preference for repair over ligation in good-risk patients, arterial repair before venous repair for combined injuries, use of intraluminal shunts for the arterial injuries, use of contralateral saphenous conduit, a low threshold for performing fasciotomies, postoperative lower extremity compression, and therapeutic anticoagulation throughout the postoperative period. Successful repair was documented in 85% of the patients by ultrasonography performed on the same day as the CT. However, it is conceivable that the vein thrombosis rate and the incidence of pulmonary emboli could have actually been greater if serial imaging studies had been performed. These findings suggest that the current treatment algorithm after popliteal vein repair is ineffective and needs to be changed. The alternatives include additional anticoagulation with a higher target partial thromboplastin time (or heparin units) or the placement of an inferior vena caval filter. However, it is worth emphasizing that the anticoagulation regimen used in the current study (18 U/kg/h, aPTT 2– 2.5 times control) was appropriate, suggesting that additional anticoagulation would put patients in the supratherapeutic range. Furthermore, the current dosing schedule was already associated with a 47% incidence of bleeding complications. The placement of a filter at the time of the venous repair appears to be the best option and should likely become the new standard of care, particularly given their expanding indications in trauma patients and the availability of retrievable devices.

T. S. Huber, MD, PhD

Miscellaneous

Transcatheter versus Surgical Aortic-Valve Replacement in High-Risk Patients

Smith CR, for the PARTNER Trial Investigators (Columbia Univ Med Ctr—New York Presbyterian Hosp, et al)
N Engl J Med 364:2187-2198, 2011

Background.—The use of transcatheter aortic-valve replacement has been shown to reduce mortality among high-risk patients with aortic stenosis who are not candidates for surgical replacement. However, the two procedures have not been compared in a randomized trial involving high-risk patients who are still candidates for surgical replacement.

Methods.—At 25 centers, we randomly assigned 699 high-risk patients with severe aortic stenosis to undergo either transcatheter aortic-valve replacement with a balloon-expandable bovine pericardial valve (either a transfemoral or a transapical approach) or surgical replacement. The primary end point was death from any cause at 1 year. The primary hypothesis was that transcatheter replacement is not inferior to surgical replacement.

Results.—The rates of death from any cause were 3.4% in the transcatheter group and 6.5% in the surgical group at 30 days (P = 0.07) and 24.2% and 26.8%, respectively, at 1 year (P = 0.44), a reduction of 2.6 percentage points in the transcatheter group (upper limit of the 95% confidence interval, 3.0 percentage points; predefined margin, 7.5 percentage points; P = 0.001 for noninferiority). The rates of major stroke were 3.8% in the transcatheter group and 2.1% in the surgical group at 30 days (P = 0.20) and 5.1% and 2.4%, respectively, at 1 year (P = 0.07). At 30 days, major vascular complications were significantly more frequent with transcatheter replacement (11.0% vs. 3.2%, P < 0.001); adverse events that were more frequent after surgical replacement included major bleeding (9.3% vs. 19.5%, P < 0.001) and new-onset atrial fibrillation (8.6% vs. 16.0%, P = 0.006). More patients undergoing transcatheter replacement had an improvement in symptoms at 30 days, but by 1 year, there was not a significant between-group difference.

Conclusions.—In high-risk patients with severe aortic stenosis, transcatheter and surgical procedures for aortic-valve replacement were associated with similar rates of survival at 1 year, although there were important differences in periprocedural risks. (Funded by Edwards Lifesciences; ClinicalTrials.gov number, NCT00530894.)

▶ The result of the randomized, controlled Partners Trial comparing transcatheter aortic valve replacement with open surgical repair in patients deemed to be high risk for open repair are presented. Notably, the 30-day operative mortality for the open repair was estimated to be at least 10% by the Society for Thoracic Surgery risk prediction model. The authors found no differences in either mortality or stroke at both 30 days and 1 year, although there was a trend toward a lower mortality rate and a higher stroke rate for the transcatheter group at the early time point (*P* = .07). There was a significantly higher incidence of vascular complications in the transcatheter group as might have been predicted based on the size of the delivery system that ranges from 22 to 24 French. It is noteworthy that the valve-related outcomes (eg, New York Heart Association congestive heart symptoms, 6-minute walk distance, aortic valve gradient, incidence of severe valvular regurgitation) were equivocal between the groups at 1 year, further supporting the "noninferiority" of the transcatheter approach. Similar to endovascular aneurysm repair, the overall hospital and intensive care unit lengths of stay favored the catheter-based approach over open repair. Taken together, the results seem to justify the transcatheter approach for high-risk patients given the comparable outcomes and the less invasive nature of the procedure. However, it is important to remember that the outcome assessments were relatively short term, and there was no consideration of the overall costs of the 2 approaches. I would suspect that the cost of the transcatheter valve itself likely negates any savings to the health care system from the shorter length of stay, similar to the case with endovascular aneurysm repairs. Additionally, the findings are limited to this defined group of high-risk patients and should not be used to justify a more widespread application of the technique to a lower risk patient population. Although transcatheter aortic valve repair is likely outside the scope of practice of most vascular surgeons, the study merits inclusion among the other articles abstracted because of its potential significance. The transcatheter approach may change practice patterns similar to endovascular aneurysm repair for both abdominal and thoracic aneurysms. The magnitude of the procedure and the potential adverse outcomes are both significant and make endovascular repair of abdominal aortic aneurysms look fairly pedestrian by comparison. I suspect that many vascular surgeons will be asked to help manage the access-related complications given the large sheath sizes. Furthermore, I would contend that vascular surgeons should be involved in the early implementation of the transcatheter aortic programs given our skill sets and the many important lessons that we have learned from our collective abdominal and thoracic endovascular aneurysm experiences.

T. S. Huber, MD, PhD

Reinterventions for stent restenosis in patients treated for atherosclerotic mesenteric artery disease
Tallarita T, Oderich GS, Macedo TA, et al (Mayo Clinic, Rochester, MN)
J Vasc Surg 54:1422-1429, 2011

Objective.—Mesenteric artery angioplasty and stenting (MAS) has been plagued by high restenosis and reintervention rates. The purpose of this study was to review the outcomes of patients treated for mesenteric artery in-stent restenosis (MAISR).

Methods.—The clinical data of 157 patients treated for chronic mesenteric ischemia with MAS of 170 vessels was entered into a prospective database (1998-2010). Fifty-seven patients (36%) developed MAISR after a mean follow-up of 29 months, defined by duplex ultrasound peak systolic velocity >330 cm/s and angiographic stenosis > 60%. We reviewed the clinical data, radiologic studies, and outcomes of patients who underwent reintervention for restenosis. End points were mortality and morbidity, patient survival, symptom recurrence, reintervention, and patency rates.

Results.—There were 30 patients (25 female and five male; mean age, 69 ± 14 years) treated with reintervention for MAISR. Twenty-four patients presented with recurrent symptoms (21 chronic, three acute), and six had asymptomatic preocclusive lesions. Twenty-six patients (87%) underwent redo endovascular revascularization (rER) with stent placement in 17 (13 bare metal and four covered) or percutaneous transluminal angioplasty (PTA) in nine. The other four patients (13%) had open bypass, one for acute ischemia. There was one death (3%) in a patient treated with redo stenting for acute mesenteric ischemia. Seven patients (27%) treated by rER developed complications, including access site problems in four patients, and distal embolization with bowel ischemia, congestive heart failure and stent thrombosis in one each. Symptom improvement was noted in 22 of the 24 symptomatic patients (92%). After a mean follow-up of 29 ± 12 months, 15 patients (50%) developed a second restenosis, and seven (23%) required other reintervention. Rates of symptom recurrence, restenosis, and reinterventions were 0/4, 0/4, and 0/4 for covered stents, 2/9, 3/9, and 2/9 for PTA, 5/13, 8/13, and 5/13 for bare metal stents, and 1/4, 4/4, and 0/4 for open bypass. For all patients, freedom from recurrent symptoms, restenosis, and reinterventions were 70% ± 10%, 60% ± 10% and 50% ± 10% at 2 years. For patients treated by rER, secondary patency rates were 72 ± 12 at the same interval.

Conclusions.—Nearly 40% of patients developed mesenteric artery in-stent restenosis, of which half required reintervention because of symptom recurrence or progression to an asymptomatic preocclusive lesion. Mesenteric reinterventions were associated with low mortality (3%), high complication rate (27%), and excellent symptom improvement (92%).

▶ Mesenteric angioplasty and stenting has largely replaced open surgical bypass as the first-line treatment for patients with chronic mesenteric ischemia. It is widely accepted that the periprocedure outcomes for the endovascular approach are significantly lower than those associated with bypass, although the durability in terms of recurrent symptoms and in-stent restenosis is inferior. The current study documents that 36% of the index stents required reintervention at mean follow-up of 29%, with the overwhelming majority requiring reintervention for recurrent symptoms, including a few patients with acute mesenteric ischemia. Fortunately, the outcomes after reinterventions were favorable, with recurrence, restenosis, and reintervention rates (ie, second reintervention) of 70%, 60%, and 50%, respectively, at 2 years. The incidence of recurrent symptoms, particularly acute mesenteric ischemia, is somewhat concerning and underscores the importance of close postprocedure surveillance. The authors have advocated duplex surveillance at 6 months for the first year and then yearly thereafter. We have adopted a more aggressive approach and commit patients to a 6-month schedule indefinitely. It has been our anecdotal impression that the long-term outcomes in terms of recurrent symptoms are better, but it is difficult to argue anecdote with the authors' data. It is worth emphasizing that the duplex criteria for an in-stent restenosis greater than 60% exceed those for a de novo or nonstented lesion with a peak systolic velocity of 330 cm per second used in the current study. Similar to the authors, we have been reluctant to reintervene on a truly asymptomatic, recurrent stenosis but readily concede that these lesions are worrisome and the natural history is poorly defined. Unfortunately, the selection bias in the current study prevents any real conclusions about the optimal recurrent treatment although the favorable outcomes associated with the covered stents is encouraging and appears to support their theoretic advantage. It is important to remember that the long-term outcomes after open mesenteric bypass are excellent and that it still plays a role in the treatment of mesenteric ischemia.

T. S. Huber, MD, PhD

12 General Thoracic Surgery

Esophageal Cancer

Modified Pleural Tenting for Prevention of Anastomotic Leak After Ivor Lewis Esophagogastrectomy

Asteriou C, Barbetakis N, Lalountas M, et al (Theagenio Cancer Hospi, Thessaloniki, Greece; Aristotle Univ of Thessaloniki, Greece)
Ann Surg Oncol 18:3737-3742, 2011

Background.—The most dangerous complication following esophago-gastrectomy for esophageal cancer is anastomotic leakage. Surgical interventions described did not have a major impact in reducing the risk of occurrence. On the other hand, pleural tenting has been used for more than a decade by thoracic surgeons to prevent prolonged air leak after formal upper lobectomy with excellent results.

Methods.—A retrospective analysis of 114 cases of esophagogastrectomy for cancer of esophagus or cardioesophageal junction is presented. Patients have been divided in 2 groups. In group B modified pleural tenting was used to prevent a potential anastomotic leak, while in group A, the control group, pleural tenting was not used. Evaluation of modified pleural tenting in preventing anastomotic leakage was the aim of the study.

Results.—The pleural tenting group showed a significant decrease in anastomotic leak. In 1 patient versus 8 in group without pleural tenting the complication appeared ($P = .032$). The risk for an anastomotic leakage in group without pleural tenting was almost 9 times greater (odds ratio: 9.143, 95% confidence interval: lower bound 1.104, upper bound 75.708). The 30-day mortality, although lower in pleural tenting group, was not statistically significant.

Conclusions.—Pleural tenting is a safe, fast, and effective technique for prevention of anastomotic leakage after Ivor Lewis esophagogastrectomy. Subpleural blanketing of intrathoracic anastomosis could diminish the consequences of a possible anastomotic leak.

▶ Intrathoracic leak following esophagectomy is a disastrous and potentially lethal complication. The use of pleural tenting is commonly used following lung resection to decrease the complication of air leak from the pulmonary parenchyma following upper lobectomy, with excellent results. The authors retrospectively review their single-center experience with the Ivor Lewis esophagectomy procedure and the use of pleural tenting as an intervention to prevent leak. As with all retrospective reviews, there may be a selection bias in that the authors may select the pleural tent in times of higher risk for leak. However, in this review, that logic strengthens the argument that perhaps the patient selection was biased against the pleural tent group. The main disadvantage of surgical treatment (in comparison with chemotherapy and radiation therapy) for either palliation or long-term survival is the morbidity and mortality associated with anastomotic leak.

As described in the article, the technique of pleural tenting is fast, safe, easy, and efficient. The buttressing material (pleura) is already present and does not require relocation from the abdomen. In this study, the mean difference in operating time was 10 minutes, suggesting the addition of the pleural tent procedure was not particularly onerous. The authors demonstrated a decrease in the leak rate in those patients who received the pleural tent. Although this series is not large enough to be adequately powered to detect, it would seem logical to hypothesize that in patients who did develop leak, the consequences might be less in the pleural tent group because of better containment. Pleural tenting is relatively simple and efficient and may be considered for this and other intrathoracic buttressing applications.

C. T. Klodell, Jr, MD

Lung Transplantation

Fundoplication After Lung Transplantation Prevents the Allograft Dysfunction Associated With Reflux
Hartwig MG, Anderson DJ, Onaitis MW, et al (Duke Univ, Durham, NC)
Ann Thorac Surg 92:462-469, 2011

Background.—Gastroesophageal reflux disease (GERD) in lung recipients is associated with decreased survival and attenuated allograft function. This study evaluates fundoplication in preventing GERD-related allograft dysfunction.

Methods.—Prospectively collected data on patients who underwent transplantation between January 2001 and August 2009 were included. Lung transplant candidates underwent esophageal pH probe testing before transplantation and surveillance spirometry evaluation after transplantation. Bilateral lung transplant recipients who had pretransplant pH probe testing and posttransplant 1-year forced expiratory volume in the first second of expiration (FEV_1) data were included for analysis.

Results.—Of 297 patients who met study criteria, 222 (75%) had an abnormal pH probe study before or early after transplantation and 157 (53%) had a fundoplication performed within the first year after transplantation. Patients with total proximal acid contact times greater than 1.2% or total distal acid contact times greater than 7.0% demonstrated an absolute decrease of 9.4% (± 4.6) or 12.0% (± 5.4) in their respective mean 1-year FEV_1 values. Patients with abnormal acid contact times who did not undergo fundoplication had considerably worse predicted peak and 1-year FEV_1 results compared with recipients receiving fundoplication (peak percent predicted = 75% vs. 84%; $p = 0.004$ and 1-year percent predicted = 68% vs. 77%; $p = 0.003$, respectively).

Conclusions.—Lung transplant recipients with abnormal esophageal pH studies attain a lower peak allograft function as well as a diminished 1-year FEV_1 after transplantation. However a strategy of early fundoplication in these recipients appears to preserve lung allograft function.

▶ This important contribution to the literature retrospectively reviews a high-volume single-institutional experience with lung transplantation and the aggressive treatment of gastroesophageal reflux disease (GERD) with fundoplication. Over an 8-year period, lung transplantation candidates underwent pH testing before and surveillance spirometry after transplantation. Two hundred ninety-seven patients were identified with pretransplant pH probe testing, and posttransplant 1-year forced expiratory volume in the first second of expiration (FEV_1) data were analyzed. Of the 297 patients, 222 had abnormal pH probe testing, and ultimately 157 received fundoplication within the first year following transplantation. Those who had abnormal acid contact times and did not undergo fundoplication had considerably lower FEV_1 compared with those who did receive fundoplication. The fundoplication wraps were 360° Nissen fundoplications, except in patients noted to have abnormal esophageal motility in whom partial wraps were performed.

Although lung transplantation is an effective therapy for extending both the quality and quantity of life in patients with end-stage lung disease, it is hampered by one of the shortest graft survival times when compared with other solid organ transplants. The short graft survival is attributable to development of bronchiolitis obliterans (BO), and the clinical correlate of BO is BO syndrome (BOS). No therapeutic interventions thus far have been successful in mitigating the deleterious effects of BOS. Gastroesophageal reflux is common after lung transplant (up to 75% of recipients) and has been shown to be associated with increased rates of BOS and worse actuarial survival.

The authors should be commended for their ongoing work in this area. They have previously highlighted the association between GERD and BOS and now demonstrate that fundoplication may reduce the risk of BOS following transplantation. Most patients in this study received fundoplication within 3 months of transplantation, and it should be noted that 15% to 20% of patients developed abnormal pH testing after transplantation. With the information brought forth by this study, it would seem reasonable to suggest that all lung transplant candidates have pH testing prior to and following transplantation. Strong consideration of fundoplication may be appropriate in those with abnormal testing in hopes of reducing the development of the devastating BOS.

C. T. Klodell, Jr, MD

Intra-Operative Concerns

Intrathoracic Anastomotic Leakage and Mortality After Esophageal Cancer Resection: A Population-Based Study

Rutegård M, Lagergren P, Rouvelas I, et al (Karolinska Institutet, Stockholm, Sweden)
Ann Surg Oncol 19:99-103, 2012

Background.—Results are conflicting and no population-based studies are available regarding the postoperative mortality after intrathoracic anastomotic leakage. The current study addressed the unselected and independent fatality rate of intrathoracic esophageal anastomotic leaks after resection for cancer.

Methods.—A prospective, nationwide study was conducted in Sweden in April 2001 through December 2005. Details concerning patient and tumor characteristics, surgical procedures, postoperative anastomotic leakage, and mortality were collected prospectively. Logistic regression was performed to estimate odds ratios (ORs) and 95% confidence intervals (95% CIs), adjusted for age, tumor stage, comorbidity, and hospital volume.

Results.—Among 559 resected patients with an intrathoracic anastomosis, 44 patients (7.9%) sustained an anastomotic leak within 30 days of surgery. Of these, 8 patients (18.2%) died within 90 days of surgery, compared with 32 of the 515 patients without leakage (6.2%) ($P = .003$). The adjusted OR of postoperative death following intrathoracic anastomotic leakage was increased 3-fold compared with those without such a complication (OR 3.0, 95% CI 1.2—7.2).

Conclusion.—Intrathoracic anastomotic leakage after esophageal resection for cancer remains a major risk factor for short-term postoperative death in an unselected, population-based setting.

▶ The authors performed a prospective nationwide study over a 4-year period to better elucidate the postoperative mortality after intrathoracic anastomotic leakage following esophageal cancer resection. Over the 4-year period, there were 559 patients with intrathoracic anastomosis, and 8% sustained a leak from their anastomosis. The patients who developed leak following resection and intrathoracic anastomosis had an adjusted odds ratio of postoperative death that increased 3-fold compared with those patients without leak.

Esophageal resection has long been associated with relatively high morbidity and mortality, especially following anastomotic leak. As the practice has evolved to fewer centers doing higher volumes, these numbers have slowly improved, with many centers now reporting in-hospital mortality rates of 5% or less following esophageal resection for cancer. The reported mortality rate from major esophageal leaks has been in the range of 21% to 35% in most studies, with very little improvement over time.

This population-based study indicates that intrathoracic anastomotic leakage after esophageal resection for cancer remains a major risk factor for postoperative death. This particular study was not adequately powered to differentiate between leaks of different magnitudes or if the leaks required operative management or could be controlled with more conservative measures. This study serves to further heighten our awareness of the devastating consequences of intrathoracic esophageal anastomotic leakage. It emphasizes the need to perform any additional buttressing of the anastomosis in the surgical armamentarium, such as pleural tent or other vascularized pedicle, in efforts to decrease the incidence of esophageal leak and eliminate the devastating consequences.

C. T. Klodell, Jr, MD

Appropriate Use of Emergency Department Thoracotomy: Implications for the Thoracic Surgeon
Mollberg NM, Glenn C, John J, et al (Mount Sinai Hosp and the Univ of Illinois at Chicago)
Ann Thorac Surg 92:455-461, 2011

Background.—Practice guidelines for the appropriate use of emergency department thoracotomy (EDT) according to current national resuscitative guidelines have been developed by the American College of Surgeons Committee on Trauma (ACS-COT) and published. At an urban level I trauma center we analyzed how closely these guidelines were followed and their ability to predict mortality.

Methods.—Between January 2003 and July 2010, 120 patients with penetrating thoracic trauma underwent EDT at Mount Sinai Hospital (MSH). Patients were separated based on adherence (group 1, n = 70) and nonadherence (group 2, n = 50) to current resuscitative guidelines, and group survival rates were determined. These 2 groups were analyzed based on outcome to determine the effect of a strict policy of adherence on survival.

Results.—Of EDTs performed during the study period, 41.7% (50/120) were considered outside current guidelines. Patients in group 2 were less likely to have traditional predictors of survival. There were 6 survivors in group 1 (8.7%), all of whom were neurologically intact; there were no neurologically intact survivors in group 2 ($p = 0.04$). The presence of a thoracic surgeon in the operating room (OR) was associated with increased survival ($p = 0.039$).

Conclusions.—A policy of strict adherence to EDT guidelines based on current national guidelines would have accounted for all potential survivors while avoiding the harmful exposure of health care personnel to blood-borne pathogens and the futile use of resources for trauma victims unable to benefit from them. Cardiothoracic surgeons should be familiar with current EDT guidelines because they are often asked to contribute their operative skills for those patients who survive to reach the OR.

▶ The survival rates for emergency department thoracotomy (EDT) have varied significantly in the literature and range from 2% to 31%. Some of the variance in outcomes is based on variable indications and variable adherence to the guidelines for appropriate indications for the procedure. There are competing interests in that no physician wants to exclude any possible survivor, while inappropriate use of EDT may expose health care workers to unnecessary risk and the health care system to unwarranted expense.

The authors report on outcomes of EDT at their institution over a 7-year period with the purpose of determining if a policy based on current resuscitative guidelines can predict mortality for patients arriving at the hospital in extremis from penetrating trauma. In addition, they wished to retrospectively review if the presence of a thoracic surgeon in the operating room was associated with increased survival. They included only patients who received EDT for penetrating trauma in the analysis. The authors retrospectively reviewed the records for adherence to current indications for EDT, which are patients sustaining witnessed cardiac arrest from penetrating thoracic trauma and with signs of life in the field and less than 15 minutes of unsuccessful cardiopulmonary resuscitation. All patients had EDT via a left anterolateral thoracotomy in the fourth or fifth interspace with selective transternal extension. Consultation with a thoracic surgeon was determined by clinical judgment of the on-call general trauma surgeon.

All survivors were in the group that met the guidelines and indications (8.7% survivors), and all survivors were neurologically intact. The presence of a thoracic surgeon in the operating room was noted to be associated with increased survival. No survivors would have been excluded by strict adherence to current guidelines and indications. These are very important findings, as they may allow health care workers to avoid the inherent risks involved with the performance of EDT in those patients falling outside the guidelines without excluding any potential survivors. Furthermore, although it is well known that trauma surgeons are capable of rendering definitive surgical care for major thoracic injuries secondary to penetrating trauma, it may still be beneficial in selected cases to seek the intraoperative consultation of a thoracic surgeon.

C. T. Klodell, Jr, MD

Ten-Year Results of Thoracoscopic Unilateral Extended Thymectomy Performed in Nonthymomatous Myasthenia Gravis
Tomulescu V, Sgarbura O, Stanescu C, et al (Fundeni Clinical Inst, Bucharest, Romania)
Ann Surg 254:761-766, 2011

Objective.—The aim of this study was to analyze the 10-year results of thoracoscopic unilateral extended thymectomy (TUET) performed in nontumoral myasthenia gravis according to the Myasthenia Gravis Foundation of America recommendations.

Background Data.—Thoracoscopic unilateral extended thymectomy has the benefits of a minimally invasive approach. Previous data have shown promising midterm results but long-term results were lacking.

Methods.—Two hundred forty patients with nontumoral myasthenia gravis who underwent surgery between 1999 and 2009 were eligible for the study. The mean follow-up was of 67 months (range: 12–125), 134 patients completed follow-up assessments more than 60 months after TUET.

Results.—There were 39 males (16.3%) and 201 females (83.7%), with an age range from 8 to 60 years. The mean preoperative disease duration was 21.5 months. All patients underwent preoperative steroid therapy. Anticholinesterase drugs were required for 123 patients (51.3%), and immunosuppressive drugs were required for 87 (36.3%) patients. The pathologic findings were as follows: normal thymus in 13 patients (5.5%), involuted thymus in 65 patients (27%), and hyperplastic thymus in 162 patients (67.5%). The average weight of the thymus was 110 ± 45 g. Ectopic thymic tissue was found in 147 patients (61.3%). There was no mortality, and morbidity consisted of 12 patients (5%). Complete stable remission was achieved in 61% of the patients, and the cumulative probability of achieving complete stable remission was 0.88 at 10 years.

Conclusions.—With zero mortality, low morbidity, and comparable long-term results to open surgery, TUET can be regarded as the best treatment option for patients undergoing surgery for myasthenia gravis.

▶ The thymus gland is known to play a central role in the pathogenesis of myasthenia gravis (MG). Thymectomy is an accepted option in the treatment algorithm of MG as part of a multifaceted treatment plan, which includes immunosuppression and surgical therapy. Extended thymectomy has been the accepted practice in MG, although previous data have shown reasonable midterm results with thoracoscopic unilateral extended thymectomy (TUET). There are very few studies that examine the long-term outcomes after surgical therapy for nonthymomatous MG.

The authors examined the long-term outcomes in 240 patients who underwent TUET for nonthymomatous MG at their center and reported an average of 67 months of follow-up per patient. They reported zero mortality and low morbidity in these patients, as well as an impressive 61% of patients with stable complete remission. They concluded that TUET may be the best treatment option for patients selected for surgery with nonthymomatous MG.

The current clinical consensus is patients with generalized MG between the ages of puberty and 60 years should undergo surgery. However, the best technique for thymectomy has not been clearly established. The surgical goal is to remove as much thymic tissue as possible, with the current thought perhaps favoring a unilateral approach for less morbidity and better cosmetic results.

We have utilized this technique for the last decade and agree with the authors as to the technical aspects of the procedure. Often the procedure can be accomplished with two 5-mm ports and a single 12-mm port in the anterior axillary line at the inframammary crease. The larger port is not required for the actual dissection but allows for a specimen bag to be inserted and removal of the thymus after resection. I favor the use of cautery for the bulk of the dissection and then harmonic scalpel or similar device for the dissection of the innominate vein and caval recess. Often, the small thymic veins encountered can be adequately managed, but a 5-mm laparoscopic clip applier is occasionally used. The addition of CO_2 insufflation to 8 mm Hg pressure allows enhanced visualization. Dissection of the contralateral side must be meticulous and careful, as it is easy to pull hard enough on the specimen to prolapse the left phrenic up toward the operative field. A single small-caliber drain or chest tube should be left overnight, and the patient can often be discharged the next morning if the MG stays well controlled.

C. T. Klodell, Jr, MD

Thoracoscopic Sympathicotomy for Disabling Palmar Hyperhidrosis: A Prospective Randomized Comparison Between Two Levels

Baumgartner FJ, Reyes M, Sarkisyan GG, et al (Doctors Outpatient Surgery Ctr, Fountain Valley, CA)
Ann Thorac Surg 92:2015-2019, 2011

Background.—Thoracoscopic sympathicotomy is highly effective in treating disabling palmar hyperhidrosis. The ideal level to maximize efficacy and minimize the side effect of compensatory hyperhidrosis (CH) is controversial. This study compared sympathicotomy over the second (R2) vs third (R3) costal head relative to these variables in patients with massive palmar hyperhidrosis.

Methods.—This prospective, randomized study enrolled 121 patients with disabling palmoplantar hyperhidrosis assigned to bilateral sympathicotomy (sympathetic transection), which was done over R2 in 61 (n = 122 extremities) or R3 in 60 (n = 120 extremities). Patients were questioned at 6 months and at 1 year or more to assess efficacy, side effects, and satisfaction with the procedure.

Results.—Sympathicotomy at R2 failed to cure palmar hyperhidrosis in 5 of 122 (4.1%) extremities, but only 2 (1.6%) were to a truly profound dripping level of recurrence. Sympathicotomy at R3 failed to cure palmar hyperhidrosis in 5 of 120 extremities (4.2%), and all were dramatic failures with dripping recurrent sweating. The patients whose palmar hyperhidrosis was not completely cured were aged 19.7 ± 2.5 vs 26.4 ± 8.0 years ($p = 0.04$). Two R3 patients with failure underwent three redo R2 sympathicotomies, with curative results. R2 patients showed a trend toward a higher level of CH vs R3 patients at 6 months and after 1 year. The CH severity scale was 4.7 ± 2.7 (n = 38) for R2 vs 3.8 ± 2.8 (n = 36) for R3 ($p = $ NS) at 6 months and 4.7 ± 2.5 (n = 43) for R2 vs 3.7 ± 2.8 (n = 37) for R3 ($p = $ NS) after 1 year. Younger age, male sex, and higher levels of preoperative and postoperative plantar sweating were predictors of failed sympathicotomy. Increased age was associated with increased CH.

Conclusions.—R2 and R3 sympathicotomy for massive palmoplantar hyperhidrosis are highly effective, with low recurrence and incidences of severe CH. R2 tends to have a higher level of CH vs R3, and a higher incidence of dramatic failures is suggested in R3 patients, for which reoperation at the R2 level will likely be curative.

▶ The authors present their experience with endoscopic thoracic sympathectomy (ETS) in 121 patients in an attempt to better elucidate the impact of the level of sympathotomy (second thoracic sympathetic ganglion [T2] vs third thoracic sympathetic ganglion [T3]) on both successful resolution of palmar hyperhidrosis as well as the subsequent development of compensatory sweating. As the authors more fully describe in the article, there is much controversy over which levels should be addressed, as well as the method of addressing them. The literature is full of reports detailing various combinations of levels and sympathotomy (cutting, clipping, or cautery) vs sympathectomy (resecting part of the chain). Many have felt that the resection of a segment of the chain leads to greater compensatory sweating, as does the T2 lesion. In this study, the authors find that the T3 lesion is equally efficacious in their experience but that the failures were more dramatic when they did occur. They did note an increased incidence of compensatory sweating with the T2 lesion.

We have used a similar strategy of micro-ETS using 3-mm ports and sympathotomy of the T3 and T4 ganglion for patients with palmar and pedal hyperhidrosis. The addition of the T2 ganglion is performed only in patients with facial symptoms. We have also used the pulsatility index of a standard pulse oximeter probe as an indicator of adequate sympathectomy. Although there still exists controversy over the exact conduct of ETS, given the propensity for increased compensatory sweating with the T2 lesion, it would seem prudent to reserve its application for only those cases with facial symptoms given ample evidence of equal efficacy of the T3 lesion. Additionally, it would seem the methods of sympathotomy (either clipping or cautery) should be used preferentially in an effort to limit compensatory sweating, which is the most common side effect of the procedure and has been shown to lessen postoperative patient satisfaction.

C. T. Klodell, Jr, MD

Oncologic Efficacy of Anatomic Segmentectomy in Stage IA Lung Cancer Patients With T1a Tumors
Donahue JM, Morse CR, Wigle DA, et al (Mayo Clinic, Rochester, MN)
Ann Thorac Surg 93:381-388, 2012

Background.—Segmentectomy provides an anatomic, parenchymal-sparing strategy for patients with limited lung function. Recently, interest has been renewed in segmentectomy for the treatment of early stage lung cancer.

Methods.—We reviewed the medical records of all patients undergoing segmentectomy from January 1999 through December 2004. Survival curves were estimated using the Kaplan-Meier method.

Results.—There were 113 consecutive patients (58 men, 55 women); median age was 72.5 years (range, 30 to 94 years). Median forced expiratory volume in 1 second was 1.53 L (range, 0.5 L to 3.27 L). Median diffusion capacity of lung for carbon monoxide was 69% predicted (range, 23% to 129%). Significant comorbidities were present in 62 patients (55%). There was no perioperative mortality. Major morbidity occurred in 28 patients (25%). Mean tumor size was 2.1 cm. Resection margins were negative in all cases. Ninety-two patients (81%) were stage I. Overall

5-year survival was 79% for stage IA patients. Current smoking, diffusion capacity of lung for carbon monoxide less than 69%, tumor size greater than 2 cm, N2 disease, and advanced histology grade were associated with decreased survival by univariate analysis. In a multivariate model, only tumor size greater than 2 cm remained significant. Tumor recurrence was observed in 39 patients (35%): local in 17 patients (15%) and distant only in 22 (20%). For stage IA patients with T1a lesions, local recurrence was 5% and distant recurrence was 13%. Five-year recurrence-free survival of these patients was 69%.

Conclusions.—Pulmonary segmentectomy can be performed safely in selected patients with preoperative reduced lung function and comorbidities. For stage IA disease, survival approximates that seen after lobectomy, with similar local recurrence rates for patients with T1a tumors.

▶ The authors review their extensive experience with segmentectomy for stage IA lung cancer at their institution. The Lung Cancer Study Group reported the only prospective, randomized study to compare limited, sublobar resections (segmentectomy and wedge resections) with lobectomy for stage IA non–small cell lung cancer. Based on the increased incidence of local recurrence (3× increase) in the sublobar resection group, it became standard of care for formal anatomic lobectomy for stage IA lung cancer. However, this study considered wedge resection and segmentectomy together, which might have biased the result against segmentectomy. Even with the grouping of wedge resection and segmentectomy together, there was no survival disadvantage when compared with the lobectomy group.

Several reports in the contemporary literature have supported the consideration of segmentectomy for early-stage lung cancer. The local recurrence rates reported in these contemporary series are much less than those observed in the prior study in which wedge resection and segmentectomy were grouped.

Although there is a current ongoing randomized trial comparing the results of lobar and sublobar resection for peripheral lung cancer greater than 2 cm in diameter, this retrospective review gives us some insight as to the potential of anatomic segmentectomy for treatment of stage IA lesions. The authors demonstrated excellent local control and survival with segmentectomy for T1a lesions in carefully selected patients. This may be considered an excellent option for patients with lesions amenable to this technique, especially in patients with limited pulmonary reserve. As the population continues to age and medicine supports people far beyond what was possible in years past, the patients presenting for surgical consideration continue to become higher risk. Perhaps with appropriate consideration of anatomic segmentectomy, patients with limited pulmonary reserve who would poorly tolerate lobectomy can still benefit from the advantage of surgical extirpation.

C. T. Klodell, Jr, MD

Clinical Ramifications of Bronchial Kink After Upper Lobectomy

Ueda K, Tanaka T, Hayashi M, et al (Yamaguchi Univ Graduate School of Medicine, Japan; Nagasaki Univ Graduate School of Biomedical Science, Japan)
Ann Thorac Surg 93:259-265, 2012

Background.—Bronchial kink is caused by upward displacement of the remaining lower lobe of the lung after upper lobectomy, which can cause an intractable cough or shortness of breath. However, bronchial kink is often overlooked because of the difficulty in the simultaneous diagnosis of bronchial curvature and narrowing.

Methods.—Screening for bronchial kink with three-dimensional computed tomography (CT)-based bronchography was done on 50 patients who had undergone hemilateral upper lobectomy for cancer. Bronchial kink was confirmed if there was airway angulation and resultant stenosis exceeding 80%. We compared postoperative changes in spirometry-based ventilatory capacity with CT-based functional lung volume (FLV) in patients with and without bronchial kink.

Results.—Bronchial kink was confirmed in 21 patients (42%). Postoperative FLV and ventilatory capacity were significantly greater in patients without than in those with bronchial kink ($p < 0.05$ for both measures). Postoperative FLV and ventilatory capacity were also significantly greater than the estimated postoperative values for both measures in patients without bronchial kink (both, $p < 0.05$), representing favorable compensatory adaptation of the remaining lung, whereas this was not the case in patients with bronchial kink (both, $p > 0.1$). Patients with bronchial kink complained more often than those without bronchial kink of an intractable cough and shortness of breath (76% vs 21%, respectively, $p < 0.01$).

Conclusions.—Bronchial kink after upper lobectomy is a common and functionally unfavorable condition that can exacerbate postoperative shortness of breath. Computed tomography-based bronchography is a useful tool in screening for bronchial kink. Strategies for preventing bronchial kink should be explored in the clinical setting.

▶ Postoperative pulmonary function is usually predicted by calculating the proportion of remaining lung expected after the resection and adjusting the preoperative pulmonary function tests proportionally. However, it may also be influenced by the ability of the remaining lung to adapt to the new intrathoracic environment. It has been reported that the adaptive remodeling of the respiratory system can sometimes induce anatomic distortion, leading to a dissociation of structure and function and incomplete normalization of the remaining lung. The authors previously reported that adaptation of the remaining lung after upper lobectomy may be less favorable than with lower lobectomy. They hypothesized that this may be secondary to kinking of the bronchus that specifically follows upper lobectomy as a consequence of the upward displacement of the diaphragm and remaining lower lobe of the lung.

In this study, the authors utilize 3-dimensional computed tomography (3DCT)-based bronchographic images obtained with a 64-detector CT scanner and imaging software to screen for bronchial angulations and bronchial narrowing (bronchial kinking) in patients following upper lobectomy. These patients are often found to have a chronic cough and complain of ongoing (often unanticipated) shortness of breath. Interestingly, the authors noted bronchial kinking in 42% of the patients screened with this method following upper lobectomy. This may be the first systematic description of this entity in the medical literature. They report that although bronchial kink was not associated with postoperative cardiopulmonary complications, it was associated with the occurrence of persistent cough and breathlessness. They further noted that bronchial kinking exacerbated the postoperative deterioration of pulmonary function, which was accompanied by a dissociation of pulmonary structure and function.

The authors should be congratulated for this elegant description of the entity of bronchial kinking following anatomic upper lobectomy. We have all encountered patients who seemed more breathless than anticipated following upper lobectomy as well as patients with persistent pooling of secretions in the lower lobe despite adequate cough effort and mucociliary function. While shortness of breath and cough after lobectomy are known complications, this may help explain some of the unexpected breathlessness that is occasionally seen. The next challenge is to now utilize this technology of detecting bronchial kink and transform it into either preventative or therapeutic interventions.

C. T. Klodell, Jr, MD

Miscellaneous

Early VATS For Blunt Chest Trauma: A Management Technique Underutilized By Acute Care Surgeons

Smith JW, Franklin GA, Harbrecht BG, et al (Univ of Louisville, KY)
J Trauma 71:102-107, 2011

Background.—Retained hemothorax and/or empyema is a commonly recognized complication of penetrating chest injuries that may be treated by early video-assisted thoracoscopy (VATS). However, the use of VATS in blunt chest trauma is less well defined. Our acute care surgeon (ACS) group aggressively treats complications of penetrating chest trauma with VATS, and our results suggested that the early use of VATS by ACS should be expanded.

Materials.—A retrospective review of Trauma Center admissions between January 2007 and December 2009 was performed to identify patients with blunt thoracic injuries who underwent VATS.

Results.—Eighty-three patients underwent VATS to manage thoracic complications arising from their blunt chest trauma. All operations were performed by ACS. The majority of patients (73%, 61 of 83) were treated with VATS for retained hemothorax, 18% for empyema (15 of 83), and 10% for persistent air leak (8 of 83). All (15) patients who developed empyema had chest tubes placed in the emergency department. No patient treated with VATS for a persistent air leak required further operation or conversion to thoracotomy. VATS performed ≤5 days after injury was associated with a lower conversion to open thoracotomy (8% vs. 29.4%, $p < 0.05$). Hospital length of stay (LOS) was significantly lower for patients receiving VATS ≤ 5 days after injury (11 ± 6 vs. 16 ± 8, $p < 0.05$). No patient treated with VATS ≤ 5 days had persistent empyema; however, five patients treated with VATS for retained hemothorax or empyema >5 days after injury required further intervention for thoracic infection. Multivariate analysis demonstrated that both a diagnosis of empyema and VATS >5 days after injury were predictors of increased LOS and increased conversion to thoracotomy.

Conclusions.—Early VATS can decrease hospital LOS and thoracotomy rate in patient suffering blunt thoracic injuries. ACS can perform this procedure safely and effectively.

▶ Although there are several reports from this and other institutions detailing the use of early video-assisted thoracoscopy (VATS) for penetrating trauma, this report details its use for blunt trauma. The authors retrospectively review their experience over a 3-year period with the use of VATS following blunt trauma and detail the outcomes of 83 patients. Most patients received VATS for retained hemothorax, although in some the indication was empyema or persistent air leak. Based on their single-institution data, the authors note that early VATS may decrease the length of stay and reduce the thoracotomy rate. Their data set was segregated by those operated at less than or greater than 5 days following injury, noting that the complications and conversion rate were lower in the subset operated earlier. All procedures were performed by the acute care surgery faculty, with the expert guidance and consultation of a senior acute care surgeon who is also board-certified in thoracic surgery (JDR). Although VATS procedures should be performed by acute care surgeons, it is important to note the institutional advantage the authors have in helping young faculty gain early experience with VATS.

This study highlights an important technique for treatment of blunt trauma patients with persistent intrathoracic abnormalities. The most common complications (retained hemothorax, empyema, and persistent posttraumatic pneumothorax) may occur in up to 20% of patients after blunt chest trauma and can lead to deleterious consequences if left untreated. Although additional chest tubes are commonly placed in these circumstances, it seldom resolves the underlying pathology. In this study of 1384 patients who sustained blunt chest trauma, only 83 required operation (6.0% operative rate). They also note that all patients who developed complications requiring VATS had an abnormal chest radiograph immediately following chest tube placement. Finally, it should be noted that for retained hemothorax and persistent air leak, the conversion rate to thoracotomy was low (4.9% and 0%) whereas for empyema, it was higher (73%). The conversion rate was higher in operations performed after 5 days compared with earlier VATS. The most common reason cited for conversion was poor visibility in the operative field.

The authors and institution should be commended for their ongoing pioneering work in thoracic surgery following blunt trauma and the early and aggressive use of VATS. Although this was a retrospective study and the 5-day breakpoint may have been somewhat arbitrary, the message is strong. Patients who have an abnormal chest radiograph following chest tube placement should be considered for early chest CT and possible early VATS. One technical point valuable during these operations is the use of sealed trocars and CO_2 insufflation if the visualization is poor. Often the pleural adhesions from early to intermediate empyema may be better visualized with 8 to 10 mm Hg CO_2 insufflation, which helps with normal lung compression and better visualization. With the combination of a pulse irrigation system and CO_2 insufflation, seemingly challenging visualization can be greatly improved and allow successful thoracoscopic surgery.

C. T. Klodell, Jr, MD

Catamenial pneumothorax and endometriosis-related pneumothorax: clinical features and risk factors
Rousset-Jablonski C, Alifano M, Plu-Bureau G, et al (Université Paris Descartes, France)
Hum Reprod 26:2322-2329, 2011

Background.—Catamenial pneumothorax and thoracic endometriosis (TE) are still under diagnosed. The purpose of this study is to increase the diagnostic accuracy for these conditions in patients with spontaneous pneumothorax and to identify their risk factors.

Methods.—We conducted a retrospective study on all consecutive women of reproductive age referred to our Centre for surgical treatment of spontaneous pneumothorax between July 2000 and January 2009.

Results.—The study population comprised 156 premenopausal women of whom 49 (31.4) had catamenial and/or TE-related pneumothorax. Over a quarter of these 49 patients had a previous history of recurrent thoracic or scapular catamenial pain. They experienced their first pneumothorax episode at an older age (mean ± SD) (34.0 years ± 6.7) than women with idiopathic pneumothorax (28.7 ± 6.1 years, $P < 0.001$). Pelvic endometriosis was found in 51 of women with catamenial and/or TE-related pneumothorax. After adjustment for confounding factors by multiple logistic regression analysis, the Results show that, infertility [odd ratio (OR) = 4.21, 95 confidence interval (CI) = 1.28–13.88] and a history of pelvic surgery with a uterine procedure and/or uterine scraping (OR = 2.85, 95 CI = 1.12–7.26) were the strongest predictors of catamenial and/or TE-related pneumothorax.

Conclusions.—Infertility and uterine procedures are significantly associated with catamenial and/or TE-related pneumothorax. Scapular or thoracic pain during menses often precedes the occurrence of pneumothorax and is highly specific for the diagnosis of TE. Our Results suggest that in women with pelvic endometriosis, these symptoms should be systematically investigated for an earlier diagnosis of TE.

▶ The authors present an excellent retrospective review of 156 premenopausal women who presented to their institution with pneumothorax over a 9-year period, finding 31.4% had catamenial or thoracic endometriosis—related pneumothorax. This report highlights a condition that remains both underdiagnosed and likely undertreated by the surgical community.

Catamenial pneumothorax is defined as recurrent episodes of pneumothorax (at least 2) occurring between the day before and within 72 hours from the onset on menses. Often patients may experience recurrent thoracic or scapular catamenial pain before the first episode of pneumothorax. This pain usually started several months before the onset of the first pneumothorax and in some cases up to a year prior.

Nearly all cases are right sided, although the authors noted a few patients with bilateral presentation and a single patient with left sided presentation. The presenting symptoms are typical and include chest pain, shortness of breath, and cough. The right-sided predominance is theorized to be from the transdiaphragmatic passage of air from the genital tract through diaphragmatic perforations caused by endometrial implants. These implants are most commonly found on the right hemidiaphragm, related to the circulation from the pelvis up the right paracolic gutter. Over time, the implants lead to small perforations in the diaphragm.

As surgeons, we are called upon to evaluate and treat young women with recurrent pneumothorax, making it imperative that a proper evaluation and therapeutic intervention are performed. A history of scapular pain or thoracic pain during menses before presentation with pneumothorax is suggestive, as is right-sided presentation.

At thoracoscopy, a diligent search of the visceral and parietal pleura should be conducted to detect nodular brown lesions. Similarly, the diaphragm should be inspected closely for holes or endometrial implants. When abnormalities are found, they must be corrected or resected. Those resected should be sent for pathology, where the presence of endometrial glands or stroma will confirm the diagnosis. Further conduct of the operation should be routine, including any blebs resected and mechanical pleurodesis as well as excellent tube drainage. A reminder to the anesthesiologist and postoperative care team to avoid anti-inflammatory drugs following pleurodesis is often helpful.

C. T. Klodell, Jr, MD

Percutaneous Tracheostomy: To Bronch or Not to Bronch—That Is the Question
Jackson LSM, Davis JW, Kaups KL, et al (UCSF/Fresno, CA)
J Trauma 71:1553-1556, 2011

Background.—Percutaneous tracheostomy is a routine procedure in the intensive care unit (ICU). Some surgeons perform percutaneous tracheostomies using bronchoscopy believing that it increases safety. The purpose of this study was to evaluate percutaneous tracheostomy in the trauma population and to determine whether the use of a bronchoscope decreases the complication rate and improves safety.

Methods.—A retrospective review was completed from January 2007 to November 2010. Inclusion criteria were trauma patients undergoing percutaneous tracheostomy. Data collected included age, Abbreviated Injury Score by region, Injury Severity Score, ventilator days, and outcomes. Complications were classified as early (occurring within <24 hours) or late (>24 hours after the procedure).

Results.—During the study period, 9,663 trauma patients were admitted, with 1,587 undergoing intubation and admission to the ICU. Tracheostomies were performed in 266 patients and 243 of these were percutaneous; 78 (32%) were performed with the bronchoscope (Bronch) and 168 (68%) without bronchoscope (No Bronch). There were no differences between the groups in Abbreviated Injury Score by region, Injury Severity Score, probability of survival, ventilator days, and length of ICU or overall hospital stay. There were 16 complications, 5 (Bronch) and 11 (No Bronch). Early complications were primarily bleeding (Bronch 3% vs. No Bronch 4%, not statistically significant). Late complications included tracheomalacia, tracheal granulation tissue, bleeding, and stenosis; Bronch 4% versus No Bronch 3%, (not statistically significant). One major complication occurred, with loss of airway and cardiac arrest, in the bronchoscopy group.

Conclusion.—Percutaneous tracheostomy was safely and effectively performed by an experienced surgical team both with and without bronchoscopic guidance with no difference in the complication rates. This study suggests that the use of bronchoscopic guidance during tracheostomy is not routinely required but may be used as an important adjunct in selected patients, such as those with HALO cervical fixation, obesity, or difficult anatomy.

▶ In this report, the authors examine their experience with percutaneous tracheostomy in an effort to compare the complication rate between procedures performed with and without bronchoscopic guidance. In the authors' center, there were 7 attending physicians who performed the procedure and varied in the use of bronchoscopy. Four used bronchoscopy selectively, such as in patients in HALO fixation, obese patients, or known surgical injury. Of the remaining 3 physicians, 2 used bronchoscopy in the majority of procedures, and 1 used it routinely.

Interestingly, the authors describe their technique as dissecting to the pretracheal fascia and either direct puncture of the trachea based on palpation or puncture based on bronchoscopic guidance. In their series, they discovered no difference in complications between patients who did and did not have bronchoscopy at the time of tracheostomy.

Other authors have reported that the use of bronchoscopy may not reduce the number of complications but may lessen the severity by avoiding disastrous complications, such as posterior membranous tracheal puncture. Yet others have insisted that the routine use of tracheostomy is required for procedural safety.

Some of the disparity of opinion may be from not comparing "apples to apples." I would suggest that the author's description of dissecting to the pretracheal fascia and visualizing the trachea is not a percutaneous tracheostomy but rather an open tracheostomy performed with a percutaneous tracheostomy kit, which would seem feasible with or without bronchoscopy as the authors suggest. Other authors' technique descriptions focus more on a pure percutaneous approach.

I favor a bronchoscopically guided percutaneous approach and have used it exclusively for over 10 years. With placing the bronchoscope down to the right main stem bronchus, the endotracheal tube can be safely withdrawn to 16 cm. The cuff on the endotracheal tube remains inflated and usually sits just below the larynx. With this technique, the airway is always secure as the tube can easily be advanced back over the bronchoscope as a guide if accidentally withdrawn too far. Once secure at this level, the bronchoscope is carefully withdrawn to the tip of the endotracheal tube to protect it from accidental puncture. A small skin incision is made at the intended site, and the remainder of the procedure is performed using the contents of the kit totally percutaneously. The use of the bronchoscope allows access to the trachea and assurance of the correct site of entry without the need for additional dissection. Once the tracheostomy is placed, the bronchoscope is quickly removed from the endotracheal tube and advanced through the tracheostomy to confirm correct placement. Only after this maneuver, the ventilation is moved to the tracheostomy and the endotracheal tube removed. When performed in this manner, the airway is never at risk for loss, nor is the bronchoscope vulnerable to accidental puncture. Because the procedure is done without additional dissection, it is also very efficient and safely performed in a short time, typically less than 5 minutes.

C. T. Klodell, Jr, MD

Thoracic Epidural or Paravertebral Catheter for Analgesia After Lung Resection: Is the Outcome Different?
Elsayed H, McKevith J, McShane J, et al (Liverpool Heart and Chest Hosp, UK)
J Cardiothorac Vasc Anesth 26:78-82, 2012

Objective.—The aim of this study was to determine whether thoracic epidural analgesia (TEA) or a paravertebral catheter block (PVB) with morphine patient-controlled analgesia influenced outcome in patients undergoing thoracotomy for lung resection.

Design.—A retrospective analysis.

Setting.—A tertiary referral center.

Participants.—The study population consisted of 1,592 patients who had undergone thoracotomy for lung resection between May 2000 and April 2008.

Interventions.—Not applicable.

Measurements and Main Results.—Patients who received PVBs were younger, had a higher forced expiratory volume in 1 second, had a higher body mass index, a higher incidence of cardiac comorbidity, fewer pneumonectomies, and more wedge resections. A multivariable logistic regression model was used to develop a propensity-matched score for the probability of patients receiving an epidural or a paravertebral catheter. Four patients with an epidural to one with a paravertebral catheter were matched, with 488 patients and 122 patients, respectively. Postmatching analysis now showed no difference between the groups for preoperative characteristics or operative extent. Postmatching analysis showed no significant difference in outcome between the two groups for the incidence of postoperative respiratory complication ($p = 0.67$), intensive therapy unit (ITU) stay ($p = 0.51$), ITU readmission ($p = 0.66$), or in-hospital mortality ($p = 0.67$). There was a significant reduction in the hospital length of stay in favor of the paravertebral group (6 v 7 days, $p = 0.008$).

Conclusions.—Paravertebral catheter analgesia with morphine patient-controlled analgesia seems as effective as thoracic epidural for reducing the risk of postoperative complications. The authors additionally found that paravertebral catheter use is associated with a shorter hospital stay and may be a better form of analgesia for fast-track thoracic surgery.

▶ The thoracotomy incision is known to be one of the more painful procedures patients must endure, related to both the anatomy of muscles and ribs as well as potential entrapment of intercostal nerves. The authors sought to compare paravertebral and epidural catheters in terms of outcomes. The patients in the paravertebral group were also given morphine as patient-controlled analgesia (PCA).

In this retrospective study, there may be considerable selection bias in that the decision between catheter choices was based on discussions with the patient and allowing choice. This may introduce bias based on different personality types and a predilection for choosing one therapy type over another. These same personality traits may also impact the perception of pain. Additionally, it should be noted that there was a higher incidence of wedge resections in the paravertebral group.

One nuance of this study is the surgical placement of the paravertebral catheters under direct vision at the end of the procedure. This is in contradistinction to the traditional method of loss of resistance placement by anesthesiology. Some would argue that this method of placement allows greater control over the final location of the catheter and more predictable pain relief when compared with catheters placed without direct vision.

The authors use propensity matching to attenuate the differences between groups. They conclude that the combination of paravertebral catheter and morphine PCA was as effective and may be associated with decreased length of stay. Unfortunately, the article contains very little with respect to hemodynamics. Many would argue that the biggest advantage of paravertebral catheters when compared with epidural is the decreased sympathectomy, less vasodilation, and less consequent hypotension.

The authors should be commended for this study, and particularly for the intraoperative placement of the paravertebral catheters by the surgeons. While this technique is relatively easy to perform, it does consume some time in the operating room. Many of us instead select the more classic route of having them placed preoperatively in the block room by the anesthesiology team. This method, although more efficient for the flow of the day when trying to perform multiple thoracic operations, is unlikely to be as efficacious as directly placed catheters.

C. T. Klodell, Jr, MD

Pre- and Postoperative Management

Comparison of Continuous Thoracic Epidural With Paravertebral Block on Perioperative Analgesia and Hemodynamic Stability in Patients Having Open Lung Surgery

Pintaric TS, Potocnik I, Hadzic A, et al (Univ Med Centre Ljubljana, Slovenia; Columbia Univ, NY; et al)
Reg Anesth Pain Med 36:256-260, 2011

Background.—Epidural analgesia can result in perioperative hypotension in patients having thoracotomy. This randomized prospective study assessed the effects of epidural and paravertebral analgesia on hemodynamics during thoracotomy.

Methods.—Thirty-two patients were randomized to receive either epidural analgesia (n = 16, 0.25% levobupivacaine and 30 µg/kg morphine) or paravertebral block (n = 16; 0.5% levobupivacaine and 30 µg/kg morphine). Oxygen delivery, stroke volume and systemic vascular resistance indices, heart rate, and mean arterial pressure measurements were performed before administration of local anesthetic, after induction of general anesthesia, institution of 1-lung ventilation, first skin incision, retractor placement, lung-inflation maneuver, and at last skin suture. The primary end point was the volume of the colloid infusion necessary to maintain oxygen delivery index of 500 mL/min per squared meter or higher. Postoperative analgesia was provided immediately after surgery by an infusion of 0.125% levobupivacaine and 20 µg/mL morphine in epidural/paravertebral infusion. Pain, rescue-analgesia consumption, arterial pressure, and heart rate were recorded at 6, 24, and 48 hrs after surgery. Administration of anesthesia and data collection were done by research staff blinded to the regional analgesia technique.

Results.—The groups did not differ significantly in heart rate, mean arterial blood pressure, or systemic vascular resistance indices. However, to maintain the targeted oxygen delivery index, a greater volume of colloid infusion and phenylephrine were required, respectively, in the epidural than in the paravertebral group (554 ± 50 vs 196 ± 75 mL, $P = 0.04$; and 40 ± 10 vs 17 ± 4 µg, $P = 0.04$). Pain intensity before and after respiratory physiotherapy as well as 24 hr rescue piritramide consumption was similar in the epidural (4.1 ± 3.1 mg) and the paravertebral (2.5 ± 1.5 mg) groups ($P = 0.14$). Systolic blood pressure after 24 and 48 hrs was lower in the epidural group.

Conclusions.—Under the conditions of our study, continuous paravertebral block resulted in similar analgesia but greater hemodynamic stability than epidural analgesia in patients having thoracotomy. Paravertebral block also required smaller volume of colloids and vasopressors to maintain the target oxygen delivery index (DO_2I).

▶ The authors present 32 patients randomized to either thoracic epidural of paravertebral catheter for regional analgesia at the time of anterolateral thoracotomy.

The objective of this randomized trial was to compare their respective effects on hemodynamics using a goal-directed therapy approach to achieve a target oxygen delivery. They also compared the analgesia the patients experienced and the need for rescue therapy for adequate pain control.

Their technique involved either epidural or paravertebral catheter placement targeted at the T6-7 interspace. All the thoracic procedures were anterolateral thoracotomy approach, in contrast to the more common posterolateral approach used in the United States, but this should still allow some generalizations of the results.

Interestingly, they reported only a single failure of analgesia in the paravertebral arm (1/12 or 8% failure, 92% success) and no failures in the epidural arm (12/12, 100% success). All patients also received nonsteroidal anti-inflammatory drugs and rescue analgesics as required.

The authors reported that epidural and paravertebral approaches provided similar quality of postoperative analgesia after open lung surgery. However, the paravertebral approach resulted in greater cardiovascular stability as evidenced by lower volume of colloids and vasopressor use to maintain the targeted parameters. This correlates well with other authors who have reported a better adverse-effect profile with paravertebral approach and is likely related to the more peripheral and unilateral sympathetic blockade achieved with the paravertebral approach.

The difference in fluid requirement and hemodynamic stability can be of great importance during major lung resections. Optimal fluid management is critical in mitigating the risk for developing acute lung injury and especially post pneumonectomy pulmonary edema. Although this complication occurs in less than 5% of patients in the absence of left ventricular dysfunction or infection, the mortality is exceedingly high.

This comparison is timely; as surgeons our input is solicited in block selection. Although I prefer the paravertebral block for the reasons nicely elucidated by the authors, anecdotally there seems to be a higher failure rate when compared with the epidural block. To mitigate these shortcomings, our center uses a multifaceted approach. The patients receive pharmacotherapy to include gabapentin, acetaminophen, nonsteroidal anti-inflammatory drugs, as well as paravertebral catheters at 2 levels. Like the authors, we place 1 catheter at the anticipated level of the incision in the interspace. Additionally, we place a second catheter a few interspaces lower at the approximate level of the anticipated chest tube. Additionally, as advocated by Cerfolio et al, intraoperative dissection of the intercostal muscle and nerve away from the underside of the rib prior to placing the retractor will greatly reduce postoperative intercostal neuralgia. Finally, for patients not yet tolerating oral intake at 4 to 6 hours postoperatively, it is helpful to give a supplemental dose of acetaminophen intravenously.

C. T. Klodell, Jr, MD

Daily Chest Roentgenograms Are Unnecessary in Nonhypoxic Patients Who Have Undergone Pulmonary Resection by Thoracotomy

Cerfolio RJ, Bryant AS (Univ of Alabama at Birmingham)
Ann Thorac Surg 92:440-444, 2011

Background.—The purpose of this study is to assess the clinical benefit of performing a daily chest roentgenogram (CXR) on patients who have had a pulmonary resection.

Methods.—Patients underwent thoracotomy and pulmonary resection, and all had a daily CXR. The impact the CXR had on their care was evaluated. Hypoxia was defined as a sustained decrease in oxygen saturation of 6% or greater from patient's baseline.

Results.—Between January 2006 and December 2009, 1,037 patients met the eligibility criteria for this study. Types of resection were wedge in 282 patients, segmentectomy in 146, and lobectomy in 609. Only 20 of the 834 patients (2%) who did not have a pneumothorax on the recovery room CXR had hypoxia, compared with 42 patients (21%) who had a recovery room pneumothorax (odds ratio 10.6, 95% confidence interval: 6.1 to 18.5, $p < 0.001$). Daily CXR changed the care of only 268 of 975 patients (27%) who never had hypoxia compared with 49 of the 62 patients (79%) who were hypoxic (odds ratio 9.2, 95% confidence interval: 4.3 to 13.7, $p < 0.001$). Moreover, the changes in care made by the CXR in the 268 nonhypoxic patients were for small pneumothoraces, and the impact of these changes is dubious.

Conclusions.—Daily CXRs are not needed in the vast majority of patients who undergo elective pulmonary resection after thoracotomy. It is of little benefit for patients who do not have a pneumothorax on their recovery room CXR or for patients who do not become hypoxic.

▶ In this interesting study, the authors describe the impact (or lack of impact) of daily postoperative chest x-rays in patients who underwent pulmonary resection over a 4-year period. The study focused only on patients who underwent resection via thoracotomy.

The authors demonstrated that the management of patients was affected 72% of the time if the patients had either hypoxia or a pneumothorax on the immediate postoperative x-ray. In contrast, 27% of patients (268/975) had a change in clinical management in the absence of hypoxia. The authors then conclude that daily chest x-rays provide little benefit in patients who are not hypoxic and did not have a pneumothorax on their immediate postoperative x-ray.

While the authors seemed to suggest broader conclusions, I believe they demonstrated that patients with no pneumothorax who are not hypoxic may not benefit from daily chest x-ray. Although even in this subset of patients the x-ray did lead to a change in clinical management in 27%, the authors note that the changes were minor and unimportant. They further suggest that this finding may be possible to generalize to lesser resections such as thoracoscopic lobectomy and wedge resections.

One main caveat is that we do not fully understand how the minor changes affected the length of stay, duration of air leak, duration of chest tube drainage, and many other factors. While this study certainly questions the surgical dogma that the presence of a chest tube requires a daily x-ray, it may be a bit early to generalize this practice to all pulmonary resections. Perhaps the authors or some other similar volume institution will consider a randomized trial of daily chest x-rays versus x-rays only when hypoxic or following tube removal. This may allow us to better access the impact on length of stay, duration of chest tube drainage, need for chest tube reinsertion, lobar collapse, retained blood, and other more subtle findings.

The authors should be congratulated for challenging the surgical dogma and questioning the common practice of daily chest x-rays in these patient subsets. Furthermore, perhaps this will allow us all to question our current practice as to the number and frequency of x-rays we require to provide excellent care to our patients.

C. T. Klodell, Jr, MD

Perioperative Management of Patients on Clopidogrel (Plavix) Undergoing Major Lung Resection
Ceppa DKP, Welsby IJ, Wang TY, et al (Duke Univ Med Ctr, Durham, NC)
Ann Thorac Surg 92:1971-1976, 2011

Background.—Management of patients requiring antiplatelet therapy with clopidogrel (Plavix) and major lung resection must balance the risks of bleeding and cardiovascular events. We reviewed our experience with patients treated with clopidogrel perioperatively to examine outcomes, including results of a new strategy for high-risk patients.

Methods.—Patients who underwent major lung resection and received perioperative clopidogrel between January 2005 and September 2010 were reviewed. Initially, clopidogrel management consisted of discontinuation approximately 5 days before surgery and resumption immediately after surgery. After July 2010, high-risk patients (drug-eluting coronary stent placement within prior year or previous coronary event after clopidogrel discontinuation) were admitted 2 to 3 days preoperatively and bridged with the intravenous glycoprotein IIb/IIIa receptor inhibitor eptifibatide (Integrilin) according to a multidisciplinary cardiology/anesthesiology/thoracic surgery protocol. Outcomes were compared with control patients (matched for preoperative risk factors and extent of pulmonary resection) who did not receive perioperative clopidogrel.

Results.—Fifty-four patients who had major lung resection between January 2005 and September 2010 and received clopidogrel perioperatively were matched with 108 control subjects. Both groups had similar mortality, postoperative length of stay, and no differences in the rates of perioperative transfusions, reoperations for bleeding, myocardial infarctions, and strokes. Seven of the 54 clopidogrel patients were admitted preoperatively for an eptifibatide bridge. Two of these patients received perioperative transfusions, but there were no deaths, reoperations, myocardial infarctions, or stroke.

Conclusions.—Patients taking clopidogrel can safely undergo major lung resection. Treatment with an eptifibatide bridge may minimize the risk of cardiovascular events in higher risk patients.

▶ With the near ubiquitous use of drug-eluting coronary stents (DES), the decision of how to manage antiplatelet therapy at the time of noncardiac surgery has become commonplace. The risks of cardiovascular events from stent thrombosis due to cessation of antiplatelet therapy and the procoagulant response of surgery must be carefully weighed with the accelerated bleeding often seen if these agents are continued through surgery. Data and guidelines covering this topic are limited, and perhaps even more so for the subset of patients known to have lung cancer and its ramifications.

The authors describe their initial management strategy, consisting of discontinuation of clopidogrel (but not aspirin) 5 days before surgery and reinitiation 12 to 72 hours after surgery at the daily maintenance dose of 75 mg per day. However, in the later subset of their retrospective study, they implemented a multidisciplinary approach for high-risk patients in which the clopidogrel was stopped 5 days before surgery, and the patients were admitted 2 to 3 days earlier for eptifibatide (Integrilin) bridging therapy. The eptifibatide was discontinued 8 hours before surgery, and the clopidogrel was reinitiated postoperatively in identical fashion to the early group. The high-risk patients who received this method of eptifibatide bridging were selected based on DES placed within a year, off label use of coronary stent, critical location, or previous coronary event with discontinuation of clopidogrel.

Laboratory evaluation of platelet function was not performed in any patients. Procedures and chest tube management was performed in routine fashion. Of note, the patients who received eptifibatide bridging did not receive perioperative epidural catheters for pain control.

The authors are to be congratulated for helping to better define a strategy for this difficult patient population. It is well known that premature cessation of platelet therapy is a significant contributor to in-stent thrombosis. The guidelines following DES placement recommend dual antiplatelet therapy not be interrupted for a year if at all possible. The use of heparin as a bridge has not been shown to be beneficial as the antiplatelet effect is limited.

The summation of these factors makes the use of a glycoprotein IIb/IIIa inhibitor attractive because it binds to the pivotal mediator for platelet aggregation and thrombus formation. Eptifibatide is the most attractive option because of its pharmacokinetics and short half-life, allowing a brief period of withdrawal and safe surgery.

This report details the use of this strategy with 54 patients. Interestingly, we independently and simultaneously moved to a similar strategy at our institution and have applied it for the past 2.5 years. Our results have been similar, and we have used the same protocol for bridging patients who require either cardiac or noncardiac surgery with excellent results.

Although further study and better delineation of guidelines will drive future directions, the authors have given us an excellent starting point for managing high-risk patients receiving clopidogrel who require antiplatelet management during the perioperative period.

C. T. Klodell, Jr, MD

Early results of a highly selective algorithm for surgery on patients with neurogenic thoracic outlet syndrome
Chandra V, Olcott C IV, Lee JT (Stanford Univ Med Ctr, CA)
J Vasc Surg 54:1698-1705, 2011

Objective.—Neurogenic thoracic outlet syndrome (nTOS) encompasses a wide spectrum of disabling symptoms that are often vague and difficult to diagnose and treat. We developed and prospectively analyzed a treatment algorithm for nTOS utilizing objective disability criteria, thoracic outlet syndrome (TOS)-specific physical therapy, radiographic evaluation of the thoracic outlet, and selective surgical decompression.

Methods.—Patients treated for nTOS from 2000-2009 were reviewed (n = 93). In period 1, most patients were offered surgery with documentation of appropriate symptoms. A prospective observational study began in 2007 (period 2) and was aimed at determining which patients benefited most from surgical intervention. Evaluation began with a validated mini-*Quick*DASH (QD) quality-of-life scale (0-100, 100 = worse) and duplex imaging of the thoracic outlet. Patients then participated in TOS-specific physical therapy (PT) for 2 to 4 months and were offered surgery based on response to PT and improvement in symptoms.

Results.—Thirty-four patients underwent first rib resection in period 1 (68% female, mean age 39, 18% athletes, 15% workers comp). In operated patients undergoing duplex imaging, 47% showed compression of their thoracic outlet arterial flow on provocative positioning. Based on subjective improvement of symptoms, 56% of patients at 1 year had a positive outcome. In period 2 during the prospective cohort, 59 consecutive patients were evaluated for nTOS (64% female, mean age 36, 32% athletes, 12% workers comp) with a mean pre-PT QD disability score of 55.1. All patients were prescribed PT, and 24 (41%) were eventually offered surgical decompression based on compliance with PT, interval improvement on QD score, and duplex compression of the thoracic outlet. Twenty-one patients underwent surgery (SURG group) consisting of first rib resection, middle and anterior scalenectomy, and brachial plexus neurolysis. There were significant differences between the SURG and non-SURG cohorts with respect to age, participation in competitive athletics, history of trauma, and symptom improvement with PT. At 1-year follow-up, 90% of patients expressed symptomatic improvement with the mean post-op QD disability score decreasing to 24.9 ($P = .005$) and 1-year QD scores improving down to 20.5 ($P = .014$).

Conclusions.—This highly-selective algorithm for nTOS surgery leads to improvement in overall success rates documented subjectively and objectively. Compliance with TOS-specific PT, improvement in QD scores after PT, young age, and competitive athletics are associated with improved surgical outcomes. Long-term follow-up will be necessary to document sustained symptom relief and to determine who the optimal surgical candidates are.

▶ The authors should be commended for this report, detailing their management algorithm over 2 periods in evaluation and therapeutic choice decisions for patients with suspected neurogenic thoracic outlet syndrome (nTOS). Thoracic outlet syndrome (TOS) can result from various causes including cervical ribs, anomalous fascial bands, and abnormalities of the anterior and middle scalene muscles. It is thought that nTOS may account for 95% of all cases of TOS. Neurogenic TOS may present with a wide range of symptoms but usually includes some form of upper extremity pain and paresthesias. The etiology of these symptoms may be related to antecedent history of trauma, particularly hyperextension injuries to the neck. Repetitive work, vocational work, and sports overuse injuries are also implicated.

The authors' algorithm in period 2 has several interesting components, including the use of duplex ultrasound scan in multiple provocative positions to better evaluate for arterial compression. They additionally utilize the miniQuick Disability of the Arm, Shoulder, and Hand (QuickDASH), which has been well validated in the orthopedic and hand surgery literature in relation to TOS. They then subselect the patients who are not only compliant with physical therapy, but additionally those who improve with physical therapy. This commitment to a physical therapy program likely selects patients who are willing to continue with rigorous physical therapy after surgery, leading to better long-term outcomes. In period 2, 45% of the evaluated patients were offered surgical decompression for nTOS and 90% of those operated had successful outcomes.

The authors should be commended for adhering to this rigorous selection process for the treatment of nTOS. While previous reports have advocated surgery for patients who fail to improve with physical therapy, this report suggests that by selecting patients who are motivated for physical therapy and have some improvement, perhaps better long-term outcomes can be obtained. The 90% success rate in period 2 certainly warrants careful consideration. Furthermore, the authors should be commended for the use of valid quality-of-life measurement tools in the selection of treatment options. In the current era of evidence-based practice, it is essential that valid and reproducible measurement tools be utilized to allow standardization of results, and perhaps we can all find ways to emulate the authors' example.

C. T. Klodell, Jr, MD

Preoperative left atrial dysfunction and risk of postoperative atrial
fibrillation complicating thoracic surgery
Raman T, Roistacher N, Liu J, et al (Memorial Sloan-Kettering Cancer Ctr, NY)
J Thorac Cardiovasc Surg 143:482-487, 2012

Objective.—Postoperative atrial fibrillation complicating general thoracic
surgery increases morbidity and stroke risk. We aimed to determine whether
preoperative atrial dysfunction or other echocardiographic markers are associated with postoperative atrial fibrillation.

Methods.—In 191 patients who had undergone anatomic lung or esophageal resection, preoperative clinical and echocardiographic data were
compared between patients with and without postoperative atrial fibrillation. Presence of postoperative atrial fibrillation lasting more than 5 minutes
during hospitalization was detected using continuous telemetry or 12-lead
electrocardiography. Maximal left atrial volume and indices of left atrial
function were assessed.

Results.—Patients with postoperative atrial fibrillation (33/191, 17%)
were older (71 ± 5 years vs 64 ± 12 years, $P < .0001$), were taking
β-blockers more often, had greater left atrial volume, had decreased left
atrial emptying fraction, and had lower E' and A' septal velocities compared
with patients without postoperative atrial fibrillation. The incidence of postoperative atrial fibrillation in patients with left atrial volume 32 mL/m^2 or
greater was 37% (11/30) and greater than in those with left atrial volume
less than 32 mL/m^2 (14%, 22/160, $P = .002$). Length of hospital stay was
significantly increased in patients with postoperative atrial fibrillation
compared with patients without ($P = .04$). Older age was significantly associated with greater β-blocker use and left atrial volume and lower left atrial
emptying fraction. On multivariate analysis, lower left atrial emptying fraction (odds ratio, 1.03 per unit decrement; 95% confidence interval,
1.002–1.065; $P = .04$) and preoperative use of β-blockers (odds ratio,
2.82; 95% confidence interval, 1.18–6.77; $P = .02$) were the only independent risk factors associated with postoperative atrial fibrillation.

Conclusions.—These data show that an echocardiogram before major
thoracic surgery, increased use of preoperative β-blockers, and decreased
left atrial emptying fraction were associated with postoperative atrial fibrillation. Echocardiographic predictors of left atrial mechanical dysfunction
may prove clinically useful in risk stratifying patients in whom postoperative atrial fibrillation is more likely to develop and to benefit from prevention strategies aimed at mitigating atrial function before surgery.

▶ Atrial fibrillation is a common postoperative complication in general thoracic
surgery and is known to increase length of stay as well as other deleterious
consequences. Increasing age has long been associated with the development
of postoperative atrial fibrillation (POAF), whereas other risk factors have been
inconsistently confirmed. Identification of higher risk patients preoperatively
could allow for more targeted prophylactic therapies intended to mitigate the

elevated risk while reducing the number of patients receiving the treatment unnecessarily.

The authors recognize that recent literature has noted the predictive value of the maximal left atrial volume (LAV) and supports the idea that left atrial enlargement and increased ventricular filling pressures may be linked to the development of POAF. The authors studied patients who required general thoracic surgery procedures such as esophageal surgery or anatomic lung resection and also had adequate preoperative echocardiographic data available. They noted that patients who developed POAF had a length of stay that was 1.29 times longer than those who did not develop POAF. Additionally, a greater maximal LAV, as well as decreased left atrial ejection fraction and lower inflow velocities to the left ventricle were associated with POAF. The finding of β-blocker use being associated with POAF is likely related to use as a prophylactic measure and as such is a surrogate for higher risk patients.

This study demonstrates that perhaps a preoperative echocardiogram could help better delineate which patients are at the highest risk for POAF following general thoracic surgical procedures. However, the next challenge is to develop strategies to mitigate the increased risk. The selective use of measures potentially including prophylactic administration of antiarrhythmic drugs such as amiodarone would require careful study. This clinical problem seems well suited to a randomized prospective trial in which patients deemed high risk for POAF by echocardiographic findings could be randomized to receive drug prophylaxis or current standard therapy. Nevertheless, this report serves to remind us of the relatively common occurrence of POAF and may encourage us to continue developing strategies to reduce the incidence.

C. T. Klodell, Jr, MD

Routine Anticoagulation Is Not Indicated for Postoperative General Thoracic Surgical Patients With New-Onset Atrial Fibrillation

Makhija Z, Allen MS, Wigle DA, et al (Mayo Clinic, Rochester, MN)
Ann Thorac Surg 92:421-427, 2011

Background.—Current guidelines suggest anticoagulation for patients with new-onset atrial fibrillation (AF). Little evidence exists for the risk/benefit ratio in postoperative general thoracic surgical patients. We analyzed new-onset AF in patients after a general thoracic operation to determine the benefit of anticoagulation on prevention of stroke and its impact on postoperative outcome.

Methods.—New-onset postoperative AF developed in 759 patients (527 men, 237 women) who underwent thoracic surgical procedures between 1994 and 2009. Demographic data, clinical presentation, operative findings, and postoperative outcomes were analyzed.

Results.—The median age was 71 years (range, 31 to 92 years). We compared 228 patients anticoagulated for new-onset postoperative AF with 531 non-anticoagulated patients. The anticoagulated group had a higher incidence of male sex, pulmonary hypertension, congestive heart failure, and peripheral vascular disease. Median postoperative hospitalization was 9 days (range, 1 to 306 days) in those not anticoagulated and 11 days (range, 1 to 97 days) in those anticoagulated for AF ($p = 0.704$). Stroke occurred in 0.56% of the non-anticoagulated patients vs 2.2% of the anticoagulated patients ($p = 0.057$). Bleeding occurred in 22 patients (9.7%) who were anticoagulated and in 27 (5.1%) who were not ($p = 0.009$). Anticoagulated patients had a higher incidence of at least one complication other than stroke or bleeding (43.4%) vs non-anticoagulated patients (30.9%; $p = 0.001$). Operative mortality in anticoagulated patients was 3.1% vs 6.6% in patients not anticoagulated ($p = 0.057$).

Conclusions.—Anticoagulation did not lower the risk of stroke or transient ischemic attacks in postoperative general thoracic surgery patients with new-onset AF but did increase the incidence of postoperative bleeding and other complications. Patients with new-onset AF after a general thoracic surgical procedure should not be routinely anticoagulated.

▶ Atrial arrhythmias are a well-known and common complication following general thoracic operations. Heart rate control and possible cardioversion back to normal sinus rhythm are the central focus of treatment. However, there is little evidence offering guidance as to whether patients who have postoperative atrial fibrillation following a thoracic procedure require anticoagulation. The most feared complication of atrial fibrillation is stroke, making this decision of paramount importance.

The risk of developing stroke may be estimated using the CHADS2 score. The CHADS2 score is calculated by assigning 1 point each for congestive heart failure (CHF), hypertension (HTN), age 70 years or older, diabetes mellitus, and 2 points for a prior stroke or transient ischemic attack. The bulk of the patients in the study presented by the authors had a CHADS2 score of 2 or less.

The authors concluded that the stroke risk was not affected by the use of Coumadin (wafarin) but that the risk of bleeding complications was essentially doubled in postoperative thoracic patients who received Coumadin. They further concluded that patients who develop postoperative atrial fibrillation after a general thoracic operation should not be routinely anticoagulated.

In the newest Society of Thoracic Surgeons guidelines addressing the issue of postoperative atrial fibrillation following general thoracic surgical operations, it is suggested that the CHADS2 score should first be calculated and that patients with a score of 2 or lower be treated with aspirin alone. Controversy may still exist in patients with higher CHADS2 scores. The authors suggested future directions that may include the use of direct thrombin inhibitors. Dabigatran has been shown to have similar efficacy as Coumadin for stroke prevention and lowered the incidence of major hemorrhage, although it has not been studied on postoperative patients and was not randomized. It is unknown whether the results of this patient population can be translated into postoperative thoracic patients.

With the current paucity of evidence, the newest guideline suggestion of aspirin alone for postoperative thoracic surgical patients with CHADS2 score of 2 or lower seems reasonable, especially when considering the elevated risk for bleeding complications the authors noted.

C. T. Klodell, Jr, MD

Staging of Non-small Cell Lung Cancer

A Comparative Analysis of Video-Assisted Mediastinoscopy and Conventional Mediastinoscopy

Cho JH, Kim J, Kim K, et al (Sungkyunkwan Univ School of Medicine, Seoul, Republic of Korea)
Ann Thorac Surg 92:1007-1011, 2011

Background.—The objective of this study was to compare outcomes of video-assisted mediastinoscopic lymph node biopsy in patients with non-small cell lung cancer (NSCLC) with outcomes of conventional mediastinoscopic lymph node biopsy in this same patient population.

Methods.—All mediastinoscopies at one medical center from January 2008 to December 2009 were analyzed. Numbers of lymph nodes dissected, stations biopsied, remnant lymph nodes when major lung resection was performed after mediastinoscopic lymph node biopsy, and complications were recorded.

Results.—Of 521 mediastinoscopies, 222 were in the conventional mediastinoscopic lymph node biopsy group (CM group) and 299 were in the video-assisted mediastinoscopic lymph node biopsy group (VAM group). Eleven complications (2.11%) occurred, with more occurring in the CM group (3.6%) than in the VAM group (1.6%; $p = 0.030$). The total number of dissected nodes was higher in the VAM group (mean, 8.53 ± 5.8) than in the CM group (mean, 7.13 ± 4.9; $p = 0.004$), and there was no statistically significant difference between the average number of stations sampled in the CM group (2.98 ± 0.7) and in the VAM group (3.06 ± 0.75; $p =$ not significant). The number of remnant lymph nodes when major lung surgery was performed after mediastinoscopy was lower in the VAM group (mean, 5.05 ± 4.5) than in the CM group (mean, 7.67 ± 6.5; $p < 0.001$).

Conclusions.—This study found that video-assisted mediastinoscopic lymph node biopsy had fewer complications than did the conventional method. More lymph nodes were examined and fewer lymph nodes remained after mediastinoscopy by video-assisted mediastinoscopy (VAM) than by conventional mediastinoscopy.

▶ Lung cancer remains the leading cause of cancer-related deaths worldwide. The staging of lung cancer is of paramount importance as the benefit of neoadjuvant therapy for patients with Stage IIIa lung cancer has become better elucidated. The staging of mediastinal lymph nodes may first involve positron emission tomography/computed tomography (PET-CT) or ultrasonographically assisted endobronchial needle aspiration (EBUS). However, mediastinoscopy remains the gold standard for the preoperative evaluation of the mediastinum.

Potential advantages of the video-based mediastinoscopy (VAM) include enhanced and magnified views, simplified teaching, and a more comfortable working environment. VAM also allows bimanual operating and much better visualization and dissection. VAM improves the identification of anatomic structures such as the trachea bronchial angle, the azygos vein, and the left recurrent laryngeal nerve.

The authors reviewed all mediastinoscopy procedures over a nearly 2-year period in hope of comparing conventional mediastinoscopy (CM) with VAM. They found that VAM had fewer complications compared with CM. Additionally, it was noted that more lymph nodes were examined, and fewer lymph nodes remained after mediastinoscopy by VAM than CM.

The addition of video to conventional mediastinoscopy has yielded myriad benefits. It has allowed greater standardization of the procedure, and now the operative field is clear to all and procedural variation can be minimized. Additionally, the impact of education and learning of the procedure cannot be overstated. As mediastinoscopy has drifted to the last and most invasive staging modality, we now apply to supplement EBUS and PET/CT as well as endoscopic ultrasound, and the opportunities to train new surgeons on the procedure have become limited. Even in thoracic training programs, the mediastinoscopy procedures are in high demand as residents carefully ensure they acquire the required numbers. As opposed to conventional mediastinoscopy, multiple learners can observe the same procedure, and although each may not actually perform it, all can gain experience simultaneously. Additionally, as an attending surgeon, the comfort level is much higher when the procedure can be observed in real time on the monitor. The magnification and illumination of the technique are far superior and allow better delineation of the anatomy and safer dissection. It is my strong suggestion that anyone involved in mediastinoscopy procedures ensure that the VAM equipment is made available for your use.

C. T. Klodell, Jr, MD

Tumor Biology and Prognostic Variables

Bilobectomy for Lung Cancer: Analysis of Indications, Postoperative Results, and Long-Term Outcomes

Galetta D, Solli P, Borri A, et al (European Inst of Oncology, Milan, Italy; Univ of Milan School of Medicine, Italy)
Ann Thorac Surg 93:251-258, 2012

Background.—Bilobectomy for lung cancer is considered a high-risk procedure for the increased postoperative complication rate and the negative impact on survival. We analyzed the safety and the oncologic results of this procedure.

Methods.—We retrospectively reviewed patients who underwent bilobectomy for lung cancer between October 1998 and August 2009. Age, gender, bilobectomy type and indication, complications, pathology, stage, and survival were analyzed.

Results.—Bilobectomy was performed on 146 patients (101 men; mean age, 62 years). There were 77 uppermiddle and 69 middle-lower bilobectomies. Indications were tumor extending across the fissure in 27 (18.5%) patients, endobronchial tumor in 39 (26.7%), extrinsic tumor or nodal invasion of bronchus intermedius in 66 (45.2%), and vascular invasion in 14 (9.6%). An extended resection was performed in 24 patients (16.4%). Induction therapy was performed in 43 patients (29.4%). Thirty-day mortality was 1.4% (n = 2). Overall morbidity was 47.2%. Mean chest tube persistence was 7 days (range, 6 to 46 days). Overall 5-year survival was 58%. Significance differences in survival were observed among different stages (stage I, 70%; stage II, 55%; stage III, 40%; $p = 0.0003$) and the N status (N0, 69%; N1, 56%; N2, 40%; $p = 0.0005$). Extended procedure ($p = 0.0003$) and superior bilobectomy ($p = 0.0008$) adversely influenced survival. Multivariate analysis demonstrated that an extended resection ($p = 0.01$), an advanced N disease ($p = 0.02$), and an upper-mild lobectomy ($p = 0.02$) adversely affected prognosis.

Conclusions.—Bilobectomy is associated with a low mortality and an increased morbidity. Survival relates to disease stage and N factor. Optimal prognosis is obtained in patients with lower-middle lobectomy without extension of the resection.

▶ The removal of 2 pulmonary lobes on the right side (bilobectomy) is accepted as a standard radical procedure used in the surgical treatment of non–small cell lung cancer. This bilobectomy involves either a upper and middle lobectomy or lower and middle lobectomy (never upper and lower, leaving only the middle lobe). Few centers have high-volume experience or have reported outcomes with this procedure, and the outcomes as well as place in the surgical armamentarium remains less well defined. The authors set out to answer 2 questions based on their single-institution experience. First, they scrutinized the safety of the procedure with respect to morbidity and mortality. Second, they reviewed oncologic efficacy of the procedure in the hopes of legitimizing this type of resection for specific clinical circumstances.

The authors report that bilobectomy is associated with a low mortality but an increased morbidity, and those patients with middle and lower bilobectomy seemed to fare better. It has certainly been suggested that bilobectomy may be associated with increased morbidity and mortality because of the increased technical complexity of the procedure. Interestingly, in this study, the use of induction therapy and sleeve resections were not associated with a higher incidence of complications.

A technical aspect not mentioned in the article is that bilobectomy often sets up a space problem, with inadequate residual pulmonary tissue to fill the thoracic cavity. In these cases, consideration should be given to a pleural tent and perhaps pneumoperitoneum to facilitate resolution of air leaks and any space problems. The authors mentioned the use of a phrenic scratch to temporarily elevate the unilateral hemidiaphragm, which may have a similar effect. Surgeons routinely performing pulmonary resections must be prepared for the unanticipated need for bilobectomy, as well as various strategies to mitigate the negative effects of loss of 2 lobes on the residual thoracic space.

C. T. Klodell, Jr, MD

Pulmonary Resection of Metastatic Sarcoma: Prognostic Factors Associated With Improved Outcomes

Kim S, Ott HC, Wright CD, et al (Massachusetts General Hosp, Boston)
Ann Thorac Surg 92:1780-1787, 2011

Background.—There are few data to predict the benefit of pulmonary metastasectomy in patients with extrathoracic sarcoma. This study analyzes prognostic factors associated with improved outcomes.

Methods.—Between June 2002 and December 2008, 97 patients underwent pulmonary resection for metastatic sarcoma at Massachusetts General Hospital. Eight patients were excluded because of lack of follow-up data. Analysis was performed using Kaplan-Meier estimates of survival, log-rank test, and multivariate Cox model.

Results.—Overall 5-year survival for the cohort was 50.1%. Patients who had multiple operations for recurrent pulmonary metastases had better 5-year survival compared with patients who had a single operation (69 versus 41%; $p = 0.017$). Median disease- free survival (DFS) for the reoperation group was 12.9 months compared with 9.1 months for the single-operation group ($p < 0.028$). Patients with a disease-free interval (DFI) greater than 12 months from detection of primary sarcoma to pulmonary metastasectomy had improved survival compared with those whose DFI was less than 12 months ($p < 0.0001$). Patients with bilateral metastasectomy had lower 5-year survival compared with metastasectomy for unilateral disease (22% versus 68%; $p < 0.0001$). Two or more metastases were associated with poorer outcome compared with a single metastasis ($p = 0.0007$). A positive resection margin portended worse survival compared with a negative resection margin ($p = 0.004$). Patients with lesions larger than 3 cm had decreased survival compared with patients with lesions smaller than 3 cm ($p = 0.017$) with no difference in median DFS. Histologic type, grade of tumor, and use of chemotherapy had no effect on survival. Multivariate analysis showed that patients with a DFI greater than 12 months ($p = 0.001$), single-sided metastasis ($p = 0.001$), negative margins ($p = 0.002$), and multiple operations ($p = 0.018$) had better survival.

Conclusions.—Pulmonary metastasectomy for sarcoma can be associated with prolonged survival. Tumor resectability, DFI, number of metastases, and laterality are important factors in determining patient selection for curative surgical intervention. Repeated pulmonary metastasectomy in select patients may improve survival despite recurrent disease.

► Surgical resection of sarcoma metastasis isolated to the lung is standard therapy and is associated with improved long-term survival. There are currently no robust clinical guidelines to optimize patient selection for pulmonary metastasectomy. The authors retrospectively reviewed a 6-year period at their institution with the goal of evaluating the clinical parameters in patients who underwent pulmonary resection for sarcoma metastases and identifying prognostic factors associated with improved survival.

Although the development of metastatic sarcoma in the lung portends a poor prognosis, metastasectomy offers long-term survival for selected patients. Given that neither chemotherapy nor radiation has shown effectiveness in the absence of prospective studies comparing resection with other treatment, patients are faced with limited options. Interestingly, in the authors' review they did not observe any difference in survival across different histologic subtypes or grades of sarcoma. The biologic behavior of the tumor and disease-free interval seems to have the greatest association with long-term survival. As noted, the patient with multiple pulmonary nodules and bilateral metastases probably reflects more extensive subclinical disease at the time of the operation, which leads to poorer survival. However, complete surgical resection has been shown to be a significant predictor of survival after pulmonary metastasectomy, despite the importance of other tumor characteristics.

From a technical aspect, the high-resolution computed tomography scanners make the planning of these operations much easier in contemporary times. Patients with few metastases limited to a single hemithorax may be considered for thoracoscopic approach. Bilateral disease may be approached either by clamshell thoracotomy or by staged posterolateral thoracotomy approach. In some patients, the latter approach may be favored in that the posterior lung is more accessible, and after the hemithorax is cleared, the oncologist may consider adjuvant treatment. The second hemithorax resection can be attempted 6 weeks later. However, if the chest cannot be cleared, and residual disease remains, the contralateral operation can be avoided. Metastatic sarcoma often presents in otherwise young and robust patients, warranting aggressive surgical treatment when the possibility of benefit exists.

C. T. Klodell, Jr, MD

Article Index

Chapter 1: General Considerations

Chapter 2: Trauma

Chapter 3: Burns

Chapter 4: Critical Care

Chapter 5: Transplantation

Chapter 6: Surgical Infections

Chapter 7: Endocrine

Chapter 8: Nutrition

Chapter 9: Gastrointestinal

Chapter 10: Oncology

Chapter 11: Vascular Surgery

Author Index